# Pseudocarcinoma
# of the Skin

# Pseudocarcinoma of the Skin

## B. A. Berenbein
*Moscow Regional Institute for Clinical Research*
*Moscow, USSR*

Translated from Russian by
## V. E. Tatarchenko

Springer Science+Business Media, LLC

Library of Congress Cataloging in Publication Data

Berenbein, B. A. (Boris Aronovich)
  Pseudocarcinoma of the skin.

  Translation of a rev. version of: Psevdorak kozhi.
  Bibliography: p.
  Includes index.
  1. Skin—Cancer. I. Title. (DNLM: 1. Diagnosis, Differential. 2. Epidermis—pathology.
3. Hyperplasia. 4. Skin Neoplasms. WR 500 B488p)
RC280.S5B4713  1985                          616.99′477                          84-24988

ISBN 978-1-4757-6321-8                ISBN 978-1-4757-6319-5 (eBook)
DOI 10.1007/978-1-4757-6319-5

This volume is a translation of a revised version of the original Russian edition,
which was published by Meditsina Publishers in 1980.
This translation is published under an agreement with the
Copyright Agency of the USSR (VAAP).

PSEVDORAK KOZHI
B. A. Berenbein

© Springer Science+Business Media New York 1985
Originally published by Plenum Publishing Corporation in 1985
Softcover reprint of the hardcover 1st edition 1985

# Preface to the English Edition

Among the circumstances that may cause a too late or erroneous diagnosis of skin cancer, a most important one is the failure to distinguish a true squamous cell carcinoma of the skin from an atypical, but benign, epidermal hyperplasia which closely mimics the carcinoma clinically and particularly histologically - so-called pseudoepitheliomatous or pseudocarcinomatous hyperplasia.

Although there are many publications describing in detail the histologic features of pseudocarcinomatous hyperplasias which arise in various dermatoses or skin tumors, this book appears to be the first attempt to cover the whole subject of pseudocarcinomatous epidermal hyperplasia by considering it not only in its clinical and histopathologic aspects, but also from cytophysiologic and cytogenetic points of view, in relation to squamous cell carcinoma.

On the basis of a review of the available literature and of my own correlative clinical, histopathologic, cytophysiologic, and cytogenetic investigations in patients and experimental animals, I propose a comprehensive set of criteria of difference and similarity between pseudocarcinoma and true carcinoma of the skin. Hopefully, these criteria will be found useful by physicians in the differential diagnosis between these conditions in cases of doubt and may likewise provide a stimulus to researchers for deliberation.

I also hope that this monograph, which is a translation of a revised version of the text originally published in Russian in 1980, will serve our common cause of the fight against cancer.

I welcome suggestions regarding the choice and treatment of the material included in the book.

In conclusion, I wish to express my deep gratitude to Dr. V.E. Tatarchenko for assistance in the preparation of this revised version of the Russian text and for its translation into English.

B. A. Berenbein
Moscow, January 1984

# Preface to the 1980 Russian Edition

Pseudocarcinoma, or pseudocarcinosis, of the skin presents a challenging problem, both theoretical and practical, to dermatologic oncology. A cardinal attribute of pseudocarcinoma is hyperplasia of the epidermis. Being an atypical inflammatory reaction, pseudo-carcinomatous epidermal hyperplasia resembles squamous cell carcinoma of the skin in clinical and especially in histologic characteristics.

The histologic appearance of pseudocarcinomatous epidermal hyperplasia and that of cutaneous squamous cell carcinoma are at times so similar that it is not possible to distinguish between these two fundamentally different disease states unless concomitant clinical findings are taken into consideration.

However, the clinical features of a number of dermatoses and skin tumors in which pseudocarcinomatous hyperplasia may arise (chronic pyoderma ulcerosum vegetans, trophic ulcers with callous margins, lichen ruber verrucosus, verrucous neurodermatosis, cutaneous tuberculosis, deep mycoses, keratoacanthoma, giant condyloma acuminatum, etc.) are not always helpful in deciding with certainty whether the presenting condition is malignant or benign. Any one of the diseases just listed, if it runs a protracted course, may develop into squamous cell carcinoma. It is not possible to ascertain either clinically or histologically the time when a reactive epidermal proliferation acquires the biologic properties of malignancy. Therefore diagnostic errors with grave consequences are liable to occur if epidermal pseudocarcinomatous hyperplasia is misinterpreted as cutaneous squamous cell carcinoma, and vice versa. Indeed, there are many reports in the literature indicating that such errors are not uncommonly made by dermatologists, pathologists, oncologists, and other specialists.

Although the morphologic characteristics of pseudocarcinomatous epidermal hyperplasia have been under investigation for many years, the possibility of establishing clear-cut clinical and histologic criteria to permit unequivocal differentiation between such hyper-plasias and squamous cell carcinomas of the skin is still debatable. Also, the appropriateness of the term "pseudoepitheliomatous hyper-

plasia" which has been used widely outside the USSR to designate
processes that simulate malignant epidermal growth is questionable.
The word "epithelioma" means literally a tumor derived from epithelium, and its use with reference to authentic malignant neoplasms
has been subjected to serious and justified criticism.  Inasmuch as
atypical reactive hyperplasia of the epidermis may bear clinical
and histologic similarities precisely to squamous cell carcinoma
of the skin, the term "pseudocarcinomatous hyperplasia" is to be
preferred.

In the past two decades or so, attempts have been made outside
the USSR to classify under "pseudocarcinoses" those dermatoses in
which pseudocarcinomatous epidermal hyperplasia is seen to arise more
frequently than in others (cutaneous tuberculosis, deep mycoses,
vegetating toxicodermas, chronic ulcerative vegetating pyoderma,
papillomatosis cutis carcinoïdes of Gottron, keratoacanthoma, etc.).

The existing classifications are, however, based on the presenting histologic features of pseudocarcinomatous hyperplasia and do not
reflect its biologic nature.  Reactive proliferative processes are
now known to depend, in large measure, on characteristics of the
genetic apparatus of the cells.  It has been demonstrated in numerous
studies that the cells of human and animal malignant tumors of various anatomic sites as well as those in tissue cultures of transplantable tumors show abnormal mitoses, disordered DNA metabolism, and
quantitative and qualitative alterations of chromosomes.  Advances
made in cytology and cytogenetics have provided new insights into the
biologic nature of neoplastic proliferation and have determined the
choice of criteria for our studies on epidermal growth.

As pointed out by N.N. Blokhin (1976), the most important lines
of research in cancer today should be those concerned with problems
involved in clarifying the genetic basis of malignant transformation,
identifying processes that control the reproduction and differentiation of cells, and developing an array of methods for early recognition of premalignant and malignant conditions.  As far as dermatology is concerned, many such problems still await solution or have
not even been considered.

It has been recognized since the publication of fundamental
studies of Garshin (1939) and Glazunov (1947, 1971) that although
they may closely resemble invasive and destructive growths, inflammatory hyperplasias of epithelium in general, and of epidermis in
particular, differ from such growths in being dependent, in a correlative manner, on the functional state of the organism.  What
alterations are undergone by the genetic apparatus of epidermal cells
in pseudocarcinomatous hyperplasia and what are the differences
between these alterations and those in squamous cell carcinoma remains to be established.  Research in this area can contribute not
only to the unraveling of mechanisms by which pseudocarcinomatous

hyperplasia and squamous cell carcinoma develop, but also to the formulation of criteria for differentiating between these two pathologic processes which, although similar in clinical and histopathologic characteristics, are radically different in biologic nature.

In the Clinic of Skin and Venereal Diseases of the M.F. Vladimirskii Moscow Regional Institute for Clinical Research (MONIKI), studies on the use of genetic methods in dermatology were initiated by Belen'kii and his associates in 1967 (Belen'kii and Berenbein, 1967; Belen'kii, 1968; Belen'kii et al., 1968), and these studies have served as a basis for the present author in his attempt to clarify some pathogenetic aspects of pseudocarcinomatous epidermal hyperplasia.

This monograph describes and compares clinicopathologic, cytophysiologic, and cytogenetic studies undertaken by the present writer and his associates in patients and experimental animals with pseudocarcinomatous hyperplasia and squamous cell carcinoma. Particular attention is given to cytophysiologic and cytogenetic investigations. The latter included study of the mitotic behavior of epidermal cells, microspectrophotometric determination of DNA content in epidermal cell nuclei, karyotypic analyses, and sex chromatin studies.

Taken together, the results of these comprehensive studies have led to the formulation of criteria for differential diagnosis between pseudocarcinomatous hyperplasia and squamous cell carcinoma. These criteria are presented in tabular form and discussed in a separate chapter.

Moreover, our observations on patients have enabled us to assess the efficacy of various therapies in the management of cutaneous disorders associated with pseudocarcinomatous epidermal hyperplasia.

I am well aware that some of the problems dealt with in this monograph still await resolution, but I hope that the book will provide a stimulus to further work on these problems.

I wish to express my deep gratitude to Professor G.G. Avtandinov, Dr. I.A. Kazantseva, and Dr. D.A. Egorkina for methodologic guidance and useful discussions during the preparation of the manuscript. I also acknowledge the cooperation and assistance of the staff of the Clinic of Skin and Venereal Diseases of the MONIKI Institute.

# Contents

# 1
# Historical Background, Terminology, and Classification

The concept of pseudocarcinosis (pseudocancerosis) is customarily considered to go back to Unna (1894) who was the first to note that the excessive proliferation of epidermis seen in lesions of lupus vulgaris may resemble squamous cell carcinoma of the skin. Unna did not find any metastases in his patients, even though the disease was of long standing. It is difficult to say in retrospect whether or not the epidermal hyperplasia observed by him was benign, although atypical, because he did not follow up the patients and because no criteria were available at that time by which inflammatory hyperplasia of the epidermis can be differentiated clinically and histologically from squamous cell carcinoma. His observations did, however, attract the attention of dermatologists to so-called atypical epidermal growths. The first to study these was Friedländer (1877) who showed that atypical epidermal proliferation was not always a sign of malignancy and that it could occur in a variety of conditions including, among others, lupus vulgaris, leprosy, fistulas, and elephantiasis. Friedländer came to the conclusion that while every atypical epidermal growth should not be regarded as necessarily cancerous, every cancer represents atypical epidermal growth. Although more than a hundred years have passed since the publication of Friedländer's book, the issues raised there still remain of current interest today.

Subsequently, numerous reports appeared in the literature describing cases with a variety of skin disorders that exhibited excessive epidermal proliferations which were so similar histologically to cutaneous squamous cell carcinoma as to be indistinguishable from it even by experienced pathologists, but nonetheless underwent spontaneous involution. Winer (1940) wrote that "competent pathologists have occasionally been surprised by the spontaneous healing of a lesion which they had diagnosed squamous cell carcinoma microscopically". Miyahara (1913), having examined histologic sections from patients with lupus tuberculosus and scrofuloderma which exhibited epidermal hyperplasias that mimicked squamous cell carcinoma, stated that such hyperplasia might be a precursor of true carcinoma. He did not, however, provide any evidence to substantiate this contention.

In 1927, White and Weidman proposed a histologic grouping of atypical epidermal proliferations which they called "pseudo-epitheliomatous hyperplasia". On the basis of clinical and histologic characteristics of the epithelial hyperplasia observed in lesions of syphilitic gummae of the tongue, furuncles of the neck, and chronic ulcers of the lower extremities, they classified the types of pseudocarcinomatous hyperplasia into three grades. In grade 1, there is acanthosis only; grade 2 is characterized by downgrowth of epidermal ridges to the level of the sweat glands, by the presence of embryonoid cells with large hyperchromic nuclei, and by rupture of the basement membrane at the dermoepidermal junction; grade 3 includes growths that are virtually identical to squamous cell carcinoma microscopically. White and Weidman emphasized that despite these histological changes, the clinical picture did not show any evidence of malignancy. Followup of the patients revealed epithelialization of the lesions, no metastases, and no cachexia.

It must be acknowledged that White and Weidman's classification played a positive role in that it drew the attention of pathologists to atypical epidermal growths and stimulated work on the development of histologic criteria by which pseudocarcinomatous hyperplasia can be recognized. Yet the grading of hyperplasias proposed by the authors was only tentative and did not resolve the difficulties involved in differentiating atypical benign hyperplasias of the epidermis from squamous cell carcinoma.

Winer (1940) attached great importance to the histologic structure of the dermis in the differential diagnosis of pseudoepitheliomatous hyperplasia. He observed that in such epidermal hyperplasias, in contrast to squamous cell carcinoma, a granulomatous inflammatory infiltrate was usually present in the dermis. More recently, similar observations were made by Sommerville (1953), Gottron (1954), Fischer (1963), Ju (1976), Thambiah (1969), Connors and Ackerman (1976), Pinkus and Mehregan (1976), and other authors. "It must be admitted", wrote Petrov in 1947, "that we are often unable to draw a clear line of demarcation between chronic inflammatory or parasitic tumors, abnormalities of embryogenesis, dyshormonal and dystrophic hyperplasia, ... on the one hand, and true tumors on the other". This view is shared by many oncologists, pathologists, and dermatologists at the present time.

The fundamental clinical and experimental studies by Fischer-Wasels (1927, 1933) and Garshin (1939) demonstrated that histologic signs of malignancy such as disorderly arrangement of epidermal cells, epidermal ingrowth into the underlying tissue, and even "un-limited" epidermal growth (which continues as long as the noxious stimulus persists) may be shown not only by tumor cells of the epithelium.  In his studies into the biologic nature of atypical epidermal proliferations, Garshin noted that these might occur in skin disorders such as lupus tuberculosus, syphilids, blastomycosis, and trophic ulcers, that is, conditions where the dermis contains a chronic inflammatory infiltrate.  He pointed out that epidermal extension deep into the underlying tissue was particularly frequent at sites of chronic inflammation.  It was observed by Garshin and other investigators that the histologic appearances of proliferating epidermis in inflammatory processes affecting man were nearly ident-ical to those seen in experimental rabbits following subcutaneous injection of scarlet red or infusorial earth (Ruchinskii, 1910; Fischer-Wasels, 1927; Garshin, 1927, 1939).

That inflammatory epithelial growths may resemble squamous cell carcinoma histologically was demonstrated not only for epidermis, but also for the epithelia of salivary glands (Iskra, 1938), bronchi and mammary glands (Golovin, 1952), gall-bladder (Golovin and Pigarevskii, 1952), and liver (Darshkevich, 1952).  These findings indicate that the problem of atypical inflammatory growth is one of general biologic importance.

Studies by Garshin (1939) showed further that infiltrative epidermal growth within inflammatory lesions is not merely a reaction to stimulation: by growing around areas of an infiltrate or granuloma and around fat droplets or infusorial earth particles, the epidermis promotes their elimination.  This enabled Garshin to designate such epithelial growths as "atypical inflammatory" or "heterotopic", using the term "heterotopia" to mean the presence of epithelium "in locations from which it is normally absent".  He showed that no infiltrative growth will occur if the epithelium "overlies a sub-stratum which is physiologically proper to it", that is to say, epithelial heterotopia can occur only in the presence of an inflam-matory infiltrate which is a backing physiologically atypical for the epithelium.  As the inflammation subsides and the inflammatory infil-trate is replaced by fibrous tissue, epithelial growth into the underlying tissue ceases also (Lazarenko, 1934, 1959; Zavarzin, 1947; Khlystova, 1960; and others).  As Lazarenko (1934) aptly put it, "the organism regulates epithelial growth by means of connective tissue".

It is by virtue of their correlative relationship to the organ-ism that heterotopic inflammatory proliferations of the epidermis differ from squamous cell carcinomas in which epidermal growth is an autonomous process (Garshin, 1939; Khlopin, 1940, 1947; Glazunov, 1947, 1971; Petrov, 1947; Shabad, 1967; Willis, 1967; Sanderson, 1979; and others).  It was stressed by Petrov (1947) that "the cardi-nal sign of malignancy is that tumor cells proliferate autonomously,

independent of the organism". He provided the following definition
of neoplasia: "a tumor, or blastoma, is the pathologic growth of a
tissue that carries a stimulus for its proliferation within its own
cells". He stated further that "a hyperplasia or malformation
becomes a tumor when it begins to develop autonomously". This definition of malignancy, given as it was by one of the founders of the
Soviet school of oncology, is still relevant today.

Atypical epidermal growth may be triggered or caused not only by
inflammatory infiltrate. There are indications in the literature
(e.g. Arning and Levandowsky, 1911; Biberstein, 1931; Arnold and
Tilden, 1943; Caro, 1959; Grzhebin and Tseraidis, 1960; R. Cramer and
H. Cramer, 1963; Mashkilleison, 1965; Belenkii, 1970; Lanné, 1970;
Niemi, 1970; Schoenfeld, 1970) that infiltrative epidermal growth
may also occur in connective tissue tumors (histiocytomas, dermatofibromas, granular cell myoblastomas, hemagiomas, melanomas); in the
process, the histologic structure of the epidermis may come to
resemble closely not only squamous cell carcinoma, but basalioma as
well. Accordingly, the term "pseudobasaliomatous epithelial hyperplasia" was proposed to designate epidermal hyperplasia simulating
basal cell carcinoma (R. Cramer and H. Cramer, 1963).

Because of the clinical and histologic similarities of benign
epidermal growths in lesions of lupus tuberculosus and at the margins
of trophic ulcers to squamous cell carcinoma, White and Weidman
(1927), as already mentioned, labeled these benign growths "pseudoepitheliomatous hyperplasia". Since then this term has come into
common use to designate benign proliferations of the epidermis that
mimic squamous cell carcinoma (Winer, 1940; Sommerville, 1953;
Wiskemann, 1955; Mashkilleison, 1965; Lever, 1967; Montgomery, 1967;
Golemba, 1968; Belen'kii, 1968, 1970; Lanné, 1970; and others).

The term "pseudoepitheliomatous hyperplasia" does not, however,
reflect the nature of the process. While "epithelioma" means
literally a tumor derived for epithelium, different authors have used
it to mean different things. Montgomery (1967) pointed out that in
the USA the word "epithelioma" has been replaced by "carcinoma" and
that "epithelioma" is used only for benign epithelial tumors. German
authors employ "epithelioma" to embrace both benign and malignant
epithelial neoplasma, while French authors have used it with reference to malignant tumors only (Civatte, 1967).

In the USSR, a malignant epithelial tumor is generally designated "cancer" (or, less commonly, "carcinoma") and a benign one,
"epithelioma" (Glazunov, 1947; Golovin, 1958; Apatenko, 1973). The
present writer agrees with those (e.g. Gottron and Nikolowski, 1960;
Fischer, 1963; Nazzario and Tosti, 1968; Apatenko, 1973; Pinkus and
Mehregan, 1976; Sanderson, 1979; Kazantseva, 1981) who designate
atypical epidermal growths by the term "pseudocarcinomatous hyperplasia" to emphasize their similarity to squamous cell carcinoma.

It should be noted that "pseudocarcinomatous hyperplasia", too, has been used in different senses by different authors. Thus, some (e.g. Gottron and Nikolowski, 1960; Fischer, 1963; Raichev and Andreev, 1965; Venkei and Sugar, 1965; Nazzario and Tosti, 1968) include under this term those epidermal growths arising at margins of irradiated skin areas following x-ray therapy for carcinoma (so-called pseudorecidiva postirradiationem), while others (e.g. Lanné, 1969) extend it to the epidermal proliferations at margins of cutaneous squamous cell carcinomas. It is difficult, however, to accept the view that the epidermal growth bordering the site of a squamous cell carcinoma treated by radiation can be identical in biologic nature to those arising in sites of chronic inflammation or of benign skin tumors.

Willis (1967) defined hyperplasia as "the proliferation of the cells of a tissue either (a) as a compensatory response to loss of tissue of the same kind or to increased functional demands which the normal amount of tissue cannot satisfy, or (b) as a result of dis-turbed hormonal control of the activity of the tissue". He stated that compensatory hyperplasia is allied to repair and differs from malignant hyperplasia in that the proliferation is limited in amount and duration of its development, and that it progresses only so long as the functional need or hormonal stimulus which evoked it persists. This view is shared by Golovin (1975) who pointed out that pre-cancerous hyperplasia should not be confused with the epithelial growths seen in inflammation or regeneration. He noted further that inflammatory hyperplasia is characterized by downward growth of epithelium into the inflamed underlying tissue, whereas regenerative hyperplasia is marked by its growth over the surface of the defect. But since the boundary between these two kinds of growth is ill defined, Golovin used one term, "inflammatory-regenerative hyper-plasia", to describe both. He wrote that such hyperplasia "is devoid of precancerous significance; at most, it is a preexisting or con-comitant process". A hyperplasia becomes malignant when the excess of proliferating cells of a given tissue has ceased to depend upon the stimulus that has given rise to the hyperplasia. As defined by Willis (1967), a malignant tumor is "an abnormal mass of tissue, the growth of which exceeds and is uncoordinated with that of the normal tissue and persists in the same excessive manner after cessation of the stimulus which evoked the change".

The above concepts of inflammatory and cancerous hyperplasia do not differ substantially from those formulated earlier by Garshin (1939), Glazunov (1947, 1971), Petrov (1947), Khlopin (1947), and other representatives of the Soviet schools of pathology and oncology. It follows from these concepts that atypical hyperplasias of the epidermis in sites of chronic inflammation and in zones of squamous cell carcinomas must not be regarded as identical processes embracable by the term "pseudocarcinomatous hyperplasia". Epidermal hyperplasia at the margin of a squamous cell carcinoma is by no means

a pseudocancerous condition, for it may become the source of a true
cancer (Shabad, 1967; Willis, 1967; Kraevskii and Smol'yanikov,
1971; Golovin, 1975; and others).

Willis (1967) formulated a concept of neoplastic field according
to which a tumor arises, not only from a single focus of tumor cells,
but also from adjacent areas of normal-looking tissue within the
tumor-formative field. Fould's (1969) theory of tumor progression
considers carcinogenesis as a multiple-stage process whereby epithelium undergoes sequential transformation from normal into hyperplastic, then into carcinoma in situ, and finally into invasive
carcinoma. Squamous cell carcinoma may therefore be thought to
develop through progressive neoplastic transformation of cells in
tissue areas adjacent to the epicenter of the tumor. This point has
far-reaching practical implications because it indicates the need for
extensive surgical excision so as to secure an adequate margin of
normal-appearing tissue beyond the visible lesion (Golovin, 1970).

The number of conditions in which atypical epidermal hyperplasia
has been found to develop, is ever increasing. Among these,
Montgomery (1967), for example, mentioned gangrenous, vegetating, and
ulcerative pyodermas; prurigo nodularis of Hyde; tuberculosis verrucosa cutis; syphilis; yaws; fourth venereal disease; granuloma
inguinale; acne keloid; condylomata acuminata; oral florid papillomatosis; North American blastomycosis; chromoblastomycosis; coccidiomy-
cosis; histoplasmosis; sporotrichosis; Norwegian scabies; lesions
arising from insect bites; the verrucose type of discoid lupus
tuberculosus; keratoacanthoma; and Abrikosoff's granular cell
myoblastoma. Pseudocarcinomatous hyperplasia has also been reported
to develop in chronic eczema, lichen ruber verrucosus, giant lichenification of Brocq and Pautrier, trophic ulcers, cutaneous leishmaniasis, lupus tuberculosus, pemphigus vegetans, epidermodysplasia
verruciformis of Lewandowsky and Lutz, dermatitides resulting from
lubricating the skin with tars or acridine dyes, papillomatosis cutis
carcinoides of Gottron, balanoposthitis, chondrodermatitis nodularis
helicis, the warty form of psoriasis, giant condyloma acuminatum of
Buschke and Loewenstein, cutaneous amebiasis, schistosomiasis, seborrheic warts, and histiocytoma (e.g. Gottron and Nikolowski, 1960;
Grzhebin and Tseraidis, 1960; Venkei and Sugar, 1965; Montgomery,
1967; Rook, 1968; Shanin, 1969; Lanné, 1970; Niemi, 1970; Seldam,
1970; Lever and Schaumburg-Lever, 1975).

This listing of skin diseases which may show pseudocarcinomatous
hyperplasia is far from complete. Indeed, it seems that atypical
epidermal hyperplasia bearing clinical and histologic similarities of
varying degrees to keratinizing squamous cell carcinoma can occur in
any skin disorder under certain circumstances (depending on the
general state of the body, duration of the disease, exposure to
adverse environmental factors, etc.).

On the other hand, true squamous cell carcinoma of the skin may arise in a variety of dermatoses.  These have been reported to include, among others, lupus vulgaris, tuberculosis verrucosa cutis, pyoderma ulcerosum vegetans and pyoderma gangrenosum, discoid erythematosis, psoriasis, lichen planus, long-standing fistulas with little tendency to heal, scars, gunshot wounds, trophic ulcers of the lower extremities, condyloma acuminatum and giant condyloma acuminatum of Buschke and Loewenstein, keratoacanthoma, deep mycoses, congenital dyskeratosis of Darier, epidermodysplasia verruciformis of Lewandowsky and Lutz, verrucous acrokeratosis, and bullous epidermolysis (e.g. Glazunov and Blinova, 1960; Belenkii, 1963; Raichev and Andreev, 1965; Venkei and Sugar, 1965; Montgomery, 1967; Jablonska et al., 1969; Shanin, 1969; Helle, 1972; Babayants et al., 1973; Lovell et al., 1980).

It can be inferred from the foregoing that the study of pseudo-carcinomatous hyperplasias arising in various dermatologic disorders is of great practical importance, as is the development of criteria for differentiating these hyperplasias from squamous cell carcinoma of the skin.

The frequent occurrence of pseudocarcinomatous hyperplasia in association with certain dermatoses and skin tumors has led a number of authors (Gottron, 1954; Gottron and Nikolowski, 1960; Civatte, 1967; Nazzario and Tosti, 1968; Pinkus and Mehregan, 1976; Tilgen, 1976) to classify these dermatoses and cutaneous neoplasms under "pseudocarcinoses of the skin".  Gottron (1957) defined cutaneous pseudocarcinosis as a "disease state whose gross or microscopic appearance, or both, so closely resembles a cancer that their differentiation, which is vitally important for the patient, is extremely difficult to make".  Gottron and Nikolowski (1960) grouped under pseudocarcinoses those skin disorders which "despite invasive epidermal growth, cannot be interpreted as carcinoma because of their biologic benignancy".  They stated that since atypical epidermal proliferations are recognized, for the most part, histologically rather than macroscopically, it is at times impossible to discard a diagnosis of carcinoma unless concomitant clinical findings are taken into consideration.  They included in the group of pseudocarcinoses a variety of skin diseases such as carcinoid papillomatosis, keratoacanthoma, pseudorecidiva postirradiationem, epidermal proliferations after topical application of tars or acridine dyes, Abrikosoff's granular cell myoblastoma, certain nevi, senile keratosis, histiocytoma, eccrine spiradenoma, and trichoepithelioma.

Review of this group shows that it is fairly heterogeneous.  Along with dermatoses and skin tumors that are separate disease entities, it includes the "pseudorecurrences" arising after radiation treatment of carcinomas (pseudorecidiva postirradiationem).  In 1947 Knierer described nodular eruptions in the form of a circle or segment arising at the margins of skin areas x-irradiated for carcinoma, and, as pointed out by Knierer and other authors (e.g. Gottron and Nikolowski, 1960; Raichev et al., 1964; Civatte, 1967), such pseudo-recurrence may disappear within 3 to 4 months without any specific treatment being given. There are, however, other reports (Mazur, 1958; Aliev, 1962) indicating that viable tumor cells may persist at the periphery of irradiated skin areas and that these cells may be responsible for tumor regrowth in 7 to 9% of cases. The inclusion of true, but treated malignant neoplasms under pseudocarcinoses is questionable.

Different authors classify cutaneous pseudocarcinoma in different ways. Raichev and Andreev (1965, for example, divided them into primary, or idiopathic, and secondary to various dermatoses. Idio-pathic pseudocarcinoses were taken by them to include keratoacanthoma and papillomatosis cutis carcinoides of Gottron.

Civatte (1967) likewise classified cutaneous pseudocarcinoses into primary and secondary (reactive). In his classification, pri-mary pseudocarcinoses include conditions to which pseudocarcinoma-tous hyperplasia is inherent (Gottron's carcinoid papillomatosis, keratoacanthoma, and micaceous balanitis), while secondary pseudo-carcinoses are those arising in sites of chronic inflammation (pyodermas, toxicodermas, deep mycoses) and of certain benign or malignant connective tissue tumors of the skin. A similar classifi-cation was proposed by Pinkus and Mehregan (1969).

Stevanović (1968) described cancerous hyperplasias as "dynamic", that is, capable of progression (e.g. in keratoacanthoma), or "static" (in Darier's disease, tuberculosis verrucosus, lupus vulgaris). It is difficult, however, to accept this classification because cases are known where pseudocarcinomatous hyperplasia was not only progressing in lesions of lupus vulgaris, trophic ulcers, Darier's disease, and other conditions, but, under certain circum-stances, provided a favorable setting for the development of true squamous cell carcinoma.

Nazzario and Tosti (1968) pointed out that the category of pseudocarcinoses is of a "hybrid nature", for it includes both dis-tinct disease entities and those conditions which cannot be described as such with any certainty. They considered keratoacanthoma, papil-lomatosis cutis carcinoides of Gottron, and pseudoneoplastic giant condyloma of Buschke and Loewenstein as diseases in which pseudo-carcinomatous hyperplasia is primary. The other group included a variety of skin disorders in which it is secondary.

Thambiah (1969), in reviewing clinical and histological errors involved in diagnosis of squamous cell carcinoma of the skin, dis-tinguished premalignant dermatoses from those which may show pseudo-carcinomatous hyperplasia. These latter were taken by him to include cutaneous tuberculosis (lupus vulgaris and lupus verrucosus),

bromoderma and iododerma, blastomycosis, venereal granuloma, keratoacanthoma, seborrheic warts, syphilis, lesions resulting from insect
bites (phlebotodermas), granular cell schwannoma, chronic ulcers,
pyoderma gangrenosum, prurigo nodularis, the hypertrophic form of
Darier's disease and of lichen ruber planus, discoid lupus erythematosus, Norwegian scabies, histiocytoma, and malignant melanoma.  He
noted also that a picture mimicking pseudocarcinomatous hyperplasia
might be seen if tissue sections for histologic study were taken
improperly.

It should be said that Thambiah considered cutaneous tuberculosis, venereal granuloma, chronic ulcers, and discoid erythematosis
as being all premalignant conditions.  Some authors (e.g. Bedner and
Stanova, 1976) include pseudocarcinomatous hyperplasia under
cutaneous precarcinoses, whereas others (e.g. Greiter, 1969) believe
that cutaneous pseudocarcinoses, while presenting a picture of pre-
carcinoma histologically, differ from it in that they never undergo
malignant transformation.  It appears, though, that one should not be
so categorical in evaluating the prognosis for pseudocarcinomatous
hyperplasia.

Although there are reports in the literature that squamous cell
carcinoma develops in association with a number of dermatoses often
included under cutaneous pseudocarcinoses (keratoacanthoma, giant
condyloma of Buschke and Loewenstein, papillomatosis cutis carcinoides of Gottron, pyoderma vegetans, trophic ulcers, etc.), it has
not been demonstrated conclusively whether it actually arises in
sites of pseudocarcinomatous hyperplasia or in other areas of the
epidermis.  It seems more likely that, as pointed out by Golovin
(1975), "... cancer begins evolving from its own, specific precancerous hyperplasia which is devoid of any adaptive significance".

Lanné (1970) has concluded from her studies that although the
processes underlying the epidermal hyperplasias ("pseudoepitheliomatous hyperplasias" according to her terminology) at sites of
chronic inflammation (as in chronic eczema, trophic ulcers of the
lower leg, leishmaniasis, chromoblastomycosis, or lupus tuberculosus)
are very different in biologic nature from those occurring in neoplastic fields (as in epithelial or connective tissue tumors or at
margins of squamous cell carcinomas), the changes that arise in these
processes are very similar morphologically.

According to Golovin (1982), "pseudoepitheliomatous hyperplasia"
is a collective term which is currently employed to mean two different hyperplasias, inflammatory and tumorous; biologically, these
differ from each other in that "the inflammatory hyperplasia is
involved in the elimination of foreign substrates and does not undergo conversion into cancer, whereas the tumorous hyperplasia may well
prove to be a stage in cancer development".  In the opinion of
Golovin, the inflammatory pseudoepitheliomatous hyperplasia corre-

sponds to grades 1-2 of the White and Weidman's classification
described above, and the tumorous hyperplasia, to grades 2-3.

Tilgen (1976) has classified under the term "pseudocarcinoses"
various cutaneous changes differing in etiology and pathogenesis, but
bearing resemblance to squamous cell carcinoma clinically and, more
commonly, histologically. He proposed the following classification
of cutaneous pseudocarcinoses: (1) keratoacanthoma; (2) papillomatosis carcinoides of Gottron; (3) giant condyloma acuminatum of
Buschke and Loewenstein; (4) carcinoid papillomatosis of the oral
mucosa; (5) seborrheic (senile) warts; (6) pseudoepitheliomatous
hyperplasia of the hands; and (7) pseudocarcinomatous hyperplasias of
miscellaneous origins. He subdivided the last category into (a)
actinic pseudocarcinoses and (b) pseudocarcinomatous hyperplasias as
possible reactive concomitants of viral, granulomatous bacterial,
granulomatous mycotic, and drug-induced conditions; of chronic pyodermas; and of granulomatous or verrucose changes arising at margins
of chronic ulcers (of various origins) or of tumors. He also singled
out basal cell hyperplasias simulating basal cell carcinomas. He
stated that it is very difficult to provide a consistent classification of pseudocarcinoses because of the great diversity of skin
diseases reported in the literature as giving rise to pseudocarcinomatous hyperplasias.

Recently, attempts have been made to work out a histologic
classification of pseudomalignant neoplasms. In particular, Connors
and Ackerman (1976) have proposed a working classification of skin
pseudomalignancies. They considered the following histological
changes as simulating malignant growth: (1) hyperplasia of epidermal
keratinocytes arising in condyloma acuminatum modified by application
of podophyllum resin, seborrheic keratosis with inflammation, and
epidermal hyperplasia simulating carcinoma (squamoid and basaloid
hyperplasias); (2) hyperplasias of melanocytes in spindle-cell,
epithelioid-cell, and melanocytic nevi; (3) hyperplasia of follicular
keratinocytes in keratoacanthoma, trichoepithelioma, and proliferating follicular cysts; (4) hyperplasia of fibroblasts in nodular
fascitis and atypical fibroxanthoma; (5) inflammatory cell infil-
trates including among others lymphoid hyperplasia simulating malignant lymphoma; and (b) vascular proliferations (angiolymphoid hyperplasia with eosinophilia).

This grouping thus includes changes in various cytologic and
histologic structures that mimic malignant neoplasms of both epithelial and mesenchymal origins. It should be noted, however, that
Connors and Ackerman's listing of pathologic conditions in which
hyperplasia of keratinocytes may be present is far from complete.
Moreover, the inclusion of basaloid hyperplasia in the group of
epidermal keratocytic hyperplasias that simulate carcinoma is open
to objection, for basaloid hyperplasia is known to simulate, not
squamous cell carcinoma, but basal cell carcinoma. The inclusion of

keratoacanthoma in the group of histologic changes due to hyperplasia
of follicular keratinocytes is likewise questionable, since there are
reports (e.g. Helshan and Buchunan, 1960; Winkelmann and Brown, 1968;
Scafield et al., 1974) that keratoacanthoma may be located on the
oral mucosa, the vermilion border of the lip, or the prepuce which
are all free from follicles.

Thus, there are still may inconsistencies and much disagreement
as regards both the classification of cutaneous pseudocarcinoses and
the evaluation of their essential morphologic and biologic characteristics.

On the basis of a review of the literature and of the personal
experience Belen'kii (1968) and the present writer have identified
two groups of cutaneous diseases associated with pseudocarcinomatous
hyperplasia: those in which such hyperplasia develops in all or
almost all cases ("obligatory pseudocarcinoses") and those in which
it may or may not develop ("facultative pseudocarcinoses").

We have included in the first group keratoacanthoma, papillomatosis cutis carcinoides of Gottron, and giant condyloma acuminatum of
Buschke and Loewenstein.  In our experience, which comprises examination of histologic specimens from 28 patients with these diseases,
pseudocarcinomatous hyperplasia was present in all instances.

The second group includes a total of 29 dermatologic entities
(discoid erythematosis, eczema, psoriasis, chronic ulcerative pyoderma, trophic ulcers of the lower extremities, lichen ruber
verrocosus, tuberculosis verrucosa cutis, dermatofibroma, deep
mycoses, etc.); in these dermatoses pseudocarcinomatous hyperplasia
was present in 36% of our 195 patients.  In some other dermatoses or
skin tumors (Devergie's disease, cutaneous vasculitis, bullous dermatoses, psoriasis, etc.) such hyperplasia was found to occur rarely,
if at all.  We believe that the separation of dermatoses in which
pseudocarcinomatous hyperplasia is obligatory from those in which it
arises facultatively is of practical value because this can contribute to better differentiation between pseudocarcinomatous epidermal
hyperplasia and squamous cell carcinoma of the skin.

It must be stressed that the vast majority of studies concerned
with cutaneous pseudocarcinoses have been, so far, of a purely
descriptive character and have not inquired into the biologic essence
of pseudocarcinomatous hyperplasia.

The biologic nature of atypical hyperplasia of the epidermis can
be adequately evaluated only on the basis of combined findings from
clinicopathologic, cytophysiologic, and cytogenetic investigations.
Such investigations are described, discussed, and evaluated in the
chapters which follow.

# 2
# Factors Predisposing to Pseudocarcinomatous Hyperplasia and to Malignant Transformation of the Epidermis

This chapter considers factors, both endogenous and exogenous, which are conducive to pseudocarcinomatous hyperplasia of the epidermis and which may also have a role to play in its premalignant and malignant transformation. While some of these factors are carcinogenic in the broad sense, they may evoke either reactive or precancerous epidermal hyperplasia depending on the duration of exposure to them and on the state of the body. For example, a single trauma may result in the formation of a trophic ulcer and promote the development of ulcerative pyoderma, in both of which conditions pseudocarcinomatous epidermal hyperplasia is often seen to arise, whereas exposure of a skin area to repetitive trauma may lead to premalignant changes; or, inappropriate topical application of drugs in certain dermatoses (lichen ruber verrucosus, psoriasis, lupus erythematosus, etc.) may bring about either changes that clinically stimulate malignant transformation or a true squamous cell carcinoma of the skin.

After Percivall Pott recognized, in 1775, coal soot as a cause of scrotal cancer in chimney sweeps (Potter, 1963), and after Yamagiwa and Ichikawa (1915) succeeded in eliciting cancer of the skin experimentally by painting rabbit ears with coal tar, an enormous number of reports have appeared in the literature to incriminate a diversity of factors in the promotion, initiation, or production of cancerous alterations in animals and humans under certain circumstances. As stated by Shabad (1967), "... we are now able to induce experimentally any malignant tumor in any body area and thus to identify and examine the various precancerous changes."

It is a well established fact that knowledge of the etiology and pathogenesis of any disorder, including hyperplasia of the epidermis, can furnish a key to its treatment. However, no systematic account

12

of factors predisposing to or promoting pseudocarcinomatous epidermal hyperplasia has appeared in the literature so far.

Here, we will discuss the following factors:  sex, age, chronic inflammation of the skin, trauma, sunlight, chemical agents, and heredity.  It should be stressed at the outset that these factors are regarded, not as being directly responsible for pseudocarcinomatous hyperplasia, but only as being conducive to the development in the body of a special biologic situation in which the epidermis becomes capable of an atypical, excessive proliferation of keratinocytes which is, however, subject to regulatory control by the organism.

## 2.1   SEX AND AGE

A review of the literature and our personal experience indicate that pseudocarcinomatous hyperplasia may be associated with the factors of sex and age in only so far as these affect or have a bearing on the dermatologic disorder in which such hyperplasias arise.

As discussed in Chapter 1, there are dermatoses and cutaneous tumors in which pseudocarcinomatous hyperplasia is seen to develop invariably or almost so (obligatory pseudocarcinoses) as well as dermatoses in which it may or may not arise (facultative pseudo-carcinoses). The range of skin ailments falling into the latter category is so wide that it seems impossible to establish any statistically meaningful sex or age predilection.

A more meaningful assessment can be made for obligatory pseudo-carcinoses, because their range is narrow and well defined.  Thus, keratoacanthoma has been reported to be more common in men aged over 40 (Torsuev, 1959; Silberberg et al., 1962; Korelenshtein, 1970; Mashkilleison, 1970; Schnitzler et al., 1977; and others).  Torsuev (1959) found from a review of some 300 reported cases that the disease affected men in 55.3% of the cases and that the average age of all the patients was 61½ years.  Silberberg et al. (1962) found that keratoacanthoma of the lip was 3 times more frequent in men than in women and that the average age of the patients was 52 years.  Giant condyloma acuminatum of Buschke and Loewenstein usually affects men, mostly between the ages of 30 and 50 (Machacek and Weakley, 1960; Nazzario and Tosti, 1968).  Predilection for men aged over 50 is also shown by the rarely encountered disease known as papillomatosis cutis carcinoides of Gottron (Adam et al., 1956).  These data indicate that obligatory pseudocarcinomatous hyperplasia tends to occur in men aged beyond 40 years, and this tendency prevailed in our patients also: of the 28 patients with such hyperplasia, 20 were men and 8 women and only 4 of the patients were under 40 (the age of the other 24 patients ranged 40 to 80 years).

A similar tendency was seen among our 195 cases of dermatoses with facultative pseudocarcinomatous hyperplasia. This group included 63 women and 132 men, and 23 patients were aged 20 to 29 years; 30,30 to 39; 52, 40 to 49; 38, 50 to 59; 33, 60 to 69; and 19, 70 to 80 years or older. Thus the age of most (72.8%) of the patients was over 40 years.

Men aged over 50 years likewise predominated among our patients with squamous cell carcinoma of the skin. Of the 36 patients in this group, 22 were men and 14 women, and 23 were aged between 50 and 83 years. Similar sex and age incidence rates have been reported by other authors (e.g. Raichev and Andreev, 1965; Venkei and Sugar, 1965; Shanin, 1969). This suggests that the factors of sex and age have a role to play in the occurrence of squamous cell carcinoma.

It seems therefore that age and sex are important factors predisposing to pseudocarcinomatous hyperplasia, particularly in skin conditions for which such hyperplasia is an essential, obligatory feature (keratoacanthoma, papillomatosis cutis carcinoides, Buschke-Loewenstein's tumor). Age, in addition, appears to be a factor inviting to pseudocarcinomatous hyperplasia in chronic pyoderma ulcerosum vegetans and in trophic ulcers of the lower extremities. Of 35 of our patients with such pyodermas, 22 were aged over 40 years, and of the 16 patients with trophic ulcers, the age of 12 was beyond 50. These data provide indirect evidence that general health and the state of individual bodily systems may be important factors in promoting or counteracting the development of atypical reactive epidermal hyperplasia.

## 2.2  CHRONIC INFLAMMATION OF THE SKIN

Gershin (1939) wrote that "... inasmuch as we recognize a given epithelial proliferation as inflammatory, we have to acknowledge that the stimulus to this proliferation is identical with that to inflammatory proliferation of the mesenchyme." However, as was rightly believed by Garshin, the recognition of epithelial proliferation as inflammatory does not yet explain why the epithelium is capable of infiltrative growth. In their fundamental investigations into inflammatory epithelial growth, Garshin (1927, 1939) and Fischer-Wasels (1927, 1933) showed experimentally that, given a suitable stimulus (such as scarlet red or formalin in oil), epithelial cells are able to destroy cartilage by growing into or even through it without, however, undergoing malignant transformation. It should be said that such observations indicate that epidermis is induced to proliferate not so much by inflammation as by the foreign material present in the subjacent tissue. The most convincing results were obtained by Garshin and his co-workers in experiments where atypical epidermal growth was induced by an infusorial earth (siliceous material derived from the remains of diatoms or sponges) injected intradermally into rabbit ears. The epidermis was observed to creep over and around the infusorial earth clumps when these were surrounded by connective tissue. But if connective tissue had not yet had enough time to surround the foreign particles, then epidermal cells were seen not only to grow around but also through these particles. It was concluded that it is the state of connective tissue which determines the ability of epidermis to undergo infiltrative (but nonmalignant) growth. On this basis, Garshin (1939) suggested, for the first time, that "epithelium will not show infiltrative growth if it overlies a medium that is proper to it physiologically"; if, on the other hand, epithelium is growing on a substratum which is physiologically improper to it, it will infiltrate the substratum.

The principal conclusion stemming from those studies, which were performed nearly half a century ago but are still relevant today, is that control over nonneoplastic epithelial growth, including infiltrative growth, is exercised by the organism through the mediacy of connective tissue. By contrast, neoplastic epithelial growth is not regulated by the organism, but occurs autonomously.

The importance of these studies for understanding the biologic nature of atypical, but benign, epithelial growth can hardly be overestimated. Garshin's observations regarding atypical epidermal growth have been confirmed by numerous clinical studies. The relationship of infiltrative epidermal growth to alterations in the subjacent connective tissue can be appreciated best by considering cases of pseudocarcinomatous hyperplasia. A majority of authors have noted that atypical invasive epidermal proliferations simulating differentiated squamous cell carcinomas occur more commonly over foci of granulomatous infiltration (e.g. Winer, 1940; Petrov, 1947; Allen, 1954; Glazunov and Blinova, 1960; Ju, 1967; Lever, 1967; Nazzario and Tosti, 1968; Apatenko, 1969, 1973; Lanné, 1969; Vikhert et al., 1973; Connors and Ackerman, 1976). In most instances, the appearance of pseudocarcinomatous hyperplasia is preceded by alterations in the dermis (Sanderson, 1968). Thambiah (1969) considers the causes of such hyperplasia to include chronic granulomatous processes and anoxia of the tissue. That the factor of anoxia can be involved in the production of hyperplasia, is indicated by experiments on animals in which epidermal hyperplasia was found to arise only above nonperforated cellophane plates embedded in the skin and to be absent above perforated plates (Thambiah, 1969).

According to Vasil'ev (1961) nonneoplastic epithelial growth is characterized by the following: (1) invasive downward proliferation of epithelium into the connective tissue in a certain phase of the inflammatory process, (2) formation of epithelial cysts around foci of necrosis or around foreign bodies, (3) subsequent transfer of the necrotic tissue and foreign body particles to the skin surface, and (4) complete regression of the epithelial proliferation once the inflammation has ceased. It was reported by Vasil'ev (1961) that the

epithelium adjacent to implanted foreign bodies (small celloidin
tubes) was invariably growing out to infiltrate the young connective
tissue that had developed around the celloidin tubes.  These features
of inflammatory growth are fully consistent with the results of
studies by Garshin referred to above.

Ju (1967), in discussing mechanisms of reactive epidermal proliferation, mentioned the following three possible situations which
illustrate the relationship between epidermis and dermis: (1) after
an acute loss of tissue caused by a physical, chemical, mechanical,
or other injurious agent, connective tissue elements and vascular
capillaries proliferate and fill the gap, followed by proliferation
of epidermal cells which gradually line up the wound surface, with
the proliferation of connective tissue ceasing once the new epidermis
has covered the center of the wound; (b) in lesions due to chronic
irritation of skin by chemicals, bacterial or fungal infection, or so
on, the tissue responds by a process of chronic inflammation, and the
epidermal proliferation leads to hyperplasia in which the interpapillary growth of the acanthotic epidermis occurs in an orderly
manner; and (c) in cases of pseudocarcinomatous hyperplasia, epidermal cells and those of the chronic granulomatous infiltrate proliferate simultaneously in the dermis.

It is evident that the above author considers some aspects of
the relationship between epithelium and connective tissue in regenerative and inflammatory hyperplasia.  It should be noted, however,
that the proliferation of epidermal cells in pseudocarcinomatous
hyperplasia does not necessarily occur simultaneously with that of
the cells of a granulomatous inflammatory infiltrate.  Indeed, evidence in the literature (e.g. Winer, 1940; Sommerville, 1953; Lever,
1967; Montgomery, 1967; Lanné, 1969; Vikhert et al., 1973; Connors
and Ackerman, 1976) and our own observations indicate that pseudocarcinomatous hyperplasia often arises in sites of chronic inflammation in the absence of granulomatous infiltrate (as in trophic
ulcers, lichen ruber verrucosus, chilitis, giant condyloma acuminatum, giant lichenification of Brocq and Pautrier, etc.).

Atypical epidermal hyperplasia occurs not only at sites of
inflammation but also over benign connective tissue tumors of the
skin, in particular histiocytomas.  Such a hyperplasia simulates
basalioma (basal cell carcinoma) and has been designated pseudobasaloid (e.g. R. Cramer and H. Cramer, 1963).  Pseudobasaloid hyperplasia may arise not only over a histiocytoma but also on the adjacent skin (Thies and Hennies, 1968), and it may be so similar in
appearance to basal cell carcinoma as to be misdiagnosed as such.
For example, although Tolpi and Ellen (cited in Thies and Hennies,
1968) reported histiocytoma to be associated with basal cell carcinoma in 9 out of 114 histiocytoma cases, it may well be that in some
of these cases pseudobasaloid hyperplasia was actually present.
Niemi (1970), in reviewing the literature and personal experience,

described cases of striking pseudobasaloid hyperplasia developing over benign fibrohistiocytic tumors of the skin. Goette and Helwig (1975) believe that acanthosis, pseudoepitheliomatous hyperplasia, and basal cell proliferation on the surface of dermatofibromas all represent reactive changes in the epidermis. Clinical observations have thus confirmed Garshin's observations regarding the patterns of invasive epidermal growth in cases where the connective tissue underlying the epidermis had developed a chronic inflammatory infiltrate or a tumor which altered the normal physiologic substratum of the epidermis.

Precancerous hyperplasia and squamous cell carcinoma are characterized by epidermis-dermis relationships that are different in principle from those in benign epidermal hyperplasia. Pinkus (1968) discussed the following four possible forms of relationship between epithelium and underlying connective tissue in epithelial malignancy: (1) the preformed connective tissue is invaded and destroyed by the epithelim; (2) the preformed connective tissue shows a defensive response by developing inflammation; (3) the connective tissue is induced by the tumor to supply a supporting vascular stroma for the tumor; and (4) the connective tissue interacts with, and possibly induces, epithelial growth, being part of the tumor. It should be noted that the first and fourth of these phenomena have some features in common with pseudocarcinomatous hyperplasia. Indeed, as shown by experimental (e.g. Ruchinskii, 1910; Garshin, 1939; Ou Bau-syan, 1961) and clinicopathologic studies (e.g. Winer, 1940; Sommerville, 1953; Lever, 1967; Sanderson, 1968), in pseudocarcinomatous hyperplasia there may occur infiltrative and destructive growth accompanied in some cases by destruction of connective tissue elements, and epidermal proliferation may be induced by the chronic infiltrate present in the dermis. As regards the second and third phenomena, there are no profound biologic differences between them, and they both represent a single mechanism of response in carcinogenesis.

Vasil'ev and Gel'stein (1962) emphasize that the changes taking place in tissues during carcinogenesis differ from those in the case of ordinary reactive proliferation mainly in that in the course of carcinogenic influences there occurs selection of a cell population with enhanced responsiveness to proliferative stimuli which leads eventually to autonomous replication of cells. According to Vasil'ev (1961), what predisposes to certain kinds of human cancer is not so much chronic inflammation per se as the trophic changes in the tissue which arise because of the atypical course followed by the inflammation.

It was considered by Monacelli (1967) that precancerous epidermal changes that may eventually lead to carcinoma are precipitated by chronic disease involving atrophy and scarring (such as lupus vulgaris or lichen sclerosus et atrophicus of the genitalia), and by burn scars, chronic fistulas in osteomyelitis, and some other dis-

orders.  In the above author's view, of great significance in the
promotion of pretumorous and tumorous conditions of the skin are
injury to the mesenchyme in superficial areas of the corium and an
altered state of the circulation.

Chronic inflammation is thus a principal determinant of pseudocarcinomatous epidermal hyperplasia.  By contrast, inflammation is
not a sine qua non for the development of precancerous changes
(Shabad, 1962).  Malignant transformation occurs under the influence
of exogenous and endogenous carcinogenous factors which bring about a
sequence of processes ranging from diffuse hyperplasia through circumscribed hyperplasia and benign tumors to malignant transformation
of the epithelium (Shabad, 1977).

## 2.3  TRAUMA

As early as 1910, Ruchinskii concluded from his experimental
studies that wherever the epidermis has a propensity for proliferation, a severe mechanical trauma is bound to enhance epidermal
growth, imparting to it a similarity with the atypical epidermal
proliferation seen in cancer.  Particularly abundant epidermal
growths with horn pearl formation and numerous mitotic figures,
including abnormal ones, were found by Ruchinskii (1910) to occur
in rabbit ears exposed to a strong blow followed by an injection of
scarlet red.  There are many indications in the literature to implicate mechanical trauma in the development of several dermatoses
accompanied by pseudocarcinomatous hyperplasia (e.g. Winer, 1940;
Sommerville, 1953; Sanderson, 1968; Thambiah, 1969; Tilgen, 1976).
Sommerville (1953) described a case of chronic ulcerative pyoderma
arising in a farm laborer who had suffered an accidental puncture
from barbed wire to his left ring finger.  That single traumatic
incident eventually made it necessary to amputate the upper extremity
and to undertake, over a period of 10 years, repeated surgical exci-
sions of the areas showing excessive, though benign, epidermal proliferation.  Kopf (1968) considers mechanical trauma as an important
causative factor in keratoacanthoma in which pseudocarcinomatous
hyperplasia is known to be singularly striking.  He suggested that
keratoacanthomas may arise at sites of trauma as Kobner's phenomenon.
That trauma is a factor inciting to keratoacanthoma has been pointed
out by Elscher (1956), Stevanović (1968), Tilgen (1976), and other
authors.  Civatte et al. (1973) suggested that mechanical trauma and
exposure to sunlight are implicated in the origin of "pseudoepitheliomatous hyperplasia of the hands."

Tilgen (1976) emphasizes that among the causes of carcinoid
papillomatosis of the oral mucosa, a disease classified under pseudocarcinoses, are trauma and the smoking and chewing of tobacco.  These
factors are widely recognized as important contributors to precancerous changes.  In particular, repetitive trauma may predispose to

cancerous changes in various parts of the body (Petrov, 1947;
Belisario, 1963; Raichev and Andreev, 1965; Willis, 1967; Shanin,
1969; Mashkilleison, 1970; and others).

Smoking as a possible cause of pseudocarcinomatous hyperplasia
and precancerous lesions occurring in the oral mucosa and the
vermilion border of the lip is important primarily inasmuch as it
involves repetitive exposure to heat.  It has been shown by
Scassellati and Mastrandria (1963) that the burning tip of a cigarette
has a temperature of 500 to 650°C on the average, and that the temperature decreases to only 480–490°C during the interval following an
inhalation of tobacco fume.  Apart from the direct thermal effects on
the oral mucosa, substances are formed during smoking (such as 3,4-
benzpyrene, other polycyclic hydrocarbons, and trivalent arsenic)
which are known to be obligatory precarcinogens (Shabad, 1967).

As reported by Mashkilleison (1970) from his personal experience, of 874 patients with precancerous conditions of the oral mucosa
or the vermilion border of the lip, single trauma preceded precancer
in 24 patients (2.7%) and repeated or persistent traumas, in 304
(34.7%); 61% of the 874 patients were habitual smokers, as were 434
of 536 patients with leukoplakia (81%) seen by that author.

## 2.4  EXPOSURE TO SUNLIGHT

Excessive insolation has a highly important role to play in the
causation of precancerous changes and of certain dermatoses attended
by pseudocarcinomatous epidermal hyperplasia.  The carcinogenic
component of solar ultraviolet radiation has been considered the
major predisposing factor to carcinoma and also to solar keratosis,
keratoacanthoma, and basal cell carcinoma (Belisario, 1963).  The
most important histologic finding confirming the involvement of
ultraviolet radiation in the origin of skin tumors is collagen degeneration.  Thambiah (1969) mentioned solar radiation as the most
important single environmental factor in the induction of precancerous conditions, noting that harmful effects of excessive solar exposure had been recognized since ancient times; he referred to the
Book of Psalms in the Bible, where Psalm 121 says: "The sun shall not
smite thee by day."  Prolonged exposure to sunlight is believed by
many to be decisive in the causation of keratoacanthoma, chrondro-
dermatitis helicis, and the warty form of lupus erythematosus
(Gottron and Nikolowski, 1960; Montgomery, 1967; Sanderson, 1968),
which all show pseudocarcinomatous epidermal hyperplasia as a concomitant feature.

## 2.5  EXPOSURE TO CHEMICAL AGENTS

The development of pseudocarcinomatous hyperplasia is promoted
by certain chemicals and drugs, including among others iodides and

bromides, and by viral, bacterial, and fungal infections (e.g. White
and Weidman, 1927; Montgomery and Holman, 1938; Winer, 1940; Gottron
and Nikolowski, 1960; Porters and Zantkuyl, 1975; Perroud and
Delacretaz, 1977). It is significant that chemical stimulants and
some drugs are capable of inducing atypical epidermal growth both
when acting on the skin directly and when ingested. The most typical
examples of the latter are iododerma and bromoderma which at times
closely mimic cutaneous squamous cell carcinoma in clinical and
histopathologic appearances. Porters and Zantkuyl (1975) reported a
case of iododerma arising in a 67-year-old woman following long-term
(2 years) ingestion of an iodine-containing drug. The resulting
tumors with ulcerations were thought to be malignant and were
removed. The correct diagnosis was not made until after a nonspecific granulomatous infiltrate had been found deep in the dermis
by histologic examination and more tumors had appeared on the skin.
It may be particularly difficult to differentiate pseudocarcinomatous
hyperplasia from squamous cell carcinoma following external therapy
with strongly acting drugs (those containing tar or arsenic, cytostatic agents, etc.) or exposure to potent chemical irritants (acids,
alkalis, etc.). Such therapy may modify the clinicopathologic picture of the underlying benign skin disorder to such an extent as to
make it similar to and confusable with, carcinoma, as, for example,
has repeatedly been reported to be the case with topical application
of podophyllum for condyloma acuminatum (Machacek and Weakley, 1960;
Montgomery, 1967). Warty growths in psoriasis may result from long-
continued ingestion of arsenicals, prolonged topical application of
sulfonamides, or other improper treatments (Trofimova and Mordovtsev,
1975).

In our experience, inappropriate methods of external therapy
were responsible for about 8% of the pseudocarcinomatous epidermal
hyperplasias seen to arise in various cutaneous disorders. Some of
such cases showed verrucose growths that developed ulcerations with
raised edges which aroused suspicion of malignancy while remaining
essentially benign. One example is given in Figure 1, which shows
ulcerated warty elements in a 70-year-old woman which appeared after
application of occlusive dressings containing 50% Prospidinum ointment. Histological examination (Figure 2) revealed an appearance
consistent with incipient pseudocarcinomatous hyperplasia. Inspec-
tion of this patient two years thereafter showed the presence of
atrophic scars in the lesional skin.

On the other hand, it is well established that long-continued
use of potent chemotherapeutic agents may lead to precancerous
lesions that eventuate in squamous cell cancer (Raichev and Andreev,
1965; Venkei and Sugar, 1965; Shabad, 1967; Shanin, 1969; Thambiah,
1969; Mashkilleison, 1970). Among 36 of our patients with squamous
cell carcinoma of the skin, prolonged medication (often self-
medication) with potent drugs was one of the reasons for the occurrence of cancer in six cases of lichen ruber verrucosus, trophic
ulcers, and psoriasis.

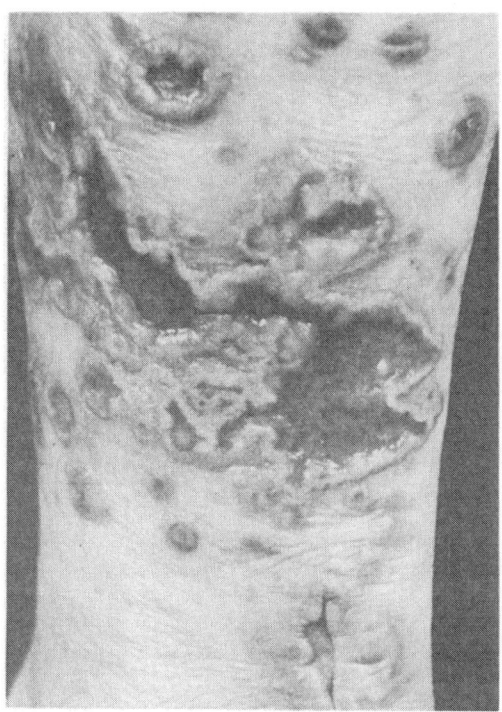

Fig. 1.   Lichen ruber verrucosus, showing ulcerations caused by
          application of 50% Prospidinum ointment.


For illustration, here is a case report.

        Patient A., a 61-year old man, was readmitted to our
department complaining of eruptions all over the skin.  He
had been suffering from psoriasis since the age 13 (i.e.
for 48 years) for which he had received, with only transient benefit, various therapies including continual treatment with Psoriasinum and chrysarobin ointments, arsenic
injections, and Asiatic pills between 1947 and 1957 and
with Antipsoriaticum and salicylic acid ointments between
1967 and 1970.  Approximately in 1972, warty growths began
appearing over psoriatic plaques in the abdominal region
and on the shins, and he continued lubricating these as
before.  In 1973 he was admitted to our department where a
diagnosis of squamous cell carcinoma supervening on
psoriasis was made.  Roentgen therapy resulted in an apparent cure, but two or three years later tumorlike lesions
began to appear again over the psoriatic plaques.

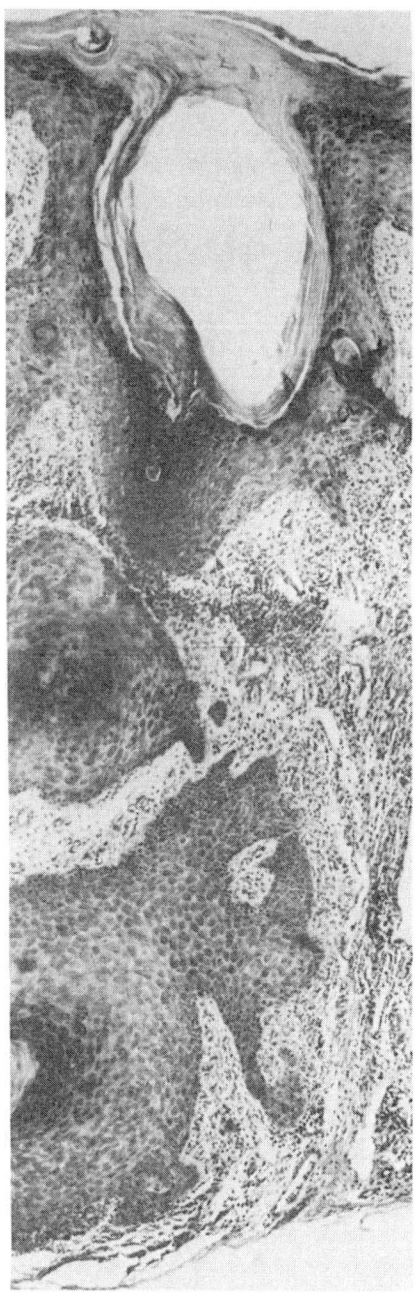

Fig. 2.  Lichen ruber verrucosus (specimen of shin skin), showing
         proliferation of the epithelium of hair follicles to produce
         an appearance of pseudocarcinomatous hyperplasia.  (75 X;
         hematoxylin and eosin. Montage.)

On physical examination large plaques of psoriasis of deep pink color showing small multilayer grayish scales on their surfaces were seen on the trunk and extremities, as were an elevated compact wartlike lesion about 1.5 cm in diameter on the abdomen (Figure 3) and a round tumor of firm consistency some 3 cm in diameter with central ulceration on the upper third of the anterolateral surface of the right leg (Figure 4); the floor of the ulcer was covered with a sanguinous exudate.

Histologic examination of the skin biopsied from the tumorlike lesion on the leg (Figure 5) revealed striking acanthosis.  The proliferating epidermis was overlaid by a loose crust consisting of a parakeratotic horn permeated by cellular detritus.  Under the crust, stratum granulosum was absent in places.  The stratum spinosum was strongly edematous, and the cytoplasm of spinous cells stained only lightly.  Strands of irregularly proliferated spinous cells penetrated deep into the dermis.  The boundary between the epidermis and dermis was indistinct in places.  Besides the

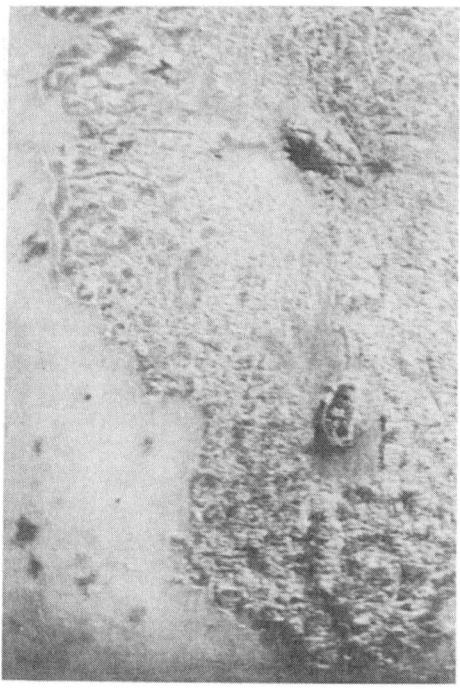

Fig. 3.  Wartlike lesion arising in psoriasis that has been long treated with Psoriasinum, Antipsoriaticum, and other topical medicaments.

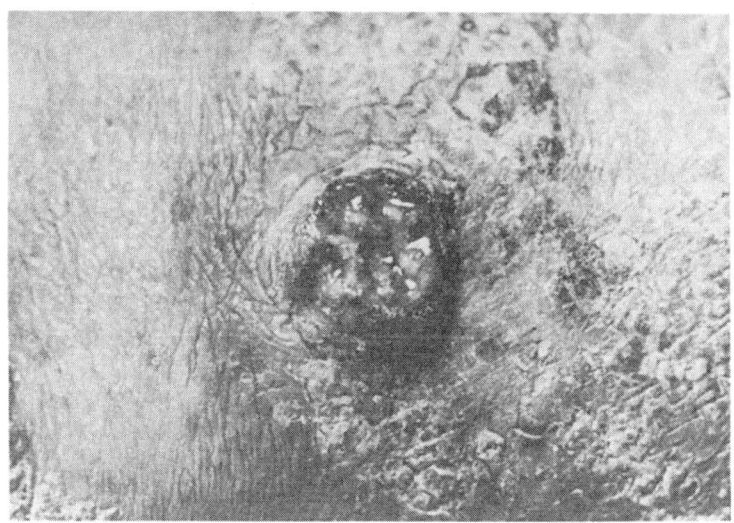

Fig. 4.  Keratinizing squamous cell carcinoma on the right shin that
         has supervened on psoriasis in same patient as in Fig. 3.


acanthotic epidermis there were groups of epidermal cells
showing disorganization and polymorphism.  Some of the
nuclei were pycnotic and lumpy, and abnormal mitotic figures were present.  Cells of a fairly dense infiltrate
consisting of lymphocytes, histiocytes, and plasma cells had
penetrated into the epidermal proliferations.

     The final diagnosis was psoriasis complicated by
squamous cell carcinoma.

     Thus, irrational topical use of potent chemotherapeutics or of
chemical stimulants may lead up to pseudocarcinomatous epidermal
hyperplasia in some cases and to squamous cell cancer in others.
Similarly, other exogenous factors (trauma, insolation, etc.) may
play important roles in the causation of atypical reactive hyperplasia, as well as of precancerous changes and squamous cancer.  In
most instances, these factors promote the development of inflammation
consequent to which an atypical reactive hyperplasia of the epidermis
may arise.  In the case of precancerous hyperplasia, such factors
first elicit dystrophic changes in epidermal cells.

     Of great importance in mediating the effects of various adverse
environmental factors on the skin appears to be the state of the
organism as a whole and of its genetic structures in particular.

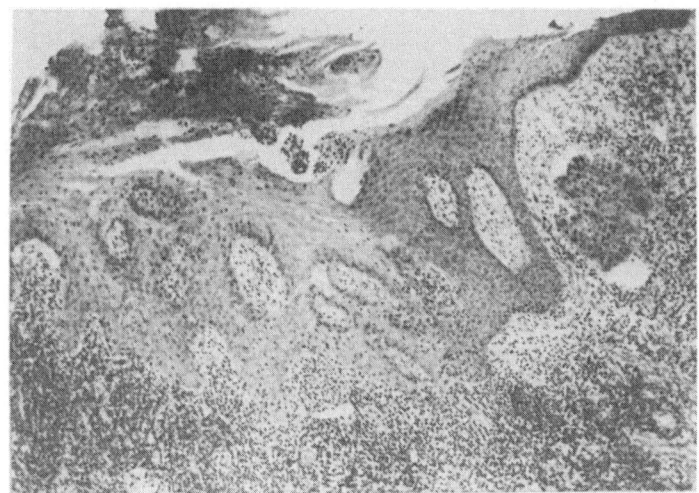

Fig. 5.   Shin skin of same patient as in Figs. 3 and 4, showing
          keratinizing squamous cell carcinoma supervening on
          psoriasis.  Note irregular epidermal proliferation, ill-
          defined border between epidermis and dermis, parakeratosis,
          and aggregates of epidermal cells exhibiting considerable
          disarray and polymorphism. (75 X; hematoxylin and eosin.)


2.6  HEREDITY

     The role of hereditary factors in the causation of various
dermatoses showing atypical reactive epidermal hyperplasia, and of
benign tumors and squamous cell carcinomas is a subject of considerable interest.  There are numerous reports incriminating these factors in the development of many cutaneous disorders (eczema,
psoriasis, atopic dermatitis, keratoderma, epidermolysis bullosa,
etc.) (e.g. Abele et al., 1963; Graciansky, 1964; Schnyder, 1966;
Lynch, 1969; Belenkii, 1970; Berenbein, 1971; Smelov et al., 1973;
Suvorova and Anton'iev, 1977) and of benign and malignant tumors in
various body areas (e.g. Martynova, 1945; Petrov, 1947; Nierman,
1964; Willis, 1967; Shevchenko, 1976; Gay Prieto, 1977).

     It should be noted that hereditary factors have much less
importance in bringing about pseudocarcinomatous hyperplasia than
they have in the production of precancerous and cancerous lesions of
the skin.  It seems more correct to speak of the etiologic importance
of hereditary factors, not in pseudocarcinomatous hyperplasia as
such, but in those dermatoses or benign cutaneous tumors in which
such hyperplasia is seen to occur more commonly.  The advances made
in genetics in general and in oncologic genetics in particular have
provided important insights into the genetic mechanisms and hereditary factors involved in production of malignancy.  Among the dis-

eases which may be classified under "pseudocancerosis", heredity has
been demonstrated to play a part in the so-called familial primary
self-healing squamous cell carcinoma of Ferguson-Smith, a condition
which resembles squamous cell carcinoma only histopathologically and
which does not produce metastases (Curric and Ferguson-Smith, 1952;
Civatte, 1967; Montgomery, 1967; Sanderson, 1968; and others).  In
the Swiss Dermatologic Center this disease was recognized in 62
patients from 11 families (Ferguson-Smith et al., 1971)  It is inherited as an autosomal dominant trait.  Ferguson-Smith suggested
that it had originated as the result of a single mutation in a
married couple in 1790.

According to  Schnitzler et al. (1977), the fact that multiple
primary self-healing squamous cell carcinoma is genetically determined is an important consideration in distinguishing it from multiple keratoacanthoma.

Pseudocarcinomatous hyperplasia may occur in the early benign
form of pigmentary and papillary dystrophy (acanthosis nigricans)
which has an autosomal dominant mode of inheritance; in the ulcerative vegetating form of epidermolysis bullosa which has autosomal
recessive inheritance; in focal epithelial hyperplasia which is
presumably inherited as a autosomal recessive trait (Bazyka and
Bashkirova, 1975); and in some other hereditary diseases of the skin.

Much more numerous are reports associating hereditary factors
with malignant neoplasms in various parts of the body, including the
skin.  Lynch (1969), in a comprehensive review Skin, Heredity, and
Cancer, presented a systematic account of all known dermatologic
conditions associated with cancer which have a definite or presumptive hereditary etiology, listing among others neurofibromatosis,
Gardner's syndrome, malignant cutaneous melanoma, giant pigmented
nevi, and generalized keratoacanthoma which all have an autosomal
dominant mode of inheritance and mentioning xeroderma pigmentosum as
an autosomal recessive condition.

According to Shevchenko (1976), the probability of malignant
neoplasms occurring among relatives of a proband affected with skin
cancer is 5 to 7 times as high as among members of families unag-
gravated by heredity.  By analyzing archival material relating to
about 2500 medical records and inquiring into the genealogies of the
persons concerned, Schevchenko has identified a total of 183 "cancer-
prone" families in which malignant tumors had occurred among kindred
of two or three generations.  In one instance, four generations of a
proband's relatives were affected by skin cancer at the same site
(the eyelid area).

Urbach (1969) and Lane-Brown and Melia (1973) reported increased
incidence rates of basal cell carcinoma, actinic keratosis, and
squamous cell carcinoma in persons of Celtic ancestry.  Urbach et al.

(1970) found that among U.S. immigrants, Irish had significantly more
and Italians significantly fewer skin tumors than non-Italians from
Central Europe.  They suggested that there may be a genetic predisposition to cancer among the Irish.

In our series of 259 cases, diseases similar to or identical
with those affecting our patients, had occurred among close relatives
of 28 patients (10.6%).  In the group of 187 patients with various
dermatoses attended by pseudocarcinomatous hyperplasia, such diseases
had affected close relatives of 16 patients (8.5%), namely those with
giant lichenification of Brocq and Pautrier, warty psoriasis,
Darier's disease, lichen ruber verrocosus, and prurigo nodularis.  In
the group of 36 patients with epithelial or connective tissue tumors
of the skin, such tumors had occurred in close relatives of 4
patients (those with seborrheic wart or senile keratoma).  Finally,
in the group of 36 patients with squamous cell carcinoma of the skin,
close relatives of 8 patients (22%) had a history of skin cancer in
various sites. One example is a patient with cutaneous squamous cell
carcinoma whose family members had all been affected with cancer; his
father had died from esophageal cancer, his mother from mammary
cancer, and his brother from gastric cancer.

The foregoing discussion shows that various exogenous and hereditary factors act as important promoters of many skin diseases involving pseudocarcinomatous epidermal hyperplasia or skin carcinogenesis.  Of importance are also concomitant cardiovascular, nervous,
or gastrointestinal disorders which make the skin more vulnerable to
adverse environmental influences (including infectious and toxic
agents) and which are known to play an important role in many dermatologic disorders (chronic pyoderma ulcerosum vegetans, lupus
tuberculosus, cutaneous leishmaniasis, chromoblastomycosis, condyloma
acuminatum, etc.).

# 3
# Clinicopathologic Characteristics of Pseudocarcinomatous Epidermal Hyperplasia and of Squamous Cell Carcinoma

## 3.1 CLINICAL OBSERVATIONS

Although the clinicopathologic characteristics of pseudo-carcinomatous epidermal hyperplasia have much in common with those of keratinizing squamous cell carcinoma, detailed studies can reveal features that are more typical for one or the other of these conditions.

In reviewing our recent clinical experience comprising 259 cases (187 with various dermatoses accompanied by pseudocarcinomatous hyperplasia, 36 with epithelial or connective tissue tumors, and 36 with keratinizing squamous cell carcinoma), we distributed the patients in each of these three groups according to type of inflammation in lesional areas, duration of the disease process, number and distribution of lesions, and clinical and histologic appearances of these.

Type of inflammation. As early as 1938, Montgomery and Holman stated that the clinical differentiation of squamous cell carcinoma from pseudocarcinomatous hyperplasia rests primarily on the presence of a pronounced inflammatory reaction in the latter. In support of this contention, they referred to a farmer in whom a tumorlike lesion on the hand was misdiagnosed as a squamous cell carcinoma on histologic examination, and it was only the presence of inflammation around the lesion and of associated lymphangitis that enabled the clinicians to recognize sporotrichosis and thus to avoid amputation of the hand. However, the presence of an inflammatory reaction at the lesional site does not necessarily allow one to discard a diagnosis of squamous cell carcinoma in cases of doubt. Indeed, dermatologists and oncologists are well aware of instances where inflam-

mation likewise accompanied squamous cell carcinomas complicated by
secondary infection (e.g. Monastyrskaya, 1945; Shanov, 1961;
Studnitsyn, 1965). Therefore the existence of chronic inflammation
in a dermatosis in which the development of squamous cell carcinoma
is known to be a possibility, cannot be taken as conclusive clinical
evidence against malignant transformation of the hyperplastic epidermis.

Table 1 indicates the types of inflammatory process seen in our
patients. As can be found from this table, circumscribed or diffuse
inflammation was present in 198 of the 259 patients (76.4%).

Among the 187 patients with miscellaneous dermatoses, clinical
signs of inflammation were absent in only six patients (2 of them had
Darier's disease, 2 had keratodermia, and 2 had circumscribed hyperkeratosis of the lower lip). In most (155) patients of this group
chronic inflammation was unexacerbated and the lesions were markedly
infiltrated, hyperemic, firm to palpation, and somewhat edematous.
In many of the 93 patients with chronic diffuse inflammation, a considerable area of the skin was involved (especially in cases of
psoriasis, lichen planus, and disseminated neurodermatitis). Of the
26 patients in whom chronic inflammation was in a phase of exacer-
bation, the inflammation was circumscribed in 12 and diffuse in 14.
All these had heavily inflitrated, highly hyperemic, edematous lesions, some of which were oozing. The lesional surfaces were covered
with seropurulent or sanguinous exudate that had dried up to produce
crusts of exudate-impregnated scales. Of the 74 patients with circumscribed inflammation, the regional lymph nodes were firm and
enlarged but painless in 48 (most of these had chronic ulcerative
pyoderma, tuberculosis verrucosa, lichen ruber verrucosus, or cutaneous leishmaniasis) and tender to touch and inflamed in eight.
Lastly, of the 197 patients with diffuse inflammation, 22 (most of
them had neurodermatitis, psoriasis, or prurigo nodularis) had moderate polyadenitis.

In the group of 36 patients with epithelial or connective tissue
tumors, an inflammatory reaction (chronic inflammation in exacer-
bation) was present in only five cases (including one with papillomatosis cutis carcinoides of Gottron and one with angioleiomyosarcoma);
the remaining 34 patients showed no clinical signs of inflammation.

Finally, among the 36 patients with squamous cell carcinoma,
signs of inflammation (hyperemia, infiltration, edema, seropurulent
or sanguinous exudate) were observed in 12, in 11 of whom the inflammation was circumscribed; the only patient with diffuse inflammation had a squamous cell carcinoma that had superimposed on psoriasis. In this group, one patient had moderate polyadenitis and
five had enlarged regional lymph nodes.

Table 1.  Types of Inflammation in Dermatoses Accompanied by Reactive Epidermal Hyperplasis and in Skin Tumora.

| Condition | No. of patients | Inflammation | | | | |
| --- | --- | --- | --- | --- | --- | --- |
| | | Circumscribed | | Diffuse | | None |
| | | Chronic | Chronic exacerbated | Chronic | Chronic exacerbated | |
| Miscellaneous dermatoses showing epidermal hyperplasia | 187 | 62 | 12 | 93 | 14 | 6 |
| Epithelial or connective tissue tumors | 36 | - | 5 | - | - | 31 |
| Squamous cell carcinoma | 36 | 7 | 4 | 1 | - | 24 |
| Total | 259 | 69 | 21 | 94 | 14 | 61 |

In summary, chronic inflammation was present in the vase majority of our patients with dermatoses showing reactive epidermal hyperplasia.  By contrast, no inflammation was in evidence, as a rule, in
the group of epithelial and connective tissue tumors.  In the carcinoma group, chronic inflammation was present in a third of the cases,
and it should be noted that in all these cases the onset of inflammation preceded that of squamous cell carcinoma.

Duration of the disease process.  It is believed by many authors
that one of the distinctive clinical features of cutaneous pseudocarcinoses is rapid development and spontaneous resolution of the
lesions (e.g. Levi-Coblentz, 1937; Winer, 1940; Wodniansky, 1960;
Fischer, 1963; Montgomery, 1967).  These two criteria are of particular relevance for differentiating between keratoacanthoma and cutaneous squamous cell carcinoma (Rook and Whimster, 1950; Arutyunov
and Golemba, 1959; Blinova, 1959; Grzhebin and Tseraidis, 1960;
Venkei and Sugar, 1965; Fischer, 1963; Montgomery, 1967; Kopf, 1968;
Il'in, 1970; Apatenko, 1973; Connors and Ackerman, 1976) Thus, Pinkus
and Mehregan (1976) consider slow growth of tumors as an indication
of their malignancy.  Civatte (1967) took the view that a keratoacanthoma should be treated as a squamous cell carcinoma wherever the age
of the lesion is unknown.

In the literature, reports can be found, however, of cutaneous
squamous cell carcinomas showing rapid evolution (e.g. Willis, 1967;
Shanin, 1969; Apatenko, 1973; Sanderson, 1979), and of keratoacanthomas developing at a slow rate (e.g. Arutyunov and Golemba, 1959;
Glazunov and Blinova, 1960; Fischer, 1963; Raichev et al., 1964;
Isaeva et al., 1966; Montgomery, 1967; Korelenshtein, 1970; Apatenko,
1973; Miedzinski et al., 1973).

The distribution of our patients according to duration of lesions is shown in Table 2.  It can be seen that in most (70.5%) of the
patients with dermatoses accompanied by reactive epidermal hyperplasia, the lesions had been in existence for 1 to 20 years or more.
Of the longest duration were trophic ulcers, cutaneous tuberculosis,
neurodermatitis, psoriasis, lichen planus verrucosus, prurigo nodularis, and Darier's disease, that is, disorders known to follow an
indolent course and to be refractory to treatment; in about a third
of these patients the disease had lasted 5 to 20 years or longer.
The age of the lesions was under 1 year in nearly a third of patients
with such dermatoses as chronic pyoderma ulcerosum vegetans, lichen
planus, vasculitis, dermatitis herpetiformis (Duhring's disease),
vegetating iododerma, lupus erythematosus, and cutaneous
leishmaniasis.

In the group of epithelial and connective tissue tumors, the
lesions had lasted up to 1 year in 21 patients, and nearly all (19)
of these had keratoacanthoma.  Particularly long-lasting were seborrheic warts, senile keratoma, angiokeratoma, and papillomatosis cutis
carcinoides of Gottron.

Table 2.  Duration of Dermatoses Accompanied by Reactive Epidermal Hyperplasia and of Skin Tumors.

| Condition | No. of patients | Duration | | | | | | |
|---|---|---|---|---|---|---|---|---|
| | | under 6 months | 6-12 months | 1-3 years | 3-5 years | 5-10 years | 10-15 years | 15-20 years or longer |
| Miscellaneous dermatoses showing epidermal hyperplasia | 187 | 25 | 30 | 41 | 32 | 32 | 15 | 12 |
| Epithelial or connective tissue tumors | 36 | 13 | 8 | 3 | 5 | 5 | 2 | - |
| Squamous cell carcinoma | 36 | - | 7 | 13 | 8 | 4 | 4 | - |
| Total | 259 | 38 | 45 | 57 | 45 | 41 | 21 | 12 |

In the group of squamous cell carcinoma, the lesions had been present for 1 to 15 years in 29 cases and 6 to 12 months in seven.

It is noteworthy that in the groups of squamous cell carcinoma and miscellaneous dermatoses, a large proportion of patients had long-lasting disease (3-15 years or more). This suggests that duration of disease is not always a reliable criterion in differentiation of reactive epidermal hyperplasia from squamous cell cancer and also that the latter tended to go undetected for a long time (3-15 years in nearly half of our patients). It must be noted, though, that in some cases it was not possible to ascertain the duration of a squamous cell carcinoma on the basis of history because the carcinoma had supervened on a preexisting chronic dermatosis of long duration.

Among our patients, squamous cell carcinoma had arisen in traumatic lesions (3 patients), giant condyloma acuminatum of Buschke and Loewenstein (2); keratoacanthoma (2); Bowen's disease (2); scars left behind by carbuncle (1), trophic (varicose) ulcer (1), lichen ruber verrucosus (2), ulcer associated with congenital epidermolysis bullosa (1), chronic erosive balanoposthitis (1), plantar wart (1), arsenical keratosis (1), lupus tuberculosus (1), lupus erythematosus (1), and psoriasis (1). This indicates that either pseudocarcinomatous hyperplasia or squamous cell carcinoma may arise in the same dermatosis. Therefore short duration and spontaneous resolution of the lesions cannot be relied upon in the diagnosis of cutaneous pseudocarcinoses. In dermatologic practice, cases of protracted, chronic dermatoses, which frequently are unresponsive to treatment, prevail, and it is such cases (which often exhibit warty growths, vegetations, and ulcerations) that the clinician finds it particularly difficult to determine the biologic nature of the epidermal hyperplasia.

Number of lesions. It has often been observed (Raichev and Andreev, 1965; Venkei and Sugar, 1965; Shanin, 1969; and others) that squamous cell carcinoma occurs as a solitary lesion much more commonly than do the dermatoses grouped under the heading of cutaneous pseudocarcinoses, and these observations are in line with our clinical experience reported here (Table 3).

Thus, in the group of dermatoses accompanied by reactive epidermal hyperplasia, the lesions were solitary in only 60 of the 187 cases (32%), while the number of multiple lesions was more than 10 in most instances (one patient with warty tuberculosis had as many as 133 lesions).

In the group of 36 patients with epithelial or connective tissue tumors, solitary lesions occurred in 22 patients, 21 of whom had keratoacanthoma. Multiple lesions were seen in senile keratoma, seborrheic wart, and angiokeratoma. By contrast, 35 of the 36 patients with squamous cell carcinoma had one lesion each; the only

Table 3. Numbers of Lesions in Dermatoses Accompanied by Reactive Epidermal Hyperplasia and in Skin Tumors.

| Number of lesions | Miscellaneous dermatoses showing epidermal hyperplasia | Epithelial or connective tissue tumors | Squamous cell carcinoma | Total No. of patients |
|---|---|---|---|---|
| 1 | 60 | 22 | 35 | 117 |
| 2 | 18 | 2 | 1 | 21 |
| 3-5 | 24 | – | – | 24 |
| 6-10 | 22 | – | – | 22 |
| More than 10 | 63 | 12 | – | 75 |
| Total | 187 | 36 | 36 | 259 |

patient with two lesions had cancer that had developed in association with generalized psoriasis.

Distribution by anatomic site. It also seems of interest to compare the distribution of lesions by site in dermatoses, benign epithelial or connective tissue tumors, and squamous cell carcinoma (Table 4). Multiple lesions located in various areas of the skin were particularly frequent in the group of dermatoses showing epidermal hyperplasia which was often pseudocarcinomatous. The most common sites of involvement were the lower and upper extremities. This can be explained by clinical features of the dermatoses prevailing in this group (Chronic ulcerative pyoderma, trophic ulcers of the lower legs, tuberculosis verrucosa, neurodermatitis, psoriasis, lichen ruber verrucosus, and other dermatoses for which the extremities are the sites of predilection). Eruptions on the face, scalp, and neck, that is, on exposed areas of the skin, were far less frequent. In 79 patients (42.2%), the lesions were generalized, being present in various skin areas at a time.

In the group of benign tumors, the lesions were localized to the face, head, and/or neck in 22 cases, and most of these had keratoacanthoma. Widespread eruptions located on the upper and lower limbs and trunk were seen for the most part in patients with verruca seborrheica or senilis.

In the squamous cell carcinoma group, the lesions were located on the face or scalp in 15 of the 36 patients, in 10 of them on the lower lip. In the remaining 21 cases, the lesion was situated on the upper or lower extremity (13 patients), trunk (3), or genitalia (5 patients).

To sum up, the lesions were localized on the trunk and upper or lower extremities in most patients with dermatoses and on exposed areas such as the face and scalp in about a half of the patients with benign epithelial tumors and of those with squamous cell carcinoma. However, it should be pointed out that in a rather large proportion (20%) of patients in the dermatoses group, the lesions occurred on the face, scalp and/or neck and that in half of those with carcinoma the lesional site was the trunk or an extremity. This suggests that location of lesions in a particular area of the skin is not a major consideration in diagnostic differentiation between cutaneous pseudocarcinoses and squamous cell carcinoma.

3.1.1 Clinical Appearance of Lesions

The clinical features are considered by many to be of great value in the diagnosis of cutaneous pseudocarcinoses (e.g. Gottron and Nikolowski, 1960; Montgomery, 1967; Nazzario and Tosti, 1968; Tilgen, 1976). It has been noted, in particular, that the lesions

Table 4. Distribution of Lesions by Anatomic Site in Dermatoses Accompanied by Reactive Epidermal Hyperplasia and in Skin Tumors.

| Condition | No. of patients | Face | Head | Neck | Upper extrem- ities | Lower extrem- ities | Trunk | Genitalia |
|---|---|---|---|---|---|---|---|---|
| Miscellaneous dermatoses showing epidermal hyperplasia | 187 | 14 | 14 | 11 | 62 | 146 | 24 | 7 |
| Epithelial or connective tissue tumors | 36 | 17 | 4 | 1 | 5 | 3 | 9 | – |
| Squamous cell carcinoma | 36 | 13 | 2 | – | 4 | 9 | 3 | 5 |
| Total | 259 | 44 | 20 | 12 | 71 | 158 | 36 | 12 |

seen in the various dermatoses grouped under pseudocarcinoses, unlike those found in squamous cancer, are not fused with the subjacent tissues and are not very firm to palpation, but are characterized in most cases by ulcerating, vegetating, and/or wartlike tissue growths. Other authors (e.g. Winer, 1940; Sommerville, 1953; Fischer, 1963) emphasize, however, that the affected skin, for instance at the margins of trophic ulcers of the lower limbs, may be infiltrated and fused with the subjacent tissue and that the lesion may have an elevated rim and be as firm as a squamous carcinoma. This may create considerable difficulties in clinical differentiation of pseudocancer from true cancer of the skin. Even greater difficulties are liable to arise in cases where the squamous cell carcinoma is devoid of typical clinical features and resembles an eczematous process, as it did, for instance, in a case of Paget's disease (Figure 6) and a case of Bowen's disease (Figure 7) in our series. In the patient with Bowen's disease the clinical picture was characterized by hyperemia, crust formation, and itching, while histologic examination revealed changes indicating that the carcinoma in situ had transformed into an invasive growth (Figure 8).

In evaluating the clinical appearances of lesions in our patients, we separated all lesions into three types: ulcerative-in filtrative (endophytic), tumorlike (exophytic), and hyperkeratotic (Table 5).

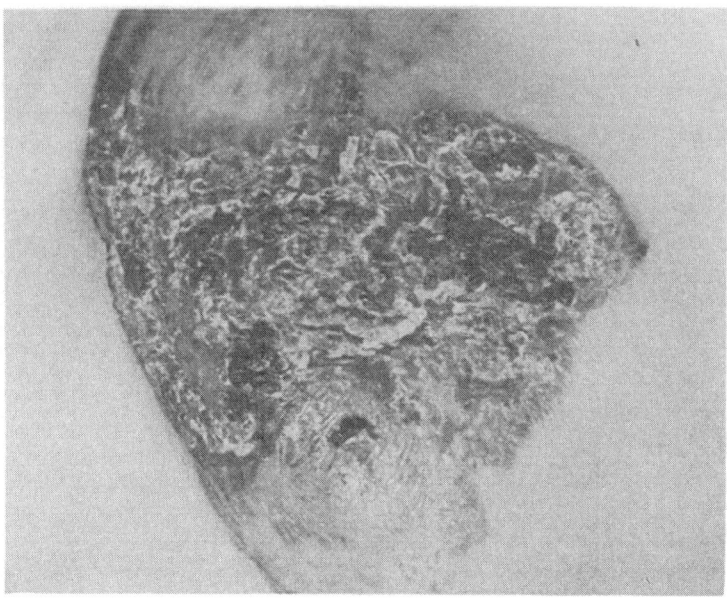

Fig. 6. Paget's disease.

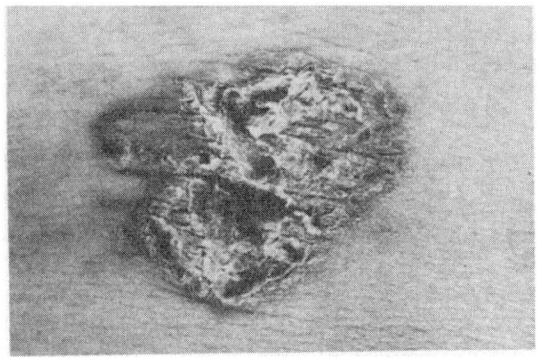

Fig. 7.  Bowen's disease.

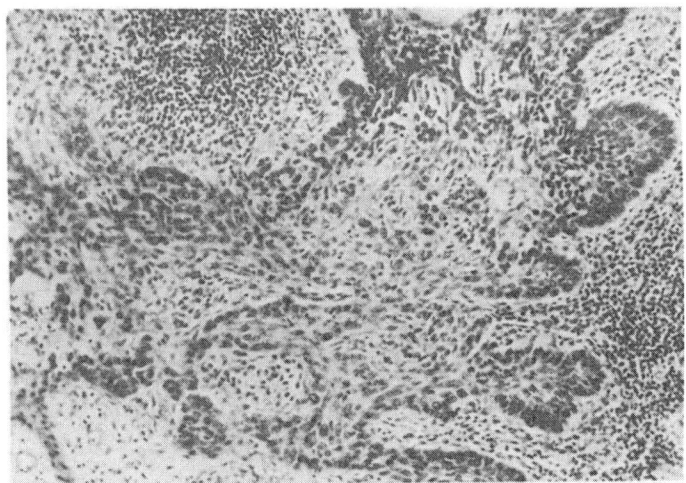

Fig. 8.  Bowen's disease that has progressed to squamous cell
carcinoma (skin of the back).  One can observe irregularly
proliferating epidermal strands, with the spinous cells
showing disorderly arrangement, polymorphism, and
penetration into dermis.  (125 X; hematoxylin and eosin.)


        It can be seen from Table 5 that ulcerative-infiltrative and
tumorlike lesions were more common than hyperkeratotic ones in all
the three groups, ulcerative-infiltrative lesions being present in
most patients in the dermatoses and carcinoma groups and tumorlike
lesions being by far the most frequent type in the group of benign
tumors.

        The ulcerative-infiltrative  type of lesion occurred in 72 of
the 187 patients (38.4%) with dermatoses accompanied by reactive

Table 5. Clinical Characteristics of Lesions in Dermatoses Accompanied by Reactive Epidermal Hyperplasia and in Skin Tumors.

| Condition | No. of patients | Type of lesion | | |
| --- | --- | --- | --- | --- |
| | | Ulcerative infiltrative | Tumorlike | Hyperkeratotic |
| Miscellaneous dermatoses showing epidermal hyperplasia | 187 | 72 | 65 | 50 |
| Epithelial or connective tissue tumors | 36 | 1 | 25 | 10 |
| Squamous cell carcinoma of the skin | 36 | 17 | 11 | 8 |
| Total | 259 | 90 | 101 | 68 |

epidermal hyperplasia that often presented as pseudocarcinomatous.
This type was more often seen in chronic ulcerative pyoderma, trophic
ulcers of the lower extremities, and leishmaniasis.  Here are two
case reports.

Patient S., a 47-year-old man, was admitted to our
clinic complaining of eruptions on the lower limbs which
had first appeared about 6 years before and followed a
contusion.  He had been repeatedly treated with various
modalities (antibiotics, autohemotherapy, vitamins, etc.),
with only temporary benefit.

On physical examination extensive areas of erosion and
ulceration alternating with atrophic scars and covered with
seropurulent or hemorrhagic crusts were seen on the lower
extremities.  On the posterior surface of the right lower
leg, a deep ulcer with a callous margin and a bright red
floor was present; it had denuded the muscles and was
discharging sanguinous material (Figure 9).

Histologic examination of a biopsy specimen from the
margin of the ulcer revealed acanthosis with irregular
epidermal proliferations.  Horny layer was absent over
extensive areas of the specimen and only remnants of horny

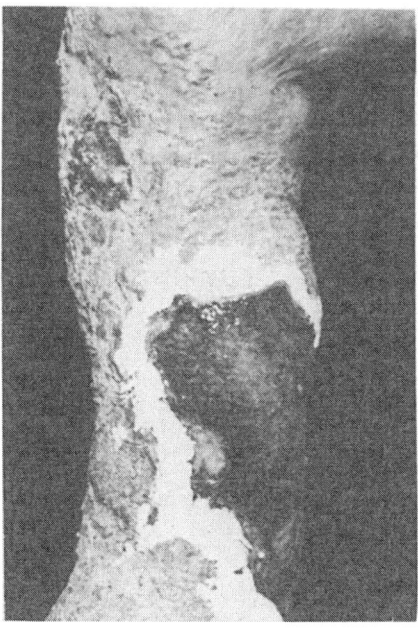

Fig. 9.  Chronic pyoderma ulcerosum.

material were present elsewhere. The cytoplasm of spinous
cells stained faintly in some areas of the downward epidermal proliferations. The basement membrane was preserved in
much of the specimen, but had indistinct borders in the
areas of acanthotic epidermal downgrowths. The dermis was
edematous and was permeated by an infiltrate composed of
lymphocytes and histiocytes with an admixture of segmented
and plasma cells whose elements had penetrated into the
epidermal strands. The histologic appearance was one of
chronic inflammation with evidence of pseudocarcinomatous
hyperplasia. The diagnosis was "chronic pyoderma ulcerosum
vegetans showing pseudocarcinomatous epidermal hyperplasia."

In this case, there was a severe, long-lasting ulcerative and
infiltrative process presenting histologically as a pronounced epidermal hyperplasia approaching pseudocarcinomatous. The clinical
doubts regarding benignity of the process were resolved by histopathologic evidence. Indeed, a combination of vigorous antiinflammatory, antibacterial, and general supportive treatments (autohemotherapy, vaccinotherapy, antibiotics, vitamins, etc.) led to a substantial improvement of the patient's condition.

Not uncommonly, trophic ulcers of the lower extremities have
hard infiltrated edges fused with the subjacent tissue and showing
hyperkeratosis, which causes such ulcers to look very much like
squamous cell cancer.

Patient A., a 48-year-old man, sought medical advice
because of painful ulcers on his left heel which had
appeared about 3 months before in the place of the scars of
several years' duration remaining after a plastic operation
for a burn. He had been unsuccessfully treated with
lotions and steroid ointments. The traumatologist had
suspected a squamous cell carcinoma.

On physical examination, two ulcers with hard inverted
edges showing striking hyperkeratosis and with floors
covered by dense grayish crusts impregnated with serous
exudate were seen on the left heel. The clinical diagnosis
was trophic ulcers of the left heel suspicious of malignant
degeneration (Figure 10).

A histologic specimen from the margin of one of the
ulcers revealed considerable hyperkeratosis of orthokeratotic structure, hypergranulosis, and acanthosis. The
spinous cells of the acanthotic epidermis stained unevenly
and were arranged disorderly in places. The boundary
between the basal epidermal layer and dermis was indistinct
in some areas (Figure 11). The dermis showed a diffuse

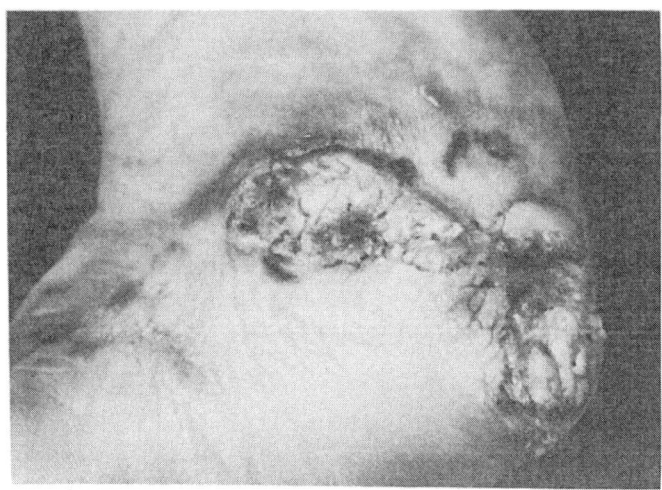

Fig. 10.  Trophic ulcers in the heel area.


infiltrate composed predominantly of lymphocytes and
histiocytes with some polymorphonuclear leukocytes, and
also a degree of exocytosis.  The blood and lymph vessels
were dilated.  On staining with the Brachet stain, the
cytoplasm of spinous cells showed diminished pyroninophilia, while the basal and suprabasal cells stained more
strongly.  On Feulgen staining, the epidermal cell nuclei
stained violet to purple, with cells of the basal and
suprabasal layers staining more deeply.  On staining with
the PAS reaction, a moderate amount of glycogen was found
in cells of the upper spinous layer, but no glycogen in the
proliferating cells of epidermal strands.  The PAS-positive
band in the basement membrane zone appeared as a fine
tortuous line that disappeared in areas where the epidermal
processes thinned out.

In this case, the tropic ulcers suspected clinically of having
undergone malignant transformation showed epidermal changes of the
reactive hyperplasia type on histologic examination.  Topical therapy
(applications of ointments containing salicylic acid and cytostatics)
combined with general supportive measures resulted in a marked improvement of the ulcers with detachment of the horny material from
the ulcer margins, followed by epithelialization of the lesionnal
areas.

The tumorlike type of lesion occurred in 65 of the 187 patients
(34.7%) with dermatoses, being more common in cases of lichen ruber
verrucosus, tuberculosis verrucosa, and prurigo nodularis.  The
tumorous structures were firm and showed warty growths and horny

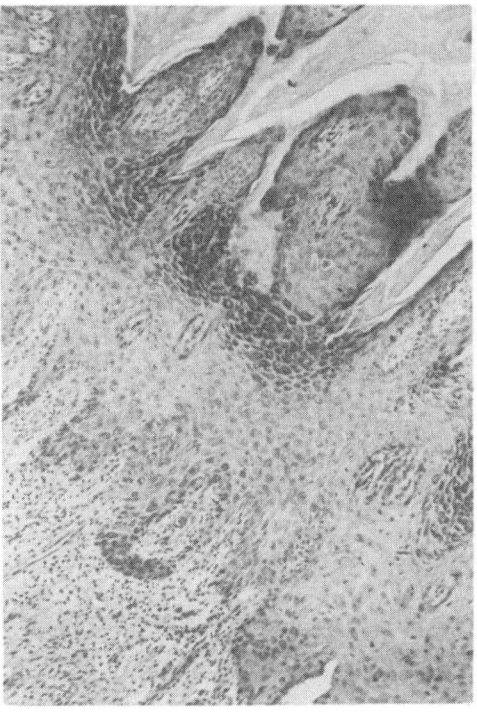

Fig. 11.  Trophic ulcer (skin from margin of one of the ulcers
          depicted in Fig. 10), showing pronounced hyperkeratosis,
          hypergranulosis, and acanthosis. (75 X; hematoxylin and
          eosin.)


material on their surfaces in most of these cases, and some of them
had an elevated rim, thus presenting an appearance similar to squamous cell carcinoma of the skin.  Here is a case report.

      Patient K., a 43-year-old man, was admitted to our
department because of tuberculosis verrucosa cutis of about
15 years' duration.

      On physical examination, a tumorlike warty lesion 5 x
3 cm in size, irregular in outline and dirty pink in color
was seen on the right shin.  The lesion was sharply delimited from the normal-looking skin and was firm to palpation; one of its edges was free from crusts and was
flattened, while the other was elevated (Figure 12).

      Histologic examination of the lesion revealed pro-
nounced acanthosis with a bizarre pattern of irregular
epidermal downgrowths that extended deep into the dermis.

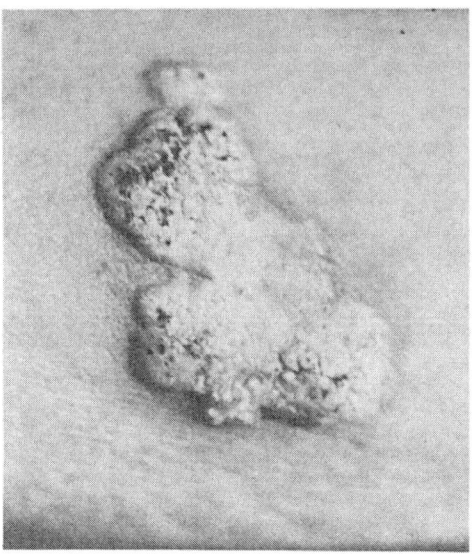

Fig. 12.   Tuberculosis cutis verrucosa.


The epidermal proliferation occurred as a proliferation of
spinous cells whose cytoplasms stained irregularly.   In
places, epidermal masses detached from the growing epidermal ridges were seen (Figure 13).   The basement membrane
was retained, but was ill-defined in some areas.

In this patient, the tumorlike lesion of warty tuberculosis
presented a picture of pronounced pseudocarcinomatous epidermal
hyperplasia.   It should be stressed that it is in cases of tumorlike
lesions that pseudocarcinomatous hyperplasia tends to be most strongly marked, so much so as to be at times indistinguishable histologically from a keratinizing squamous cell carcinoma in its initial
phase of evolution.   However, the clinical features of tumorous
growths that occur in various dermatoses showing pseudocarcinomatous
hyperplasia are in most instances basically those of the dermatosis
on which such a growth has supervened, and this facilitates the
diagnosis.

In some cases, however, the clinical characteristics, too, are
atypical of the dermatosis in question and resemble those of squamous
cell carcinoma (the lesions are of long duration, firm, fused with
subjacent tissue, painful, etc.).   In our experience, this was sometimes the case in keratoacanthoma, papillomatosis cutis carcinoides
of Gottron, and some other skin disorders.

Hyperkeratotic  lesions were present in 50 of the 187 patients
(27.6%) in the miscellaneous dermatoses group.   It should be noted,

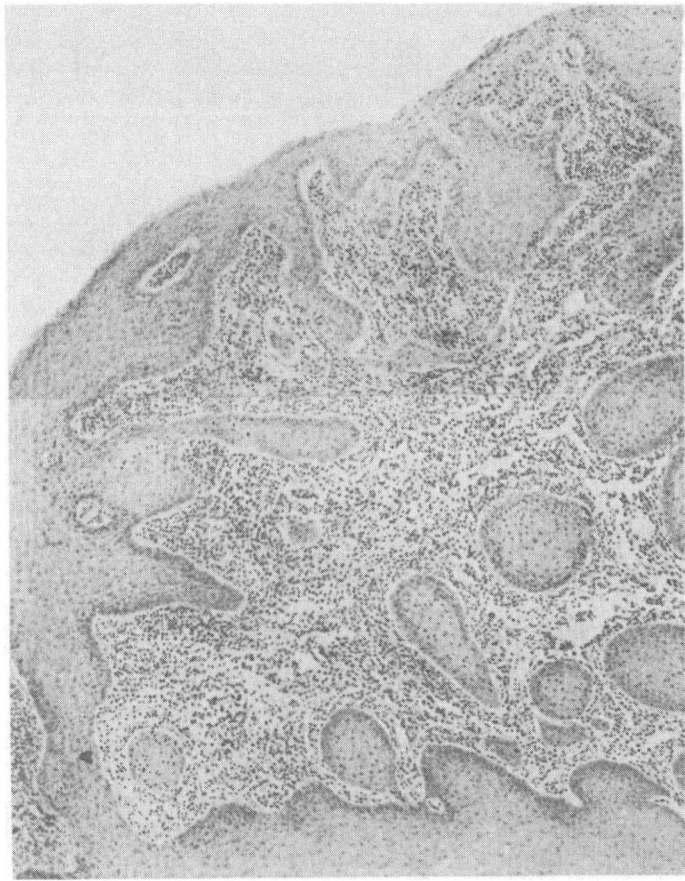

Fig. 13.  Tuberculosis cutis verrucosa (shin skin), showing
          pseudocarcinomatous epidermal hyperplasia. (75 X;
          hematoxylin and eosin. Montage.)

though, that separation of this type of lesion is rather arbitrary,
for, as shown above, the tumorlike and ulcerative-infiltrative types
likewise involved considerable hyperkeratosis in a number of cases.
For this reason, we considered under the hyperkeratotic type only
those cases in which striking hyperkeratosis was not accompanied by
ulcerative infiltrative or tumorlike changes.  The hyperkeratoic type
of lesion was more often seen in chronic eczema, psoriasis, Darier's
disease, keratodermia of the palms and soles, and circumscribed
hyperkeratosis of the lower lip.  In such cases, the reactive epidermal hyperplasia was rarely attended by changes suggestive of
possible malignancy.  In most instances, lesions of the hyperkeratotic type were unquestionably benign and had clinicopathologic
features typical of the underlying dermatosis.

In certain cases, especially those of ulcerative and infiltrative or tumorlike growths, malignancy cannot be ruled out with certainty until the patient has been followed up for a long time and
repeated histopathologic examinations have been undertaken.


### 3.1.2  Histologic Appearance of Lesions

It is generally recognized that cutaneous pseudocarcinoses
present essentially as pseudocarcinomatous hyperplasias.  White and
Weidman (1927) distinguished three stages or grades of such a hyperplasia: (1) acanthosis only; (2) pronounced acanthosis with epidermal
downgrowth, cellular atypia, and rupture of the basement membrane;
and (3) penetration of epidermal ridges deep into the dermis, cellular atypia, presence of many mitoses, and horn pearl formation.

In the opinion of Lanné (1970), the first grade is devoid of
practical importance and should not be regarded as representing
pseudocarcinomatous hyperplasia, since ordinary acanthosis bears no
similarity whatsoever to squamous cell carcinoma.

Sommerville (1953) defined pseudocarcinomatous hyperplasia as "a
prickle cell proliferation closely simulating epidermal carcinoma...,
and at times microscopically indistinguishable from it".  He stated
that none of the histologic features of cutaneous squamous cell
carcinoma (depth to which epidermal strands have penetrated into the
dermis, destruction of the basement membrane, cytologic atypia, horn
pearl formation, etc.) is by itself decisive in diagnostic differentiation of squamous carcinoma from pseudocarcinomatous hyperplasia,
for any of these features may be encountered in both conditions.
Nazzario and Tosti (1968) pointed out that psuedocarcinomatous hyperplasia tends to evolve gradually.  It does not differ from a banal
acanthosis initially, but with the course of time the dermal papillae
and epidermal ridges elongate and may impart to the lesion an appearance somewhat resembling that of a basalioma.  At this stage, however, neither the pathologist nor the clinician have the slightest
doubt that the condition is benign.  If the stimulus – the dermal
infiltrate – persists, the epidermal growth continues.  The downward
epidermal proliferation is now a proliferation of spinous cells which
show enlarged and basophilic nuclei, increased cytoplasmic volume, and
aberrant mitoses.  Because cell proliferation dominates over cell
differentiation, parakeratosis develops.  The dermis shows a diffuse
infiltrate and newly formed vessels.  Nazzario and Tosti emphasized
that confusion with squamous cell carcinoma is unlikely at this stage
too.  As the pseudocarcinomatous hyperplasia continues to progress,
irregularly arranged, racemose epithelial strands appear, with the
dermal papillae losing their typical shapes of connective tissue beds
for the epidermis.  There is pronounced cellular polymorphism.  In
places, nests of epithelial cells with faulty keratinization lie
below the sweat gland level.  These cell collections consist of

parakeratotic horns, are devoid of granular layer, and are referred to
as horn pearls.  According to the above authors, it is at this stage
that pseudocarcinomatous hyperplasia resembles most closely a true
carcinoma histologically.

What, then, are the essential histopathologic differences, if
any, between pseudocarcinomatous hyperplasia and squamous cell carcinoma?  To bring some clarity into this issue, it is useful to
review the available information regarding the more important histologic features of malignant growth.  According to most authors, these
involve (1) pattern of invasive epidermal growth (its depth and the
degree of tissue destruction which it causes), (2) features of cell
differentiation and keratinization and ability to form horn pearls,
(3) cellular relationships; (4) cytologic characteristics, (5) state
of the basement membrane, and (6) relationship between the epidermis
and dermis (e.g. Garshin, 1939; Winer, 1940; Glazunov, 1947, 1971;
Khlopin, 1947; Petrov, 1947; Allen, 1954; Golovin, 1958; Gottron and
Nikolowski, 1960; Grzhebin and Tseraidis, 1960; Studnitsyn, 1965;
Lever, 1967; Montgomery, 1967; Willis, 1967; Apatenko, 1969, 1973;
Shabad, 1967; Kraevskii and Smol'yanikov, 1971; Connors and Ackerman,
1976; Pinkus and Mehregan, 1976; Sanderson, 1979).

Pattern of invasive epidermal growth.  In pseudocarcinomatous
hyperplasia, the downward epidermal proliferation is variable.  If
the diagnosis is difficult to make, it is considered important by a
number of authors to find out whether or not epidermal cells have
proliferated below the sweat gland level: if they have, the epidermal
hyperplasia should be regarded as cancerous (e.g. White and Weidman,
1927; Gottron and Nikolowski, 1960; Melczer, 1961).  Others maintain,
however, that the epidermis may invade the lower dermis and penetrate
below sweat gland level also in sites of pseudocarcinomatous hyperplasias arising in various dermatoses (Sommerville, 1953; Fischer,
1963; Lever, 1967; Nazzario and Tosti, 1968; and others).

Glazunov and Blinova (1960), in describing the morphology of
"horny molluscum" (keratoacanthoma) of the lower lip, noted that
although the proliferative process was always benign, in 16 of the
cases observed by them the acanthotic strands had extended so deep
into the skin as to reach the arteries and salivary glands; but that
in contrast to squamous cell carcinoma, the sheets of epidermal cells
did not grow through the muscles but only compressed them, leading
eventually to their atrophy.  Accordingly, the above authors do not
believe that epidermal invasion deep to muscles is a reliable sign of
malignancy.  They write: "We have repeatedly observed spontaneous
involution of such structures to scars."  One should probably agree
with those (e.g. Sommerville, 1953; Glazunov and Blinova, 1960;
Lever, 1967) who feel that it does not matter much to what level the
epidermal strands have penetrated as long as the epidermal cells have
not invaded the lymphatic and blood vessels.  It is the invasion of
these which is considered by many to be the most important single

sign of malignant growth (Glazunov, 1947, 1971; Sommerville, 1953;
Golovin, 1958; Lever, 1967; Sanderson, 1968; Apatenko, 1969, 1973;
Shanin, 1969).

As regards the possibility of subjacent tissues being destroyed
in lesions showing pseudocarcinomatous hyperplasia, this appears to
depend on the nature of the disease in which the hyperplasia has
arisen and on the location of the lesion.  In keratoacanthoma, for
example, destructive epidermal growth is most commonly seen in lesions located in areas where subcutaneous fat is relatively scarce
(eyelids, lower lip, auricular conchae).  Such growth is not infrequently seen at sites of papillomatosis cutis carcinoides (Gottron
and Nikolowski, 1960), lupus vulgaris (Melczer, 1961), chronic
pyoderma ulcerosum vegetans (Kozhevnikov, 1946), and certain other
dermatoses.  The most striking invasion of epidermal strands into the
underlying tissues is known to occur in giant condyloma acuminatum of
Buschke and Loewenstein, in which epidermal cells may at times extend
into the cavernous bodies of the penis and cause formation of
urethral fistulas (Vulcan, 1972).

In our view, the foregoing shows clearly enough that the extent
of downward epidermal proliferation and the degree to which the
underlying tissues are damaged or destroyed do not provide a reliable
indication of whether the process involved is falsely or truly carcinomatous.

Cell differentiation and keratinization.  Patterns of cell
differentiation and keratinization in pseudocarcinomatous hyperplasia
have attracted the attention of many investigators (e.g. Garshin,
1939; Glazunov, 1947, 1971; Sommerville, 1953; Gottron and
Nikolowski, 1960; Lanné, 1969).  It has been noted (Wodniansky, 1960)
that psuedocarcinomatous hyperplasis is liable to be confused with
keratinizing squamous cell carcinoma precisely because of the pronounced hyperkeratosis shown by the vast majority of dermatoses in
which such hyperplasia arises.  Lanné (1969) stated that, unlike the
cancerous epithelial nests which contain dyskeratotic cells, the
focal proliferations seen in pseudocarcinomatous hyperplasia consist
of parakeratotic cells which are subsequently replaced by horny cells
and do not proliferate any longer.

As stated by Golovin (1982), "in tumorous pseudo-pseudoepithel-
iomatous hyperplasia, the downward epithelial proliferations, to
remain viable, have to retain association with the surface epithelium.  The epithelial nests which have lost such association
inevitably die; they are destroyed by the intruding leukocytes or
else undergo complete keratinization or necrotization."

Sommerville (1953), Lever (1967), Montgomery (1967), and
Nazzario and Tosti (1968) came to the conclusion that the most important distinctive histologic feature of cancerous as opposed to

pseudocancerous growths is individual cell keratinization. Dyskeratotic cells are found in the malpighian layer of the epidermis even in early phases of malignant growth in carcinoma in situ (Masson, 1956; Grzhebin and Tseraidis, 1960; Il'ina and Vasil'eva, 1963; Lever, 1967; Apatenko, 1969; and others), but rarely in pseudocarcinomatous hyperplasia, although individual cell keratinization in epidermal proliferations is not an uncommon finding in keratoacanthoma (Blinova, 1959; Glazunov and Blinova, 1960; Kopf, 1968; Apatenko, 1973).

According to Graham and Helwig (1963) and Montgomery (1967), it is particularly difficult to distinguish benign dyskeratotic cells from malignant ones. As pointed out by Montgomery (1967), benign dyskeratotic cells (corps ronds and grains of Darier's disease) may occur side by side with cells exhibiting a degree of individual cell keratinization in malignant transformed dyskeratosis, in Bowen's disease, and in squamous cells carcinoma; in such cases, it is almost impossible to tell whether the dyskeratotic cells are benign or malignant.

Cellular relationships. These remain normal in most cases of pseudocarcinomatous hyperplasia, even though the epidermal strands may have penetrated deep into the dermis (Sommerville, 1953; Nazzario and Tosti, 1968; Pinkus and Mehregan, 1976; and others). However, as pointed out by Sanderson (1968), cellular arrangement is disorderly in some areas of pseudocarcinomatous hyperplasia, although to a lesser extent than in squamous cell carcinoma. The cellular polarity is disturbed in foci of squamous carcinoma (Glazunov, 1947, 1971 Golovin, 1958; Raichev and Andreev, 1965; Venkei and Sugar, 1965; Willis, 1967; Apatenko, 1969, 1973; Shanin, 1969). Sommerville (1953) wrote that in cancerous hyperplasia "the normal uniform arrangement becomes distorted and lost, the individual cells assuming the character of undisciplined independent law breakers, or crowding together in ill-assorted bands." However, as indicated by Sommerville, such cellular anarchy is commonly seen only in far-advanced cancers, and it is not always possible to appreciate differences in cell behavior and interrelationship between pseudocarcinomatous hyperplasia and squamous cell carcinoma at early stages of its evolution.

Cytologic characteristics. The cytologic features of pseudocarcinomatous hyperplasia and of squamous cell carcinoma have also been given much attention by investigators. As early as 1893, Hansemann considered the following features of anaplasia as being characteristic of malignant epithelial growth: enlargement and basophilia of cell nuclei, increase in nuclear relative to cytoplasmic volume, and presence of multinucleate cells showing pathologic mitoses. McCarthy (1936) and Cowdry and Paletta (1941) reported that nucleoli, too, are increased in size and number in squamous cancer.

Whereas it is now well recognized that enlarged basophilic
nuclei, misshapen multinucleate cells, cells with abnormal mitotic
figures, and altered nucleolar-nuclear-cytoplasmic ratios are all
features of malignant epidermal transformation, the karyologic and
cytologic characteristics of pseudocarcinomatous hyperplasia have
received little study, and the information contained in the available
publications (e.g. Sommerville, 1953; Gottron and Nikolowski, 1960;
Nazzario and Tosti, 1968) is far from adequate.

It was considered by Winer (1940) that pseudocarcinomatous
hyperplasia, unlike squamous cell carcinoma of the skin is characterized by well-developed spinous cells and by the absence of atypical
dyskeratotic cells, of large hyperchromic nuclei, and of pathologic
mitoses, but this view is not shared by many.  Cowdry and Paletta
(1941) stated, for example, that malignant cells cannot be reliably
distinguished from the benign cells of hyperplastic epidermis on the
criterion of size.

Nuclear hyperchromatism, although frequently observed in growing
cancer cells, is not a constant or distinctive feature of malignant
transformation (Willis, 1967).  Also, cell size and nuclear size may
both be considerably increased not only in squamous cell cancer, but
in inflammatory processes as well (Grafova, 1965; Khesin, 1967;
Willis, 1967; Shchelkunov, 1971; and others).  The nucleoli, too, may
be as large in pseudocarcinomatous hyperplasia as in carcinoma
(Pinkus and Mehregan, 1969).

As regards the mitotic behavior of cells, which has been
attached particular importance by many investigators in the diagnosis
of malignancy, this subject is dealt with specifically in the next
chapter where a review of the relevant literature will be found.
Here, it is perhaps worth noting that more work is needed in this
area to clarify mitotic patterns in pseudocarcinomatous hyperplasia
as opposed to those in cutaneous carcinoma.

State of the basement membrane.  This is believed by many
authors to be an important consideration in histologic differentiation between pseudocarcinomatous epidermal hyperplasia and cutaneous squamous carcinoma (Gay Prieto and Cascos, 1951; Adam et al.,
1956; Melczer, 1961; Shanin, 1969; Mashkilleison, 1970; Pinkus and
Mehregan, 1969; and others).  White and Weidman (1927) emphasized the
intactness of the basement membrane in normal epidermis and in areas
of benign acanthosis, and regarded integrity of the basement membrane
as a major sign of benignity and its disruption as evidence of
malignancy.  That the basement membrane remains intact in sites of
pseudocarcinomatous hyperplasia and is defective or absent in the
invasive proliferations of squamous cell carcinoma has been noted by,
among others, Gay Prieto and Cascos (1951), Adam et al. (1956),
Raichev and Andreev (1965), Venkei and Sugai (1965) and Pinkus
(1968).  Mashkilleison (1970) reported disintegration of the basement

membrane to be a frequent finding also in precancerous lesions occurring on the vermilion border of the lip and in the oral mucosas, and
he considered the disappearance of PAS-positive material from the
basement membrane zone as a major sign of incipient malignant transformation.  Braun-Falco (1960) took the view that alterations in the
mesenchymal ground substance of basement membrane is an inconstant
but important feature of malignant growth.  Pinkus (1966, 1968),
Szodoray and Vezekenyi (1968), and a number of other authors regard
changes in the basement membrane in cancer as one of the conditions
which promote invasive epidermal growth.

     In contrast, other authors (e.g. Miescher, 1950; Sommerville,
1953; Allen, 1954; Lund, 1957; Willis, 1967; Montgomery, 1967;
Sanderson, 1968, Pinkus and Mehregan, 1969, maintain that basement
membrane destruction is not a reliable diagnostic criterion, for the
basement membrane may remain intact even in well-differentiated
squamous cell carcinomas.

     On the other hand, the basement membrane may be indefinite or
absent in some areas of pseudocarcinomatous hyperplasia arising in
keratoacanthoma, papillomatosis carcinoides of Gottron, giant condyloma acuminatum of Buschke and Loewenstein, lupus tuberculosus, the
deep mycoses, and some other conditions (Wiskemann, 1955; Degos,
1958; Arutyunov and Golemba, 1959; Torsuev, 1959; Isaeva et al.,
1966; Montgomery, 1967; Nazzario and Tosti, 1968; Pinkus and
Mehregan, 1969; and others).

     It may be inferred from the above that disrupted integrity of
the basement membrane is not a consistent or trustworthy diagnostic
histologic feature of cutaneous malignancy.

     Nature of the infiltrate and status of the stroma.  These, too,
are believed by many authors to be of considerable importance in
diagnostic differentiation between squamous cell cancer and pseudocarcinomatous hyperplasia (e.g. Allen, 1954; Lund, 1957; Glazunov
and Blinova, 1960; Glazunov, 1962; Willis, 1967; Nazzario and Tosti,
1968; Apatenko, 1969, 1973).  Usually, the presence of a specific
(tuberculoid, granulomatous, or plasmacytic) infiltrate in the dermis
speaks for a reactive epidermal hyperplasia (arising in tuberculosis,
a deep mycosis, chronic ulcerative pyoderma, syphilis, or some other
benign disorder) rather than for a squamous cell carcinoma.  Apatenko
(1973) emphasized the need for ascertaining the nature of infiltrate
in histologic examination of epithelial growths suspected of being
carcinomatous; should changes specific for tuberculosis, granuloma-
tosis, or other condition be found in the infiltrate, the hyperplasia
is very likely to be pseudocarcinomatous.

     Study of the infiltrate has also been considered of great value
by, for example, Gottron and Nikolowski (1960), Montgomery (1967),
and Nazzario and Tosti (1968).

However, in cases where pseudocarcinomatous hyperplasia has to be differentiated from a squamous cell cancer that has supervened on lupus tuberculosus, chronic pyoderma, a deep mycosis, or syphilis, specificity of the infiltrate (e.g. the presence of a tuberculous or granulomatous infiltrate) may not be helpful in establishing the correct diagnosis.

In pseudocarcinomatous hyperplasia, in contrast to squamous cancer, epithelial proliferations may contain cells of the infiltrate, mainly lymphocytes (Lever, 1967) - a point which was attached great importance by Montgomery (1967) who observed that in keratoacanthoma the nests of epithelial cells with disintegrated basement membranes tended to be invaded by cells of the infiltrate and that it was often possible to differentiate keratocanthoma from cancer on this basis. Apatenko (1973) has emphasized, though, that leukocytic infiltration may well be absent in pseudocarcinomatous hyperplasia so that the diagnosis has to be based on clinical evidence.

It has been suggested that important diagnostic information can be elicited by studying fibrous structures of the dermis, since the epidermal proliferations within cancerous lesions have been shown to penetrate through these structures and to invade, in far advanced cases, the muscle and bone. On the other hand, it has been observed that in pseudocarcinomatous hyperplasia epidermal strands only compress and displace the underlying tissues without growing through them, and this eventually leads to their death (Glazunov, 1947; Sommerville, 1953; Glazunov and Blinova, 1960; Willis, 1967; Apatenko, 1969; Sanderson, 1968). However, as clearly demonstrated in experimental studies where atypical inflammatory growths were induced in rabbit ears, the epidermal strands that have penetrated deeply into the dermis may destroy not only connective tissue fibers but even cartilage (e.g. Ruchinskii, 1910; Garshin, 1939; Prokof'eva, 1952; Vasil'ev, 1967).

Of great interest is the arrangement of infiltrate within the dermis in pseudocarcinomatous hyperplasia. It was pointed out by Garshin back in 1939 that invasive epidermal growth in experimental animals is more pronounced in areas containing a fresh infiltrate that has come up close to the basement membrane. And similar observations have been made clinically. Thus Niemi (1970) reported that in cases of histiocytoma, acanthosis was most strongly marked in areas where the tumor bordered the epidermis. Pinkus (1968) noted that atypical hyperplasia was more pronounced in those places where the inflammatory infiltrate abutted the basement membrane. In cancerous lesions, location of the infiltrate close to the basal layer of the epidermis is, according to Garshin (1939), of much lesser significance than it is in pseudocarcinomatous hyperplasia.

### 3.1.3  Conclusion

It may be concluded from the foregoing discussion that the clinical and histopathologic characteristics of the lesions do not always afford clues to unequivocal diagnostic differentiation of pseudocarcinomatous hyperplasia from differentiated squamous cell carcinoma.

## 3.2  EXPERIMENTAL STUDIES ON RABBITS

Comparative clinicopathologic studies of pseudocarcinomatous hyperplasia and keratinizing squamous cell carcinoma produced in experimental animals present considerable interest, for consideration of the findings from these studies in relation to those in patients may provide a better understanding of the more general mechanisms by which pseudocarcinomatous hyperplasia arises and may contribute to the development of reliable criteria for diagnostic differentiation between these processes which are often very similar externally but are fundamentally different in biologic nature.

The following two sections describe such comparative investigations which we have carried out on rabbits.  The domestic rabbit (Oryctolagus cuniculus) was selected because it appears to be the most suitable animal model for studying psuedocarcinomatous hyperplasia which is known to be inducible the most readily in this species.

In one series of experiments, pseudocarcinomatous inflammatory epidermal growths were induced by a single intradermal injection of a saturated solution of scarlet red (scharlach red) powder in olive oil; in the other series, obligatory precancerous tumors (papillomas, keratoacanthomas) and squamous cell carcinoma were produced by painting the skin with 9,10-dimethyl-1,2-benzanthracene (DMBA), a potent carcinogen capable of inducing squamous cell carcinoma in rabbits (Shabad, 1967; Prutkin, 1968).

Since it has been shown (Ruchinskii, 1910; Garshin, 1939; Prokof'eva, 1952) that epithelial proliferation is particularly marked when scarlet red occurs at or near the basement membrane, we injected the dye under high pressure, depositing it into 2-4 sites within each auricular concha in a dose of 0.3-0.5 ml per site.  The rabbits were killed at 5, 12, 17, 20, 180, and 360 days post-injection.

DMBA was applied as a 0.5% solution in acetone in an amount of 2-3 drops to the inner surface of the auricular concha 3-4 times per week over a 6-month period.  Overt squamous cell carcinomas were found to have developed 12 to 18 months after the start of the experiment.

### 3.2.1  Clinicopathologic Characteristics of Reactive Pseudocarcinomatous Hyperplasia

Clinicopathologic characteristics of the epidermal growths produced in rabbit ears by scarlet red were studied in 35 biopsy specimens secured from 29 lesions.  At the sites of injection, there developed tumorlike cystiform lesions of soft consistency whose configuration depended on the injected amount of the dye and on its subepidermal distribution.  The skin over the lesions showed an exaggerated pattern of the follicular structures, was tense, hot to touch, and, when palpated, caused the animals to show great anxiety. Approximately in 5 days, the edema diminished and the lesions became much better demarcated (Figure 14).

Histologic examination of such a lesion revealed striking epithelial proliferation around the altered hair follicles.  The epidermal extensions were filled by horny masses of orthokeratotic structure.  In the epidermis bordering the horny masses, the granular layer cells were prominent.  The epithelial proliferations consisted of highly differentiated elements and extended irregularly into the dermis.  One could see groups of cells breaking away from the epidermal ridges.  The basal layer was preserved everywhere.  There was no cellular disorganization or polymorphism.  The dermis was edematous and showed a diffuse infiltrate composed of segmented cells and

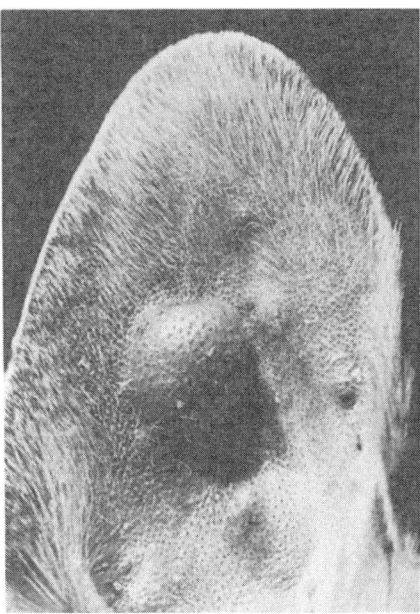

Fig. 14.   Tumorlike structures on inner surface of rabbit ear on day 5 after intradermal injection of scarlet red.

lymphocytes. Elements of the infiltrate did not penetrate into the epidermal strands (Figure 15). Some areas of the dermis contained aggregates of proliferating epithelial cells originating from the sebaceous glands and surrounded by edema and by greatly dilated blood and lymph vessels. At higher magnification, orderly arranged sheets of proliferating cells with conspicuous basal cells and numerous mitotic figures were observed around the sebaceous glands (Figure 16).

At day 12 postinjection, the inflammation was much less intense. Histologically, epidermal cells were seen to be actively proliferating around the pilosebaceous apparatus within the zone bordering the inflammatory focus. Often, the vigorous growth of hair follicles produced a picture characterized by multiple cystic structures located in the uppermost dermis and clearly showing, in their centers, concentrically oriented horny masses surrounded by rows of granular cells. In the lower dermis, epithelial proliferations were destroying the perichondrium in places (Figure 17). These epithelial sheets were sharply delimited from the surrounding tissue which was represented chiefly by fibroblastic elements. By and large, the architecture of the epithelial cells was retained, although the normal cellular relationships were disturbed in places. In many specimens, epithelial proliferations were present around the site of scarlet red injection, and in some of these specimens the epithelium, which showed pronounced keratinization and an increased number of cell

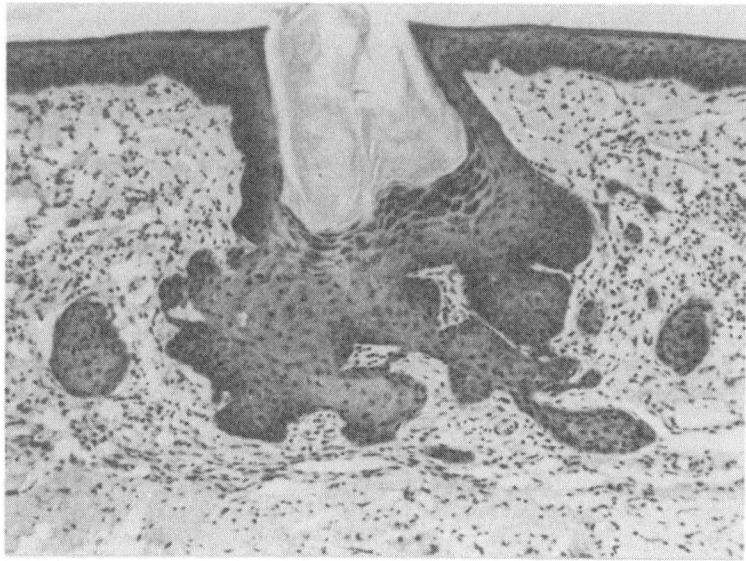

Fig. 15.  Skin of rabbit ear on day 5 after scarlet red injection, showing inflammatory epidermal proliferations at hair follicles. (80 X; hematoxylin and eosin.)

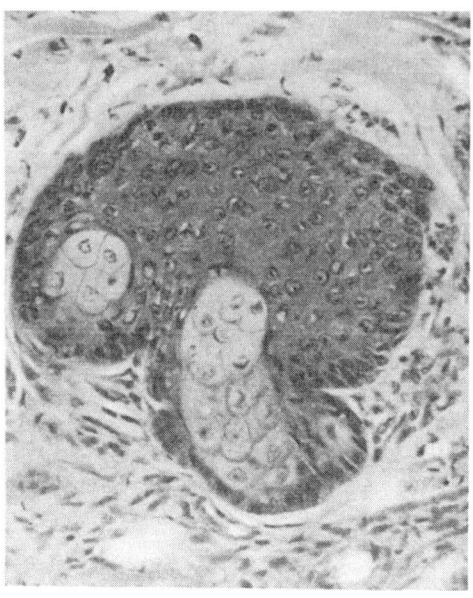

Fig. 16.  Same histologic specimen as in Fig. 15.  The dermis shows
          aggregates of epithelial cells originating from sebaceous
          glands and surrounded by edema and grossly dilated blood
          vessels and lymphatics.  (250 X; hematoxylin and eosin.)

rows, was protruding into the injection site to grow around the
cavity containing the dye and nuclear debris.  In the lower dermis,
the epithelium was proliferating around the dye-containing necrotic
masses to form cystlike structures that extended in different direct-
ions in a bizarre manner.  On staining with pyronin according to
Brachet, the strongest staining was shown by the basal cells
surrounding the epithelial strands which had not yet separated from
the epithelial mass and which contained horny material and remnants
of scarlet red in their central portions; the spinous cells located
nearer to the central parts of the epithelial proliferations, stained
more weakly.  On staining with the PAS reaction, the acanthotic
epidermal strands showed little or, in many ares, no glycogen.  The
PAS-positive, diastase-resistant material was unevenly distributed in
the basement membrane zone, being abundant in some areas and scarce
or absent in others.

     The greatest histologic changes in the epidermis were noted at
day 17 postinjection.  By that time, the lesions had not undergone
substantial alterations clinically, except that they had become
somewhat firmer and the animals no longer showed anxiety when the
intralesional skin was paplated.  Some lesions were covered by a firm
sanguinous crust impregnated with the dye.  Histologic examination of
such tumorlike structures revealed epidermal sheets proliferating

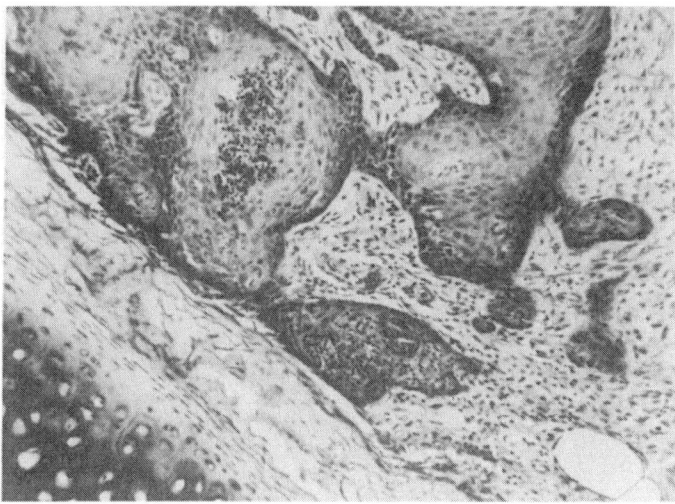

Fig. 17. Skin of rabbit ear on day 12 after scarlet red injection. Proliferating epithelial sheets have penetrated deep into the dermis destroying the perichondrium. (80 X; hematoxylin and eosin.)

downward in an irregular fashion and surrounded by an inflammatory infiltrate composed of fibroblastic elements (Figure 18a). The aggregates of proliferating cells showed pronounced architectural disarray, nuclear polymorphism, and numerous mitotic figures, including abnormal ones; in places, isolated cells detached from the epithelial proliferations had invaded the stroma (Figure 18b).

The grossly acanthotic epidermis retained glycogen only in the upper portions of the spinous layer. The epidermal downgrowths into the dermis were devoid of PAS-positive, diastase-labile granules. In the basement membrane zone, the PAS-positive substance appeared as a fine tortuous line disappearing in many places.

Six months after scarlet red injection, tumorlike lesions that were firm and freely movable to palpation were noted; some of them carried crumbly yellowish masses on their surfaces. Histologically, the epidermis consisted, over much of its extent, of 2 or 3 rows of slightly hyperkeratotic cells with a well-defined basement membrane. In some areas, the epidermis widened into small cystiform hair follicles. Some specimens contained huge cysts with horny or amorphous necrotic masses that extended to the epidermal surface (Figure 19). The walls of the cysts were lined by stratified squamous epithelium. The entire space between the epithelium and cartilage was filled with a fibrous and partly hyalinized connective tissue showing dilated and partially thrombosed vessels. With the PAS reaction, no glycogen was detectable in the epidermis. The PAS-positive substance was conspicuous in the basement membrane zone and in the blood vessel walls.

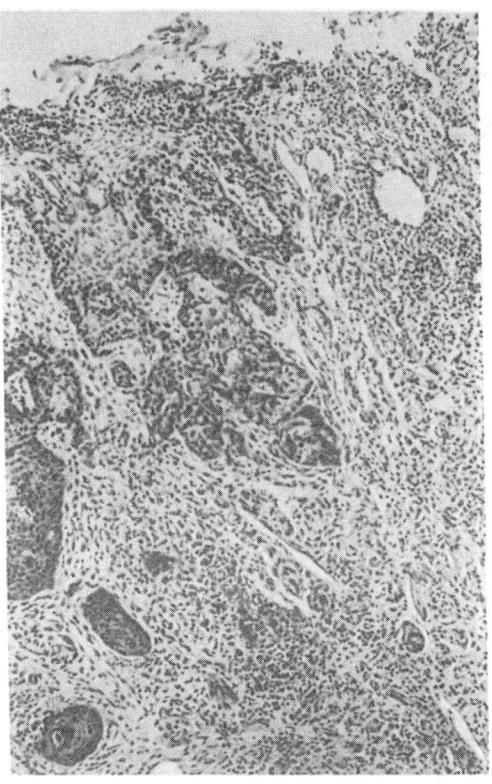

Fig. 18a.  Skin of rabbit ear.  On day 17 after scarlet red
           injection:  proliferating masses of epithelial cells
           extend deep into the dermis (75 X).


     Thus, our clinicopathologic studies of reactive pseudocarcinoma-
tous hyperplasia produced on the inner surfaces of rabbit ears by a
saturated solution of scarlet red in oil have revealed features that
resemble those characteristic of such hyperplasias seen in humans.
The epidermal proliferations at the sites of atypical inflammatory
hyperplasia had histologic similarities with the invasive proliferations occurring in cutaneous squamous cell carcinoma.

     Early during the development of reactive hyperplasia (within the
first 5 days after scarlet red injection), epidermal growth occurred
chiefly around the skin appendages (pilosebaceous units), with formation of cysts filled by horny masses.  With the course of time, the
proliferative process was expanding to involve the surface epidermis
which invaded and surrounded the sites of scarlet red injection.
Epidermal strands penetrated the dermis to the cartilage level and,
in some cases, even destroyed the perichondrium.  In general, the
epidermal proliferations retained a degree of order in cellular

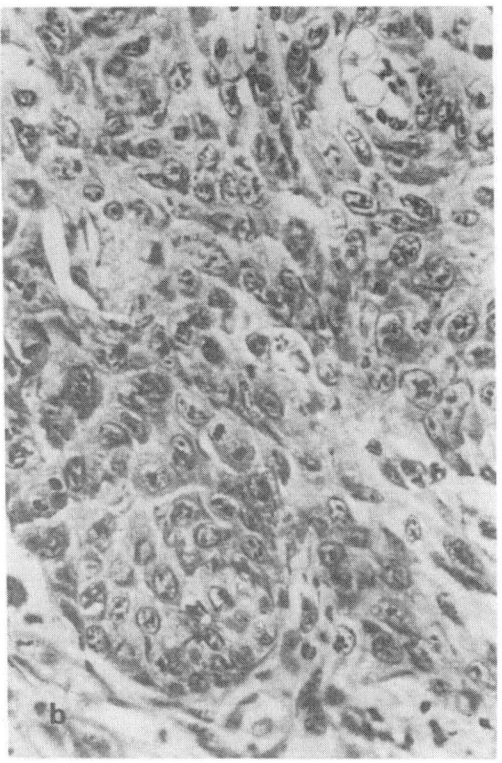

Fig. 18b.    Skin of rabbit ear.  Same specimen at 250 X magnification:
             proliferating aggregates of epithelial cells show struc-
             tural disarray, polymorphism, and numerous mitotic figures
             some of which are abnormal.  (Hematoxylin and eosin.)


arrangement, but in places disorganized cells with hyperchromic
nuclei and numerous mitotic figures, including abnormal ones, presented an appearance that was indistinguishable histologically from
cancerous proliferations.  The similarity was enhanced by the penetration into the dermis of isolated cells.  Glycogen and PAS-
positive material were absent in some areas of the basement membrane
zone within the acanthotic epidermis.  These histopathologic changes
reached their peak by days 17-20 after scarlet red injection.  Thereafter, the proliferative process subsided and by day 180 post-
injection one could see massive cysts filled with horny masses and
surrounded by uniform rows of epithelial cells that were no longer
stimulated to proliferate.

        Thus, as might be expected, the epidermal proliferations re-
sembled carcinomatous growths most closely at the height of the
inflammatory process in the dermis.  It must be emphasized that none
of the histologic specimens showing pronounced pseudocarcinomatous

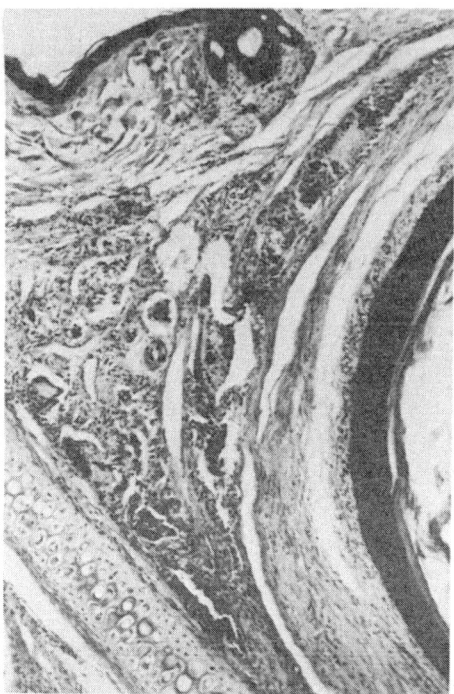

Fig. 19.  Skin of rabbit ear at 6 months after scarlet oil injection.
          The epidermis is of normal thickness and shows evidence of
          hyperkeratosis.  At right, there is a large cyst containing
          horny material surrounded by somewhat thickened epithelium.
          (75 X; hematoxylin and eosin.)

epidermal hyperplasia was found to contain either dyskeratotic cells,
cells with individual keratinization, or blood vessels and lymphatics
invaded by isolated epithelial cells.

### 3.2.2  Clinicopathologic Characteristics of Changes in Rabbit Ears during Chemical Carcinogenesis

Clinicopathologic changes occurring in rabbit ears during the
chemical carcinogenesis induced by DMBA were studied in 40 biopsy
specimens from 34 tumors.

As soon as after 5 to 6 applications of the DMBA solution, the
inner surface of the ear showed diffuse desquamation of the skin with
poorly delineated areas of mild hyperemia.  By the end of the 5th
week of painting, the hyperemia was more pronounced, with much better
delineated hyperemic areas, some edema, and infiltration of the skin.
The surfaces of such lesions displayed strongly marked follicular

hyperkeratosis. Histologic examination showed follicular hyperkeratosis and a tendency to papillomatosis. The orifices of hair follicles were plugged with horny material of orthokeratotic structure.
Throughout the surface epidermis, the number of cell rows was increased to 6-8. The epithelium of the pilosebaceous apparatus was
in a state of proliferation. The dermis was edematous and focally
infiltrated by lymphocytes and polymorphonuclear leukocytes. The
blood vessels and lymphatics were grossly dilated (Figure 20).

After 9-10 weeks of painting, the diffuse desquamation was
continuing, the follicular hyperkeratosis was more pronounced, and
there appeared circular elements slightly elevated above the plane of
the skin and containing centrally located horny masses which could be
interpreted as representing an initial phase in the development of
keratoacanthoma.

After 4 months of painting with DMBA, most of the animals
showed, along with diffuse desquamation, multiple papillomas and
keratoacanthoma-like formations appearing as roundish tumors with a
dome-shaped tip terminating in a horny spire (Figure 21). Histologic
examination revealed pronounced papillomatosis and hyperkeratosis of
orthokeratotic structure. The lower epidermis was grossly thickened,
but the spinous cells had retained their regular arrangement. The
basal cell layer was prominent. Gradually, the dermoepidermal junc-

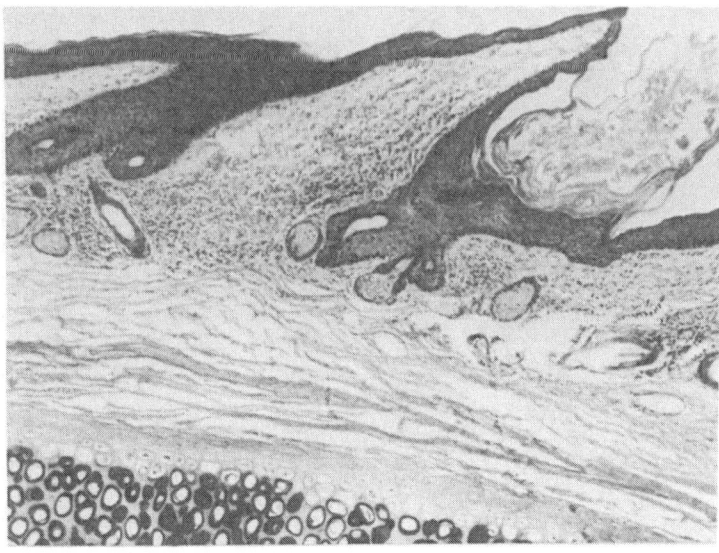

Fig. 20.  Skin of rabbit ear after 1½ months of painting with DMBA,
          showing follicular hyperkeratosis, some papillomatosis, and
          proliferating epithelium of the pilosebaceous apparatus.
          (75 X; hematoxylin and eosin.)

tion was losing its distinct outline, the acanthotic epidermal
strands were penetrating deeper and deeper into the dermis, and the
cellular arrangement within these strands was becoming increasingly
disorganized.  These processes marked the beginning of invasive
epidermal growth.  Silver impregnation by the Foot method revealed
complete absence of argyrophilic fibers in many places – not only in
the basement membrane zone but also in the underlying dermis; elsewhere, the basement membrane was still in evidence, but was fragmented and thinned out.

After 6 months of painting with DMBA, the lesional skin showed,
in some cases, a massive tumorous conglomerate that had grown through
the full thickenss of the skin which was grossly hyperkeratotic.
This clinical appearance was strongly suggestive of malignant transformation.  Histologic study of such lesions revealed striking acanthosis with massive invasive epidermal proliferations and bizarre
aggregations of cells deep in the dermis.  Among these, cystlike
structures filled with horny masses were seen.  The cytoplasm of
spinous cells within the epidermal proliferations stained faintly in
places.  Pronounced cellular disarray and individual cell keratinization were noted (Figure 22).

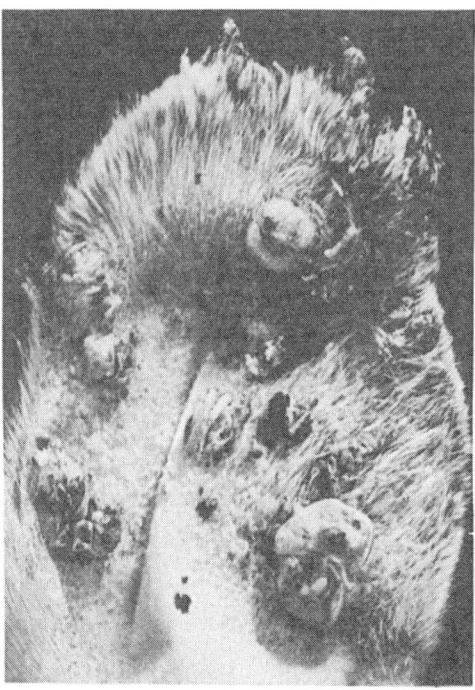

Fig. 21.   Skin of rabbit ear after 4 months of painting with DMBA,
           showing follicular hyperkeratosis, multiple papillomas, and
           keratoacanthoma-like formations.   (Same rabbit as in Fig.
           20.)

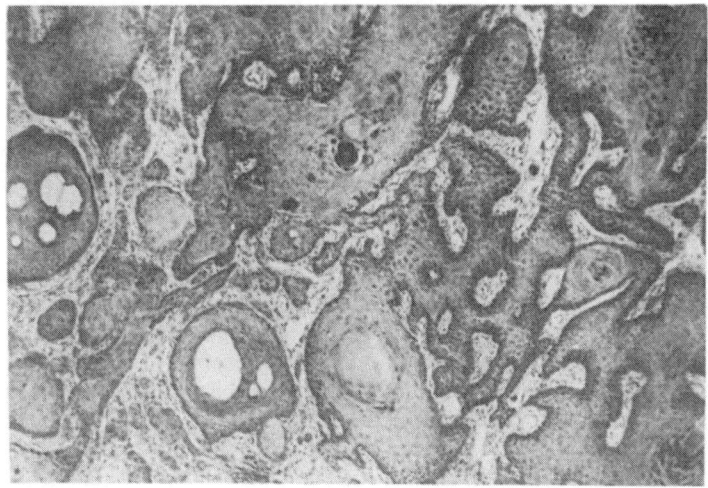

Fig. 22.  Skin of rabbit ear after 6 months of painting with DMBA, showing tumorous proliferations with areas of cellular disarray and occasional dyskeratotic cells.  Same rabbit as in Figs. 20 and 21.  (75 X; hematoxylin and eosin.)

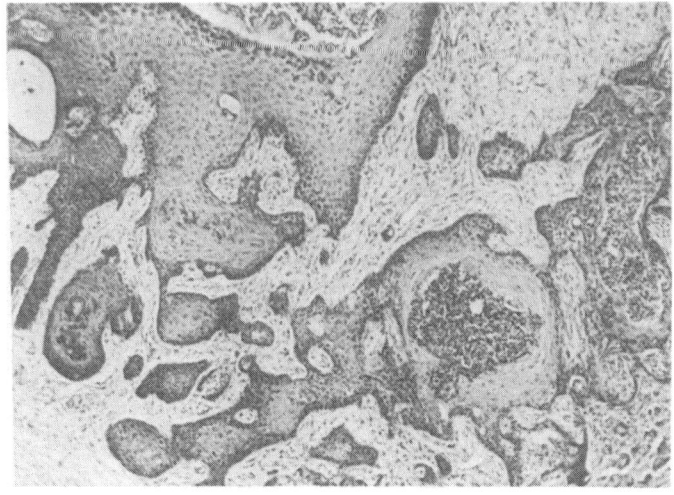

Fig. 23.  Skin of rabbit ear on day 12 after scarlet red injection. The proliferating epidermis has produced bizarre outgrowths and cystlike cavities filled with horny material and scarlet red.  Some cell aggregates have broken away from the acanthotic epidermis.  (75 X; hematoxylin and eosin.)

When one compares the above histologic picture with that of
pseudocarcinomatous reactive hyperplasia shown in Figure 23, one
cannot fail to notice their similarity.

Overtly invasive forms of squamous cell carcinoma were most
frequent 12 to 18 months after the start of the experiment.  As a
rule, a conglomerate of tumorous masses, often accompanied by tissue
breakdown, was seen at that time (Figure 24).  Histologic examination
then showed multiple nests of tumor cells exhibiting a high degree of
disorganization and nuclear polymorphism.  The central part of such a
nest consisted of larger cells with faintly stained cytoplasms, while
its peripheral part was composed of smaller cells with more intensely
stained cytoplasms and hyperchromic nuclei.  There were many grossly
dilated blood vessels around the tumorous proliferations, and some of
these vessels were arteries so restructured as to resemble end arteries.  In some areas, tumorous cells had penetrated into the lumens
of dilated blood vessels (Figure 25).

### 3.2.3  Conclusion

The experimental studies just described, in which the potent
carcinogen DMBA was applied to the skin of rabbit ears, have made it
possible to follow the process of carcinogenesis through all its

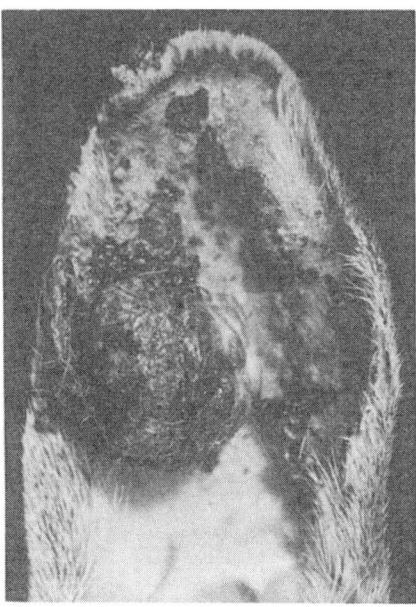

Fig. 24.   Squamous cell carcinoma of rabbit ear that has developed
           after 12 months of painting with DMBA.

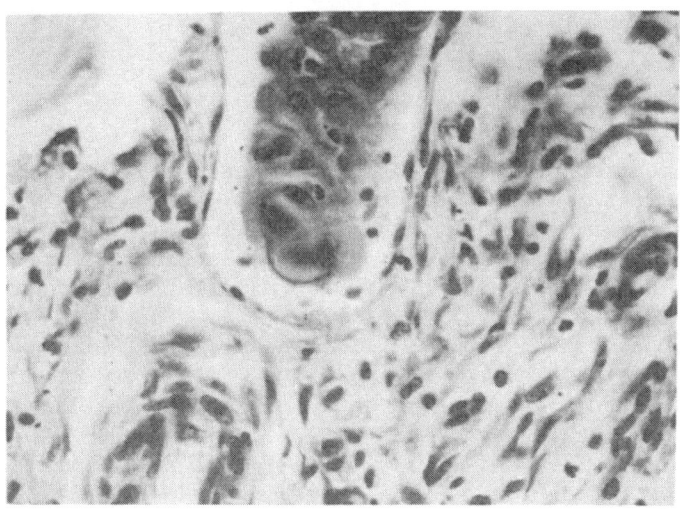

Fig. 25.  Skin of rabbit ear after 12 months of painting with DMBA.
Tumor cells have penetrated into the lumen of a blood
vessel.  (280 X; hematoxylin and eosin.)

stages from obligatory premalignant papillomas and keratoacanthomas
to an invasive squamous cell carcinoma.  A comparison of the histopathologic changes that occurred in the lesional skin shortly after
the start of DMBA application with those seen to arise in the inflammatory epidermal hyperplasia induced by the scarlet red dye, has
indicated similarities as well as differences between these two
processes.  The most important similarity is that in both the primary
changes in the epidermis involve proliferation of cells of the pilosebaceous apparatus accompanied by pronounced hyperkeratosis of
orthokeratotic structure.  Subsequently, however, painting with DMBA
leads predominantly to papillomatosis and to a degree of acanthosis
before invasive epidermal growth sets in later on.  By contrast, in
the pseudocarcinomatous epidermal hyperplasia produced by scarlet
red, there is no papillomatosis, and from the very beginning epidermal strands proliferate into the dermis toward the inflammatory
infiltrate.  In later phases of malignant transformation, epidermal
proliferation shares several features, both histologic and histochemical, with inflammatory epidermal growth.  The common histologic
features include downward epidermal growth (with destruction of
cartilage in some cases), cellular disarray, nuclear polymorphism,
numerous, including abnormal, mitotic figures, and loss of cellular
cohesion accompanied by free penetration of cells into the dermis.
The common histochemical features include sharp reduction in glycogen, absence of PAS-positive material in the basement membrane
zone, and destruction of argyrophilic elements of the basement membrane.  However, it is only in invasive carcinomas that penetration

of cells into blood vessels and lymphatics and individual cell keratinization are observed.


## 3.3  GENERAL SUMMARY

The present comparative clinicopathologic studies in three
groups of patients (with reactive epidermal hyperplasia that often
presented as pseudocarcinomatous; with benign epithelial or connective tissue tumors of the skin; and with cutaneous squamous cell
carcinoma) have demonstrated a number of similarities and differences
between these conditions.  The results are in good agreement with
those of our studies in rabbits.  In general, these studies indicate
that the considerable histopathologic and, not infrequently, clinical
similarities between, on the one hand, various dermatoses and benign
skin tumors showing atypical epidermal hyperplasia and, on the other
squamous cell carcinoma of the skin, make the differentiation of
these diseases both difficult and important from a practical point of
view.  Here, of great significance is close cooperation between the
clinician and pathologist.  Our studies, as well as those by other,
authors, have shown that the clinical suspicion of malignancy is
sometimes dispelled by histologic findings and that, conversely, a
pseudocarcinomatous hyperplasia suspected of being a malignant state
on histologic grounds may not be confirmed as such clinically.  The
most difficult cases are those where the clinical and histologic
pictures are both suggestive of carcinoma which, however, is not
actually present.  One should agree with Apatenko (1973) that
clinical and histologic criteria cannot be relied upon in such cases,
although the correct diagnosis can often be arrived at through
careful clinicopathologic correlation.

In recent years, special significance in the early recognition
of structures undergoing malignant change has been attached to
patterns of cellular proliferation, the DNA content of cell nuclei,
and cytophysiologic and cytogenetic characteristics of cells.  These,
as well as some other cytogenetic and also cytophysiologic aspects
are dealt with in the next three chapters with special reference to
pseudocarcinomatous epidermal hyperplasia.

# 4
# Mitotic Behavior of Epidermal Cells in Pseudocarcinomatous Hyperplasia and in Squamous Cell Carcinoma

A fundamental biologic characteristic of the cell is of course its ability to reproduce itself. Since the life cycle of individual cells is much shorter than the life span of a multicellular organism, the dying cells are continuously replaced by new cells. It is cell reproduction which underlies the development and regeneration of organisms (Alov, 1972). The following types of cell reproduction are recognized: mitosis (indirect division), meiosis, endomitosis (endoreduplication), and amitosis (direct division). The most widespread mode of reproduction in animals is mitosis.

Cell division is known to involve highly complex biochemical processes associated with DNA synthesis (Dubinin, 1961; Prescott, 1961; 1963; Alov, 1964, 1972; Liozner, 1966; Epifanova, 1967; Zavarzin, 1967; Davidson, 1969; Voorhees et al., 1975; and others). The life cycle of a cell (which extends from its birth to its division) consists, in terms of DNA synthesis, of four periods: presynthetic ($G_1$), synthetic (S), postsynthetic ($G_2$), and mitotic (M). Each of these periods varies in duration depending on the tissue concerned (Winder et al., 1951). For example, the life cycle of epidermal cells in tissue culture is 41h, $6\frac{1}{2}$h of which time is taken by $G_1$, 17 by S, 16 by $G_2$, and $1\frac{1}{2}$h by M (Baserga and Wiebel, 1969).

The rate of cell proliferation may be regulated through variation in the lengths of the presynthetoc and postsynthetic periods (Epifanova, 1967), with the DNA synthesis period remaining of constant duration in most epidermal cells (Gelfant and Gandelas, 1972). Cell cycle duration in normal human epidermis has been estimated to be 300 h (Gaylarde and Sarkany, 1975), of which about 284 h is spent in $G_1$ and 16 h in S (Weinstein and Frost, 1968). Allegra and De

Panfilis (1974) have shown that the basal cells of normal human
epidermis have a life cycle of some 206 h, with the S period lasting
7 h 35min.  According to Heenen et al. (1972) the duration of S in
normal human epidermis is 10.2 ± 0.5 h.

Malignant transformation is accompanied by a shortening of the
cell cycle and an increase of proliferative activity (Frankfurt,
1975).

In skin cancer the S period has been reported to increase in
duration (Weinstein and Frost, 1970).  Heenen et al. (1975) have
found this period to increase also in precancerous dermatoses.

Usually, normal human and animal epidermises show a diurnal
rhythm of mitotic activity (Broders and Dublin, 1939; Blumenfeld,
1943; Bullough, 1964; Kahn et al., 1968; Sealy et al., 1972; and
others).  No diurnal rhythm is apparent in malignant epidermis
(Blumenfeld, 1943; Sealy et al., 1972).  One of the factors con-
trolling the mitotic activity of epidermis and other tissues is the
chemical inhibitor chalone (see Chapter 7).

It has been demonstrated in numerous studies (e.g. Green and
Ghadially, 1951; Utkin, 1953; Zalkind, 1954; Vasil'ev, 1967; Kozlov,
1969) that mitotic activity can be inhibited by a wide variety of
stimuli (noise, light, pain, etc.).  At certain stages of inflammation and during the regeneration following trauma, mitotic activity
may be increased (Brodskii et al., 1969; Kozlov, 1969; Frankfurt,
1975).  It is also elevated considerably in normal epidermis in cases
of hypervitaminosis A (Logan, 1972).  However, the greatest increase
in mitotic activity occurs in malignant neoplasms (Eversen and
Iversen, 1962; Alov, 1965, 1972; Kazantseva, 1967, 1981; Manocha,
1969; Vasil'ev, 1967; Ganina and Polishchuk, 1968; Gelfant, 1977).

Malignant cells and tissues differ from their normal counterparts in a number of biochemical and genetic features as well as in
showing high mitotic activity which assures tumor growth (Sealy et
al., 1972).  According to Willis (1967), anaplastic tumors contain
many mitotic figures, and the mitotic activity of a tumor is probably
the most reliable single criterion of the degree of its malignancy.
He stated that "if several mitotic figures are found easily, then the
tumor is almost certainly a malignant one."  However, as shown in
many studies, mitotic activity is not uncommonly high in benign
cutaneous tumors as well, notably in keratoacanthoma (e.g. Blinova,
1959; Glazunov and Blinova, 1960; Apatenko, 1973), verrucae (White
and Weidman, 1927), papillomatosis cutis carcinoides of Gottron
(Schrimpf and Seller, 1963), and at sites of chronic inflammation
(Sommerville, 1953).

Another important feature of tumor cells is the presence of
abnormal mitoses. Many of them were described long ago in cancers of

various sites by Arnold (1879), Hansemann (1893), Andres and
Navaschin (1936), and others.  In 1947 Koller proposed a morphologic
classification of pathologic mitoses encountered in tumor cells.  He
divided the mitotic abnormalities which occur naturally in tumors
into three classes: (1) structural alterations in the chromosomes,
(2) numerical changes in the chromosome complement, and (3) complete
or partial suppression of the spindle.  Among pathologic mitoses he
mentioned stickiness of chromosomes, lagging of chromosomes and
fragments, multipolar mitoses, etc.  He emphasized that abnormal
mitoses account for the chromosomal variability of tumor cells.
Thus, according to Koller, the stickiness of chromosomes and their
lagging in anaphase give rise to aneuploid cells with an increased or
decreased chromosome number.

The fundamental studies on the cytophysiology and pathology of
mitosis carried out in the USSR by Alov (1964, 1965, 1972), Alov et
al. (1966), Kurilo (1970, 1973), Kazantseva and Rogachikova (1970),
Kazantseva (1981), and other investigators have led Alov to propose
the following classification of mitotic abnormalities, which is also
used here:

I. Mitotic abnormalities associated with damage to the
chromosomes: (1) mitotic delay in prophase, (2) disturbances of chromosome coiling and uncoiling, (3) early separation of chromatids, (4) fragmentation and pulverization of
chromosomes, (5) chromosome and chromatid bridges, (6)
lagging of chromosomes in metakinesis and during their
movement to opposite spindle poles, (7) formation of micro-
nuclei, (8) chromosome nondisjunction, (9) chromosome
swelling and stickiness.

II. Mitotic abnormalities associated with damage to
the mitotic apparatus: (10) mitotic delay in metaphase,
(11) C-mitosis, (12) chromosome scattering in metaphase,
(13) multipolar mitosis; (14) monocentric mitosis, (15)
asymmetric mitosis, (16) three-group metaphase and metaphase with polar chromosomes, (17) hollow metaphase.

III.  Abnormalities of cytokinesis: (18) delayed or
absent cytokinesis (dissociation between nuclear and cytoplasmic changes) and (19) premature cytokinesis.

As pointed out by Alov (1972), mitotic abnormalities associated
with chromosome damage occur when cell reproduction is disturbed at
early stages; delayed entry of cells into mitosis is most often due
to alterations in DNA synthesis resulting from exposure of the cells
to toxic chemicals or radiation; pathologic mitoses associated with
chromosome breakage are common in tumor cells and in cells exposed to
mutagens.

An important mitotic abnormality is <u>fragmentation of chromosomes</u>
which has been reported to occur in nearly 45% of cultured cells
undergoing transformation to malignancy (Levan and Biessele, 1958)
and also in cells of malignant tumors and of tissues infected by
virus (Zalkind, 1972).  A consequence of chromosome fragmentation is
the formation of bridges.  This is a fairly stable mitotic abnormality which, according to Prokof'eva-Bel'govskaya (1961), may persist
over 12-15 mitotic cycles.

Damage to chromosomes at the centromere leads to lagging of the
chromosomes in their movement in metakinesis and during their separation.  This abnormality may arise on exposure of cells to toxic
agents, but it occurs most often in tumor cells (Alov, 1972).  One
reason for the appearance of aneuploid cells may be <u>nondisjunction</u> of
chromosomes in which the two sister chromatids fail to separate and
both move to one of the poles.  A common type of mitotic abnormality
is <u>swelling</u> and <u>stickiness</u> of chromosomes; the clumpy chromosome
masses then die.

A characteristic mitotic abnormality resulting from damage to
the mitotic apparatus is <u>mitotic delay</u> in metaphase.  Such delay is a
frequent finding in tumors, and its occurrence in a high proportion
of cells is regarded by many as a sign diagnostic of malignancy
(e.g. Timonen and Therman, 1950; Scarpelli and Van Haam, 1957; Alov,
1965, 1972; Kurilo, 1973; Serov 1973; Kazantseva, 1981.  Another
mitotic abnormality of this type, which is caused by stathmokinetic
poisons and is characterized by mitotic arrest at metaphase, is
colchicine mitosis (C-mitosis).  In this common mitotic abnormality,
the chromosomes may be clumped together, be arranged in a ball-shaped
or star-shaped configuration, or be distributed all over the cytoplasm.  The outcome of C-mitosis may be death of the cell or resto-
ration of the mitotic process (Kurilo, 1973).  C-mitoses occur not
only in tumor tissues, but may also be elicited by exposure to infectious or toxic agents (Gol'tzman, 1965; Golubchik and Yakimenko,
1971; Stich et al., 1964; and others).  Less common mitotic abnormalities, which are encountered more often in malignant tissues, are
<u>multipolar, monocentric, and asymmetric mitoses</u>.  These give rise to
aneuploid cells (Alov, 1972).  Chromosome <u>scattering</u>, unlike C-
mitosis, is characterized by complete disorganization of the mitotic
apparatus and the absence of chromosome supercoiling.  This abnormality is likewise frequently seen in malignancy (Kazantseva and
Rogachikova, 1970; Kazantseva, 1981).  Yet another mitotic abnormality, which is often found in early stages of cervical cancer (Kurilo,
1970), is the so-called <u>three-group metaphase</u> resulting from metaphase lagging of chromosomes and from changes in the thiol mechanism
of mitosis (Alov et al., 1966).  A rare mitotic abnormality is the
<u>hollow metaphase</u> in which metaphase chromosomes are distributed at the
cell periphery.

Pathologic mitoses represent one of the mechanisms of mutation, in particular of somatic aneuploidy, and may occur in normal tissues as well as in various disease processes resulting from viral infection, exposure to ionizing radiation, etc. (Alov, 1965, 1972). However, as pointed out by Alov, by far the largest number of pathologic mitoses occurs in cancer. The question of whether abnormal mitoses are a cause or effect of malignant transformation of the epithelium is debatable. In the opinion of Davydovskii (1969), Cowdry (1958), and Policard and Bassis (1970), they are a consequence of malignant change. However, experiments with chemically induced malignant transformation of the epidermis in mice have shown that mitotic activity and the number of pathologic mitoses both increase in parallel with tumor progression (Skjaeggestad, 1964; Vasil'eva, 1966; and others). That mitotic abnormalities have an important bearing on the development of malignancy has been emphasized by many investigators (e.g. Koller, 1947; Zalkind, 1954; Levan and Biessele, 1958; Dubinin, 1961; G. G. Tinyakov and Yu. G. Tinyakov, 1963; Alov, 1965, 1972; Baserga, 1965; Vasil'ev, 1967; Kaiser and Schneider, 1968; Kurilo, 1970, 1973; Serov, 1973; Kazantseva, 1981).

It must be noted that while the mitotic behavior of cells in squamous cells carcinomas of various anatomic sites has been studied in great detail, there are only a few reports dealing with mitotic activity and pattern in hyperplastic epidermis, and the information presented therein is fragmentary and, as a rule, amounts to little more than the statement that the foci of squamous cell carcinomas show more mitoses than do those of reactive epidermal proliferation (e.g. Willis, 1967; Sanderson, 1968). But, as already indicated, it has been shown repeatedly that the number of mitoses in, for instance, growing keratoacanthomas, may be the same as in cancer (e.g. Blinova, 1959; Glazunov and Blinova, 1960; Montgomery, 1967; Apatenko, 1969, 1971). Sommerville (1953) observed large numbers of mitoses, including aberrant ones, in pyoderma ulcerosum vegetans. In giant condyloma of Buschke and Loewenstein, the presence of many mitoses is regarded by some authors as one of the reasons why this tumor is difficult to distinguish from squamous cell carcinoma (Vulcan, 1972). Machacek and Weakley (1960), however, took the opposite view that the absence of frequent mitoses in giant condyloma acuminatum is the major point of its differentiation from carcinoma.

The lack of consensus regarding the possibility of using mitotic activity of epidermal cells in diagnostic differentiation between malignant and benign hyperplastic processes of the epidermis is due to the fact that these two kinds of process may both show pathologic mitoses and high mitotic activity. Khlopin wrote in 1947: "When the mitotic activity of cells increases, as it does in reparative regeneration, in tissue culture, and in inflammation, an appreciable amount of mitotic irregularity also appears in the cells." However, it still remains to be established what are the mitotic patterns of cells in reactive epidermal hyperplasia and how they differ from

those in skin cancer.  The studies carried out in this area by the
present author together with Kazantseva (Berenbein and Kazantseva,
1973) suggest that analysis of epidermal mitotic patterns at sites of
pseudocarcinomatous hyperplasia and cutaneous squamous cell carcinoma
may be of considerable diagnostic aid in the differentuation between
these conditions.

## 4.1  CLINICAL STUDIES

We have studied the mitotic patterns (mitotic regimes according
to our terminology[1]) of epidermis in 53 biopsy specimens from patients
with various dermatoses accompanied by pseudocarcinomatous hyperplasia (which was often pronounced) and with squamous cell carcinoma.
As controls, 10 biopsy specimens taken from morphologically unchanged
epidermis were used.

The dermatoses showing pronounced psuedocarcinomatous hyperplasia (18 patients, 20 biopsy specimens) included chronic pyoderma
ulcerosum vegetans (4 cases), trophic ulcers of the shins (4); lupus
tuberculosus (2), tuberculosis verrucosa (2), lichen ruber verrucosus
(2), psoriasis in its warty form (1), lupus erythematosus (1), senile
keratoma (1), and papillomatosis cutis carcinoides of Gottron (1).
We classified as precancerous acanthosis (11 biopsies), the areas of
moderately proliferating epidermal ridges bordering the foci of
invasive squamous cell carcinoma and the areas of acanthosis in
certain precancerous dermatoses (senile keratoma, circumscribed
hyperkeratosis of the lower lip) and in diseases retrospectively
interpreted as precancerous because a squamous cell carcinoma had
supervened subsequently (giant condyloma acuminatum of Buschke and
Loewenstein, keratoacanthoma).  The sites of squamous cell carcinomas
(12 biopsies from 10 patients) were the upper and lower extremities,
trunk, and face (6 cases), lower lip (2), and penis (2 cases).

The results of these studies are summarized in Table 6 and
Figure 26.

In the control group, the mitotic index was low, the percentage
frequencies of the various mitotic stages were normal, and abnormal
mitoses were relatively few in number (3.6 ± 1.6%) and were represented mainly by C-mitoses (2.6%) and chromosomes and fragments
lagging in metaphase (1.4%).

---

[1]The term mitotic regime is used in Soviet literature to embrace the
following quantative characteristics of mitosis: (a) mitotic activity
as expressed by the mitotic index (number of mitoses per 1000 cells),
(b) percentage frequencies of the various mitotic stages, (c) percentage of abnormal mitoses relative to the total number of mitoses,
and (d) percentages of mitoses showing particular forms of abnormality relative to the total number of mitoses (Kazantseva, 1981,
p. 38).

Table 6. Mitotic Regime of Epidermal Cells in Different Types of Hyperplasia in Man.

| Condition | No. of specimens | Mitotic index | Percentage frequencies of various mitotic stages | | | | Percentages of abnormal mitoses | Percentages of mitoses showing particular forms of abnormality | | | | | | | | | | |
|---|---|---|---|---|---|---|---|---|---|---|---|---|---|---|---|---|---|---|
| | | | prophase | metaphase | anaphase | telophase | | lagging of chromosomes and fragments in metaphase | lagging of chromosomes and fragments in ana- & telophase | bridges | scattering of chromosomes and fragments | three-group metaphases | multipolar mitoses | monocentric mitoses | hollow metaphases | asymmetrical mitoses | C-mitoses | other forms of abnormality |
| Control (normal epidermis) | 10 | 4.6±0.6 | 31.9 | 34.0±5.0 | 11.6 | 22.5 | 3.6±1.6 | 1.4 | - | - | - | - | - | - | - | - | 2.2 | - |
| Pseudocarcinomatous hyperplasia | 20 | 12.4±1.5 | 15.5 | 52.4±2.5 | 10.5 | 21.6 | 19.5±2.5 | 6.5 | 1.8 | 0.3 | 0.3 | 0.1 | - | - | - | - | 10.5 | - |
| Precancerous acanthosis | 11 | 13.0±2.4 | 10.9 | 62.9±3.5 | 4.4 | 21.8 | 24.0±2.8 | 7.5 | 1.1 | 3.1 | 0.9 | 0.6 | - | 1.4 | 0.2 | 0.6 | 8.6 | - |
| Squamous cell carcinoma | 12 | 28.1±4.2 | 10.2 | 70.5±4.0 | 6.3 | 13.0 | 44.4±2.4 | 8.0 | 3.1 | 1.4 | 11.8 | 0.6 | 1.4 | 1.6 | 0.6 | 0.7 | 15.0 | - |

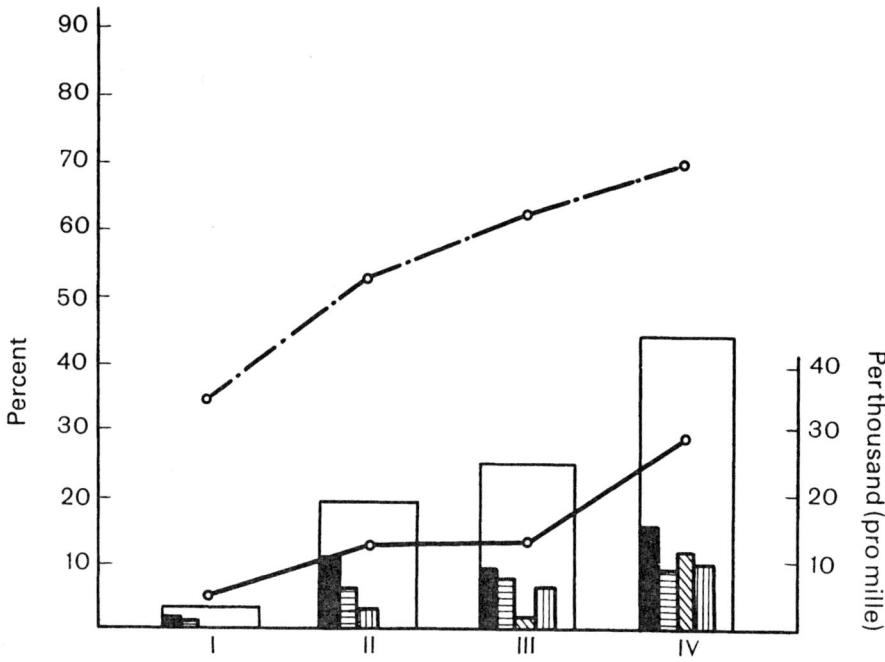

Fig. 26.  Mitotic regime of human epidermis in health (I),
          pseudocarcinomatous hyperplasia (II), precancerous
          acanthosis (III), and squamous cell carcinoma (IV).  The
          solid line shows the mitotic index and the broken line, the
          percentage of metaphases.  The large white bars represent
          the percentages of abnormal mitoses and the narrow
          variously shaded bars, the percentages of particular
          mitotic abnormalities, as follows: ■ = C-mitoses; ▤ =
          chromosome lagging; ◩ = chromosome scattering; ⬚ =
          other abnormalities.


        In the pseudocarcinomatous epidermal hyperplasia group, the
mitotic index was significantly increased as compared with the control (p<0.001), being below 10 in only 5 of the 20 biopsy specimens
examined.  The percentage ratio of the mitotic stages was likewise
abnormal, due to a decrease in the number of cells in prophase and an
increase in the number of cells in metaphase.  The percentage of
cells in metaphase averaged 52.4 ± 2.5, but it was only in 6 of the
20 specimens that this percentage was below 50.  The percentages of
anaphases and telophases did not differ significantly from the
control.  An important feature of the pseudocarcinomatous hyperplasias was a significant increase in the percentage of abnormal
mitoses as compared to the control (p<0.001).  These comprised 19.5 ±
2.5% of the mitoses, and it should be noted that they accounted for
less than 10% of all mitoses in only 4 of the 20 biopsy specimens
studied (in two specimens, no pathologic mitoses were found).  An

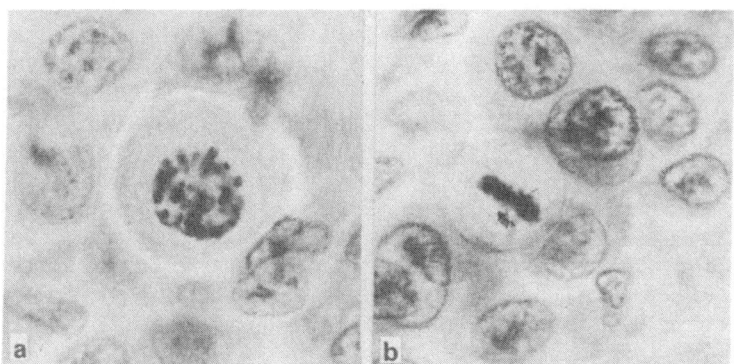

Fig. 27.   The more frequent mitotic abnormalities in pseudocarcinomatous epidermal hyperplasia.  (a) C-mitosis (ball metaphase); (b) lagging of chromosomes and fragments in
metaphase.  (1100 X; hematoxylin and eosin.)

average of 10.5% of all mitotic counts comprised C-mitoses appearing
as ball metaphases with clumped supercoiled chromosomes (Figure 27a).
Metaphases with metaphase lagging of chromosomes and their fragments
(Figure 27b) accounted for 6.5% of all mitoses.  Other mitotic abnormalities such as bridges, scattering of chromosomes and fragments,
and three-group metaphases were rare.  It must be stressed that no
mitotic patterns specific for the particular dermatoses accompanied
by pseudocarcinomatous hyperplasia were discernible in our material.

In the precancerous acanthosis group, the mitotic index was
higher than in pseudocarcinomatous hyperplasia, but the difference
was insignificant (p>0.05).  The proportion in metaphases was likewise higher and the difference was significant (p<0.05).  It should
be noted that the proportion of such cells was above 60% in all but 3
specimens, being as high as 75% in the specimen from a patient with
giant condyloma of Buschke and Loewenstein.

The precancerous acanthosis was characterized by a higher percentage of pathologic mitoses (24 ± 2.8) than the pseudocarcinomatous
hyperplasia, but the difference was again insignificant.  As in the
pseudocarcinomatous hyperplasia group, the most frequent mitotic
abnormalities were C-mitoses (8.6%) and metaphase lagging of chromosomes and fragments (7.5%).  The range of mitotic abnormalities was,
however, wider, with the appearance of such aberrant forms as monocentric mitosis, hollow metaphase, and asymmetrical mitosis.  More
frequently seen were bridges and three-group metaphases.

In the squamous cell carcinoma group, all the mitotic characteristics studied, had higher values than in the other two groups.  The
mitotic index was significantly higher than in the precancerous

acanthosis and pseudocarcinomatous hyperplasia groups (p<0.001) and ranged from 21 to 64 in most specimens. The percentage of metaphases was 70.5% ± 4 and the differences from the pseudocarcinomatous hyperplasia and precancerous acanthosis groups were significant (p<0.01). Also, the range of mitotic abnormalities was considerably wider than in the pseudocarcinomatous hyperplasia group. The most noteworthy disturbance in mitotic regime was a statistically significant (p<0.001) sharp rise in pathologic mitoses which comprised 44.4 ± 2.4% of all mitoses. The most common mitotic abnormality were C-mitoses, which accounted for 15% of all mitoses, followed in frequency by metaphases with scattered chromosomes. More frequently seen were also other forms of mitotic pathology, such as lagging of chromosomes and fragments in metaphase and ana- and telophase; bridges, three-group metaphases, multipolar mitoses, hollow metaphases, and other abnormalities were also noted (Figure 28).

These studies thus indicate that although the genetic heterogeneity of the lesional tissue may be increased even in the incipient phase of its malignant degeneration, the increase is particularly marked during the development of squamous cell carcinoma, when the spectrum of mitotic abnormalities and their frequency are far greater than in precancerous acanthosis and pseudocarcinomatous hyperplasia, as is the proportion of metaphases.

It may be concluded from the foregoing that there exist profound differences in epidermal cell mitotic behavior between squamous cell carcinoma and pseudocarcinomatous hyperplasia, and mitotic analysis may therefore be recommended for use in diagnostic differentiation between these conditions in certain difficult cases. Indeed, our studies of the epidermal mitotic regime have corroborated the biologic nature of the pathologic process in all instances. For example, in the cases of tuberculosis verrucosa and pyoderma ulcerosum showing a pronounced pseudocarcinomatous epidermal hyperplasia virtually indistinguishable histologically from a squamous cell carcinoma, the mitotic index never exceeded 10, the proportion of cells in metaphase was 48% at most, and abnormal mitoses accounted for no more than 24% of all mitoses and were even absent altogether in some cases. Followup of these patients over periods of 3 to 8 years confirmed the benign nature of the epidermal hyperplasias. By contrast, in no case of squamous cell cancer did we find a percentage of abnormal mitoses below 32 or a narrow range of mitotic abnormalities: these were represented by 4 to 7 forms in nearly all cancer patients. Generally similar results have been obtained in our experimental studies which are described below.


## 4.2  EXPERIMENTAL STUDIES

We examined 27 biopsy specimens from the lesional skin of rabbit ears with inflammatory epidermal growths induced by scarlet red (13

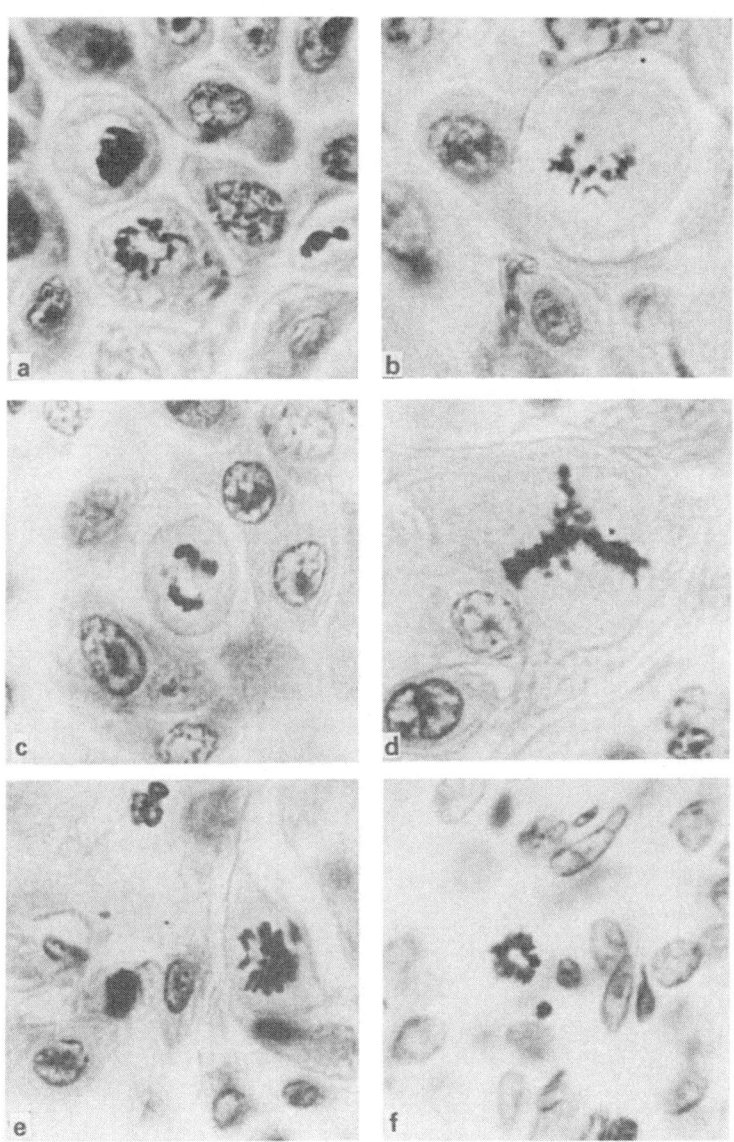

Fig. 28. The more frequent mitotic abnormalities in squamous cell carcinoma of the skin. (a) Clumpy metaphase and scattering of chromosomes; (b) chromosome scattering in metaphase; (c) lagging of chromosomes during separation; (d) three-group metaphase; (e) lagging of chromosomes in metaphase and their sticking together in prophase; (f) hollow metaphase. (1100 X; (a)-(e) hematoxylin and eosin; (f) Feulgen stain.)

Table 7.  Mitotic Regime of Epidermal Cells in Different Types of Hyperplasia Experimentally Produced in Rabbits.

| Condition | No. of specimens | Mitotic Index | Percentage frequencies of various mitotic stages | | | | Percentages of abnormal mitoses | Percentages of mitoses showing particular forms of abnormality | | | | | | | | | |
| --- | --- | --- | --- | --- | --- | --- | --- | --- | --- | --- | --- | --- | --- | --- | --- | --- | --- |
| | | | prophase | metaphase | anaphase | telophase | | lagging of chromosomes and fragments in metaphase | lagging of chromosomes and fragments in ana- & telophase | bridges | scattering of chromosomes and fragments | three-group metaphases | multipolar mitoses | monocentric mitoses | hollow metaphases | asymmetrical mitoses | C-mitoses |
| Control (normal epidermis) | 11 | 2.4±0.3 | 22.5 | 46.9±7.7 | 6.1 | 24.5 | 6.1±2.7 | 2.0 | - | - | - | - | - | - | - | - | 4.0 |
| Pseudocarcinomatous hyperplasia | 13 | 13.9±0.1 | 12.4 | 58.7±3.6 | 2.6 | 26.3 | 14.5±1.7 | 4.8 | 0.8 | 0.3 | 0.1 | - | - | - | - | - | 8.5 |
| Obligatory pre-cancerous acanthosis and squamous cell carcinoma | 14 | 16.8±1.5 | 10.6 | 68.3±2.1 | 4.0 | 17.1 | 25.3±2.7 | 5.9 | 0.7 | 0.4 | 1.5 | 0.3 | 0.3 | 1.2 | 0.3 | - | 14.7 |

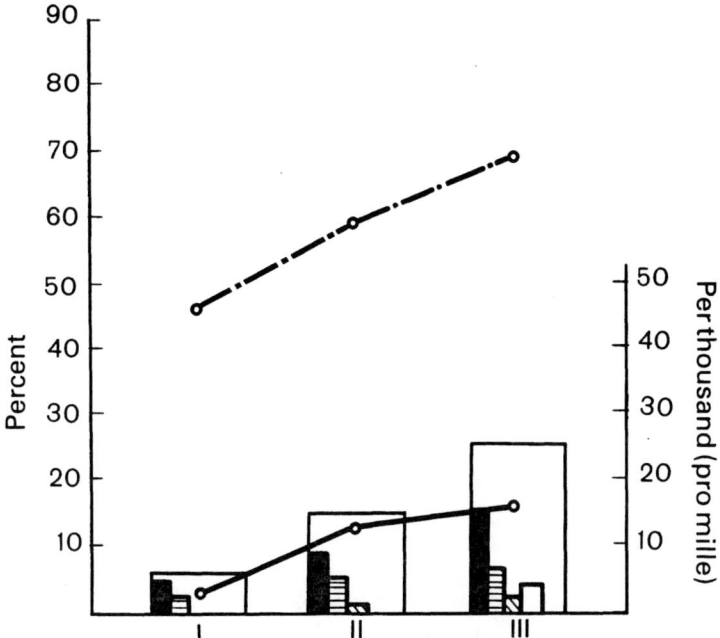

Fig. 29.  Mitotic regime of rabbit ear epidermis in health (I),
          reactive pseudocarcinomatous hyperplasia (II), and pre-
          cancerous tumors and squamous cell cancinoma (III).  The
          solid line shows the mitotic index and the broken line, the
          percentage of abnormal mitoses.  The large white bars
          represent the percentages of abnormal mitoses and the
          narrow variously shaded bars, the percentages of particular
          mitotic abnormalities, as follows: ■ = C-mitoses; ▤ =
          chromosome lagging; ◫ = chromosome scattering; ☐ = other
          abnormalities.

specimens from 3 rabbits) and of obligatory precancerous acanthosis
or squamous cell carcinoma caused by DMBA (14 specimens from 2
rabbits).  As control, 11 biopsy specimens from morphologically
unchanged rabbit ear skin were used.  The results are shown in Table
7 and Figure 29.

     In the unchanged epidermis, the mitotic indices were low, with a
mean value of 2.4, and the percentage ratio of mitotic stages was
normal and generally similar to that seen in the normal human epidermis.  The percentage frequency of abnormal mitoses was small and
these were of two types only: C- mitoses and metaphase lagging of
chromosomes and fragments.

The pseudocarcinomatous inflammatory hyperplasia was characterized by a significantly (p<0.001) increased mitotic index and an
abnormal percentage ratio of mitotic stages due to a decrease in the
number of cells in prophase and an increase in the number of cells in
metaphase. The proportion of metaphases was above 60% in 8 of the 13
specimens. The increase in the number of cells in metaphase in sites
of pseudocarcinomatous hyperplasia was, however, statistically insignificant (p>0.1), but the frequency of pathologic mitoses was
significantly higher than in the control.

The most frequent mitotic abnormality in the reactive hyperplasia were C-mitoses (ball metaphases with sticky supercoiled
chromosomes) which were present in 8.5% of all mitotic cells and
accounted for more than a half of all mitotic abnormalities. Cells
with metaphase lagging of chromosomes and fragments accounted for
4.8% of the dividing cells and one third of the abnormal mitoses.
These two forms of mitotic pathology were twice as frequent in the
reactive hyperplasia group as in the control. Occasionally, chromosomes and fragments lagging in ana- and telophase were also noted;
chromosome bridges and scattering were exceptionally rare.

In the sites of obligatory precancerous acanthosis and of squamous cell carcinoma, the changes in mitotic regime were more strongly
marked than in those of pseudocarcinomatous hyperplasia. The mitotic
index was increased to 16.8 ± 1.5, but the difference from the reactive hyperplasia group was insignificant (p>0.05). The percentage
frequency of metaphases was, however, significantly higher (p<0.05)
than in the reactive hyperplasia, being in excess of 70% in half of
the specimens. Like in the human patients, the malignant transformation of rabbit ear epidermis involved significant increases both
in the number of pathologic mitoses (p<0.01), which accounted for
some 25% of the total mitotic count, and in the spectrum of mitotic
pathology (Figure 30). The most frequent abnormality, as in the
reactive hyperplasia group, were C-mitoses, but the proportion of
these was much higher. However, the increase in the percentage of
such mitoses relative to the total number of abnormal mitoses was
insignificant. The second most frequent abnormality was metaphase
lagging of chromosomes and fragments but, again, the proportion of
these relative to the total number of pathologic mitoses was increased only insignificantly as compared to pseudocarcinomatous
hyperplasia. Metaphases with scattered chromosomes were much more
frequent, and there appeared three-group metaphases, multipolar
mitoses, and other irregularities.

In summary, our comparative mitotic analyses have indicated that
in premalignant and malignant conditions as compared to pseudocarcinomatous, reactive hyperplasia, the mitotic regime of rabbit ear
epidermis is characterized by (1) greated deviations from normal in
the percentage frequencies of cells in the various mitotic stages,
particularly as the result of a sharply increased number of cells in

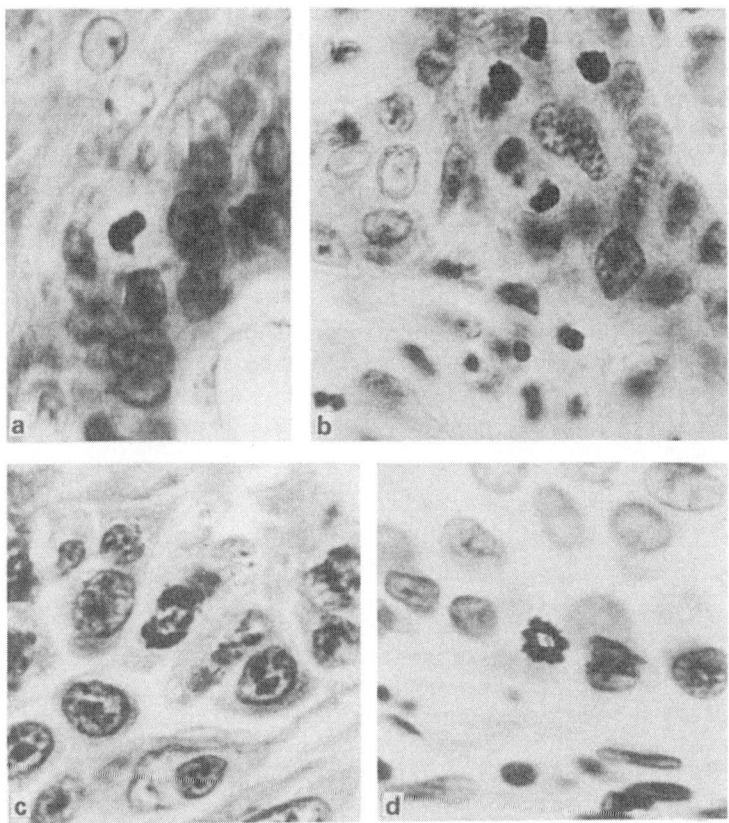

Fig. 30.  The more frequent mitotic abnormalities in rabbit ear
          epidermis after painting with DMBA.  (a) lagging of chromo-
          somes in metaphase; (b) C-mitoses and lagging of chromo-
          somes in metaphase and telophase; (c) lagging of chromo-
          somes during separation, and bridge formation; (d) hollow
          metaphase.  (1100 X; (a), (b), and (c) hematoxylin and
          eosin; (d) Feulgen stain.)

metaphase; (2) a significantly higher proportion of abnormal mitoses,
due mainly to increased numbers of cells showing C-mitoses, metaphase
lagging of chromosomes and fragments, and metaphases with scattered
chromosomes and fragments; and (3) a considerably wider spectrum of
mitotic abnormalities, with the appearance of three-group metaphases,
hollow methaphases, multipolar mitoses, etc.  As regards the mitotic
index, the difference from pseudocarcinomatous hyperplasia was
statistically insignificant.


4.3  SUMMARY

     In patients and rabbits with reactive inflammatory epidermal
hyperplasia which often presented a histologic appearance closely

mimicking that of carcinoma, the mitotic index was increased, the percentage ratio of cells at the different mitotic stages was somewhat altered due to an increase in the number of cells at metaphase, and the proportion of pathologic mitoses which were represented mainly by C-mitoses was higher than in the control. The increased frequency of C-mitoses seen in reactive epidermal hyperplasia appears to be accounted for by the action on the cells of the toxic products present in the inflammatory lesions of various dermatoses showing such hyperplasia and in those of rabbit ear skin induced by injection of the scarlet red dye.

With the conversion to malignancy, the epidermis showed a statistically significant increase in the number of metaphases as compared to pseudocarcinomatous hyperplasia, in both human patients and rabbits. GEnerally, it appears that such increases account for the high mitotic indices seen in cancer.

The most characteristic feature of epidermal "cancerization" was a sharp rise in pathologic mitoses, which were significantly higher in number (2.3-fold in patients and 1.8-fold in rabbits) than in pseudocarcinomatous hyperplasia.

It has been shown (e.g. Alov et al., 1966; Vasil'eva, 1966) that pathologic mitoses appear and increase in the course of carcinogenesis elicited by various agents, and this is considered by Alov (1972) as proof of a causal relationship between the malignant transformation of a tissue and the occurrence of abnormal mitoses therein. This view has been supported by our finding for rabbit ear epidermis that mitotic abnormalities such as chromosome scattering, monocentric mitoses, three-group metaphases, and hollow metaphases, all appear or increase in frequency during chemical carcinogenesis, but not in pseudocarcinomatous hyperplasia.

We cannot agree with those (e.g. Sommerville, 1953; Gottron and Nikolowski, 1960; Willis, 1967) who consider mitotic activity as a major criterion for diagnostic differentiation between pseudocarcinomatous epidermal hyperplasia and cutaneous squamous cell carcinoma. For, as our studies in patients and in rabbits have indicated, the mitotic index in pseudocarcinomatous hyperplasia may be even higher than in squamous cell cancer. It would therefore appear that mitotic activity may be of diagnostic value only when it is recorded in conjuction with other variables, and the most important of these seem to be the relative frequency of metaphases and the relative frequencies and range of abnormal mitoses. The results reported in this chapter warrant the use of mitotic analysis in differentiating pseudocarcinomatous hyperplasia from squamous cell carcinoma in cases of doubt, where neither clinical nor histologic clues, nor, for that matter, clinicopathologic correlation, can be relied upon in establishing a definitive diagnosis.

# 5
# The DNA Content of Epidermal Cell Nuclei in Pseudocarcinomatous Hyperplasia and in Squamous Cell Carcinoma

Proliferation of the epidermis, as of any other tissue, is inextricably linked up with the metabolism of nucleic acids, which are responsible for the storage, transfer, and translation of genetic information. The key roles in cell reproduction, genetic information transmission, and malignant transformation are played by deoxyribonucleic acid (DNA) which makes up the chromosomes. A strict correlation is now known to exist between the number of chromosomes in a cell nucleus and the amount of DNA in the nucleus (e.g. Atkin, 1962; Caspersson, 1964; Levan, 1967). As the number of chromosomes in the nucleus doubles in preparation for mitosis, so does the amount of DNA, and the variation in nuclear DNA content can therefore give an indication of variation in chromosome number (Atkin, 1962; James, 1962).

Since the karyotype of a somatic cell has twice as many chromosomes as that of a germ cell, the germ cells are generally referred to as haploid and the somatic cells as diploid. Because the amount of DNA corresponds to the number of chromosomes, the DNA content of all diploid interphase nuclei is relatively constant. A change in chromosome number results in altered ploidy of the nuclei. Although nuclear ploidy may vary within a cell population, even in normal tissues, the vast majority of cells constituting the stemline of a given cell population, have the same ploidy which persists through a number of generations (Makino, 1957; Levan and Biessele, 1958; Olenov, 1967). Along with diploid cells, normal tissues contain polyploid and aneuploid cells, that is, those containing in their nuclei, respectively a three or a higher multiple of the haploid number of chromosomes and not an exact multiple of the haploid number. The occurrence of these cells is attributable to such forms of mitotic abnormality as lagging, nondisjunction, and scattering of chromosomes and monocentric

mitosis (e.g. Alov, 1965, 1972; Bochkov et al., 1966). The progressive selection of polyploid and aneuploid cells and their pro-
liferation leads to increased genetic heterogeneity of the cell
populations forming the clonal profile of a given tissue
(Shmal'gauzen, 1946; Hsu, 1961; Gotlib-Stematsky et al., 1966;
Frankfurt, 1970; Sandberg et al., 1967; Vakhtin, 1973; and others).
Genetic heterogeneity of cell populations has been recognized as a
major attribute of malignant tissues (e.g. Pogosyants, 1969;
Pogosyants and Zakharov, 1965; Olenov, 1967; Issa et al., 1968;
Sandberg et al., 1967; Zakharov, 1970; Granberg, 1971).

It has been demonstrated in numerous experiments with tissue
cultures and transplantable tumors that malignant epithelia from
various human and animal body areas show wide variability in chromosomes and in nuclear DNA content (e.g. Leuchtenberger et al., 1954;
C. Leuchtenberger and R. Leuchtenberger, 1960; Levan, 1956, 1967;
Levan and Biessele, 1958; Sandberg et al., 1963; Sandritter et al.,
1964; Pogosyants, 1969; Zakharov, 1970; Genes, 1971; Avtandilov and
Kazantseva, 1973; Doyle and Manhold, 1975). The great majority of
tumor cells have enlarged nuclei with increased DNA content (e.g.
Leuchtenberger et al., 1954; Sandritter, 1965; Khesin, 1967; Tavares,
1968; Chervonnaya and Gladulova, 1972; Ryabinina and Benyush, 1973).
The degree of ploidy is the highest in progressing and metastatizing
tumors (e.g. Sandritter, 1965; Tavares, 1968; Avtandilov and
Chervonnaya, 1973; Shapot, 1973, 1975; Doyle and Manhold, 1975).
According to Avtandilov and Chervonnaya (1973), the most important
quantitative characteristics of malignant tumor progression, in
particular of melanomas, are increased production of DNA and altered
clonal profiles. It has been found for normal mouse epidermis that
DNA synthesis occurs in the basal cells only (Scherman et al., 1961;
Frankfurt, 1970, 1975) and that the nuclear DNA content of epidermal
cells declines as the cells undergo differentiation (De, 1963). By
contrast, tumor cells show a direct correlation between their DNA
content and degree of differentiation (Seidel and Sandritter, 1963;
Jablonska and Langner, 1968).

The fact that malignant transformation of tissues involves
increased nuclear ploidy and that improved cytophotometric methods
are now available for quantitative histochemical analysis of DNA, has
made it possible to use the characteristic of genetic heterogeneity
in the diagnosis of malignancies in various parts of the body
(Sandritter and Fischer, 1964; Ganina et al., 1968; Trutia, 1971;
Avtandilov and Kazantseva, 1973; Kazantseva, 1973; and others).

The increase in polyploidy during hyperplastic and neoplastic
processes is different in different epithelial tissues. Avtandilov
and Kazantseva (1973) reported the incidence of polyploid cells to be
highest in endometrial and gastric mucosal epithelia. In endometrial
epithelium, for example, cells in the octoploid range (paraoctoploid
cells) were found to constitute about 20% of the cell population in

ordinary hyperplasia, but as much as over 40% in atypical hyperplasia in which they become the modal class (Avtandilov and Kazantseva, 1973). In gastric polyposis the percentage of paraoctoploid cells was almost double that in gastritis (34.4% and 57.4%), while in adenocarcinoma hyperoctoploids accounted for as much as 65% of all cells and constituted the modal class (Kazantseva, 1973). These findings suggest that the increase in nuclear ploidy occurs in parallel with changes in the quality of epithelial pathologic processes from ordinary hyperplasia to malignant neoplasia. There are indications in the literature that the clonal profile varies from one stage of malignant transformation to another and that the alteration often begins to occur long before the appearance of clinical and histologic signs of malignancy (Levan and Biessele, 1958; Hauschka, 1963; Richart and Corfman, 1964; Doyle and Manhold, 1975).

The literature devoted to cytophotometric measurement of DNA in human integument is relatively scarce. Such measurements have been carried out for healthy human subjects (Freutz et al., 1980) and for patients with chromosomal disease (Lalaeva, 1972) and benign and malignant neoplasms of the skin and oral mucosa (e.g. Atkin, 1962; Ehlers, 1968, 1971; Naleskina, 1971; Schumann et al., 1971; Avtandilov, 1972; Avtandilov and Chervonnaya, 1973; Mayenburg et al., 1977).

Malignant melanomas and especially their metastases have been reported to have a much higher content of nuclear DNA than pigmented nevi or normal epidermis (Avtandilov and Chervonnaya, 1973), and the same is generally true of squamous cell carcinoma of the skin.

Ehlers (1968) found by the method of microspectrophotometry that in basal cell carcinoma the distribution pattern of DNA in epidermal cell nuclei is different from that in squamous cell carcinoma or in Bowen's disease. Whereas basal cell carcinomas of the solid and adenomatous types had a diploid amount of DNA, squamous cell carcinomas and carcinomas in situ (Bowen's disease) exhibited wide variation in DNA values extending to the hyperoctoploid range and had a hypertetraploid stemline of cells; no significant differences were observed in DNA values between the well-differentiated and poorly differentiated squamous cell tumors. Ehlers (1971) believes that quantitative determination of DNA in epidermal cell nuclei may be of value in the diagnosis of precancerous conditions. According to him, in precancerous dermatoses such as arsenical keratosis, senile keratoma, and cutaneous horn, the DNA content of epidermal cells is about 50% above normal, with no significant differences being detectable in DNA content between the individual dermatoses. He concluded from this that the separation of precanceroses into the facultative and obligatory varieties is justifiable on clinical grounds only. Schumann et al. (1971) reported the amount of DNA in epidermal cell nuclei to be substantially increased in foci of basal cell carcinoma and of squamous cell carcinoma and its metastases, and to correlate

directly with clinical and histologic characteristics of the neoplasms. Mayenburg et al. (1977), in a cytophotometric study of
biopsies from lesions of Buschke-Loewenstein's tumor and bowenoid
carcinoma of the vulva in one and the same female patient, found the
DNA content of basal cell nuclei to be similar in both these diseases. Rahrbach et al. (1972) maintain that cytophotometric studies
can demonstrate whether a given tumor is benign or malignant. However, Atkin et al. (1966) concluded that microspectrophotometry is a
poor predictor of malignant epithelial transformation, for one can
never be sure about the real implications of diploid stemlines. They
came to this conclusion from their study of 10 carcinomas, 5 of which
were found to have a diploid stemline. At the same time they emphasized that microspectrophotometric DNA measurement does allow one to
recognize the early phases of malignant transformation in specimens
which do not arouse suspicion of malignancy when viewed in the light
microscope.

In the available literature, we have not encountered any systematic studies of variation in DNA content during the various stages of
epidermal hyperplasia from reactive inflammatory all the way to
carcinomatous. Of special practical interest appear to be comparative studies of DNA content in squamous cell carcinoma and in pseudocarcinomatous hyperplasia which closely resembles this carcinoma
clinically and histologically. Such studies are described in the
following two sections.

## 5.1  DNA CONTENT IN PATIENTS

Our comparative microspectrophotometric studies of DNA content
in epidermal cell nuclei were performed in 26 Feulgen-stained histologic preparations from skin biopsies taken in patients with various
skin diseases. Nine of the specimens presented pictures of pseudocarcinomatous hyperplasia arising in trophic ulcers of the shin (3
specimens), psoriasis in its warty form (1), lichen ruber verrucosus
(3), and tuberculosis cutis verrucosa (2). Six other specimens, from
epidermal areas adjoining a cancer or from lesions retrospectively
interpreted as precancerous, were considered as representing precancerous acanthosis. Five specimens were from cutaneous squamous
cell carcinomas located on the thign, lower lip, or penis. Six
specimens of morphologically unchanged epidermis served as control.

The biopsied tissue was fixed in Carnoy's fluid, embedded in
paraffin, and prepared simultaneously for histologic examination and
for DNA determination by cutting all tissue blocks into sections of
equal thickness (7 μm) and subjecting all sections to hydrolysis in a
1% hydrochloric acid solution for 15 min at room temperature and to
staining with Schiff's reagent by the Feulgen method for 60 min. The
microspectrophotometry was done in the Laboratory of Pathologic
Anatomy of the Institute of Human Morphology under the USSR Academy

of Medical Sciences, using a single-beam integrating scanning micro-
spectrophotometer designed in that laboratory.  The procedure was
performed at a wavelength of 575 nm and a surface area of the probe
equal to 1 $\mu m^2$ or 3 $\mu m^2$ depending on the size of the nuclei.
Detailed descriptions of the method can be found elsewhere (e.g.
Agroskin, 1962; Avtandilov, 1970, 1973; Fuks, 1971; Morozov et al.,
1971; Andersson and Kjellstrand, 1972; Ryabinina and Benyush, 1973).
For each specimen, the concentration of Feulgen-positive substance was
determined in 60-100 nuclei of basal layer cells.  Only interphase
nuclei with distinct contours in which the plane of sectioning had
passed through the perinucleolar zone were used in the cytophotometric measurements.  In each histologic specimen, DNA concentration
was measured in 25 nuclei of small lymphocytes, and the mean DNA
concentration was then calculated for the epithelial cells and for
the lymphocytes.  To estimate the relative amount of DNA per nucleus,
the areas of 60-100 epithelial cell nuclei and 25 lymphocyte nuclei
were measured in the same portions of the histologic specimen where
microphotospectrometry was performed.

The results of nuclear area measurement for each specimen were
classified into groups, with each group differing from the next by 5
$\mu m^2$; the mean nuclear area was then calculated in every group and
histograms showing the percentage of nuclei in a given group relative
to the total number of nuclei were constructed.  The mean relative
content of DNA (in arbitrary units) was calculated for every group of
epithelial cell and lymphocyte nuclei.  The DNA content in epithelial
cells relative to the diploid DNA value (2C) which was given by the
lymphocytes present in the section, was taken as the final index of
epithelial cell ploidy.  For each patient group, the percentage of
nuclei with a particular ploidy index was calculated and a histogram
was prepared.  To test the usefulness of a more general indicator of
DNA variation among the various patient groups, the so-called DNA
accumulation index proposed by Avtandilov (1973)[1] was computed.

In the control, the interphase nuclei were characterized by a
specific optical density ranging from 0.24 to 0.42 (arbitrary unit)
and only a slight variation in area which varied from 7 to 15 $\mu m^2$ in
76.6% of the analyzed cells.  The microspectrophotometry showed a
definite stemline with amounts of DNA in the diploid range (diploid
and paradiploid cells); these cells constituted 72.2 ± 3.4% of the
cell population (Table 8 and Figure 31), whereas paratetraploid cells
made up 22.8 ± 3.1% and paraoctoploid ones, only 5.0 ± 1.5%.  The DNA
accumulation index was 2.2.

In the pseudocarcinomatous hyperplasia group, the mean nuclear
area had a significantly higher value of 19.8 ± 0.39 $\mu m^2$ than in the
control (p<0.001), and it was also more variable.  Values of 7 to 15

---

[1]Defined as the weighted arithmetic mean of nuclear DNA content.

Table 8.  Percentage Distribution of Human Epidermal Cells by DNA Content (As Expressed in Units of Ploidy).

| Condition | Percentage of Cells | | | | DNA Accumulation Index |
|---|---|---|---|---|---|
| | Paradiploid (2C) | Paratetraploid (4C) | Paraoctoploid (8C) | Hyperoctoploid (>8C) | |
| Pseudocarcinomatous epidermal hyper-plasia | 59.7 ± 2.9 | 28.1 ± 2.7 | 12.2 ± 1.8 | – | 2.5 |
| Precancerous acanthosis | 22.6 ± 3.4 | 52.0 ± 4.1 | 25.4 ± 3.5 | – | 3.6 |
| Squamous cell carcinoma | 6.6 ± 2.0 | 36.0 ± 3.9 | 41.4 ± 4.0 | 16.0 ± 2.9 | 5.5 |
| Normal epidermis | 72.2 ± 3.4 | 22.8 ± 3.1 | 5.0 ± 1.5 | – | 2.2 |

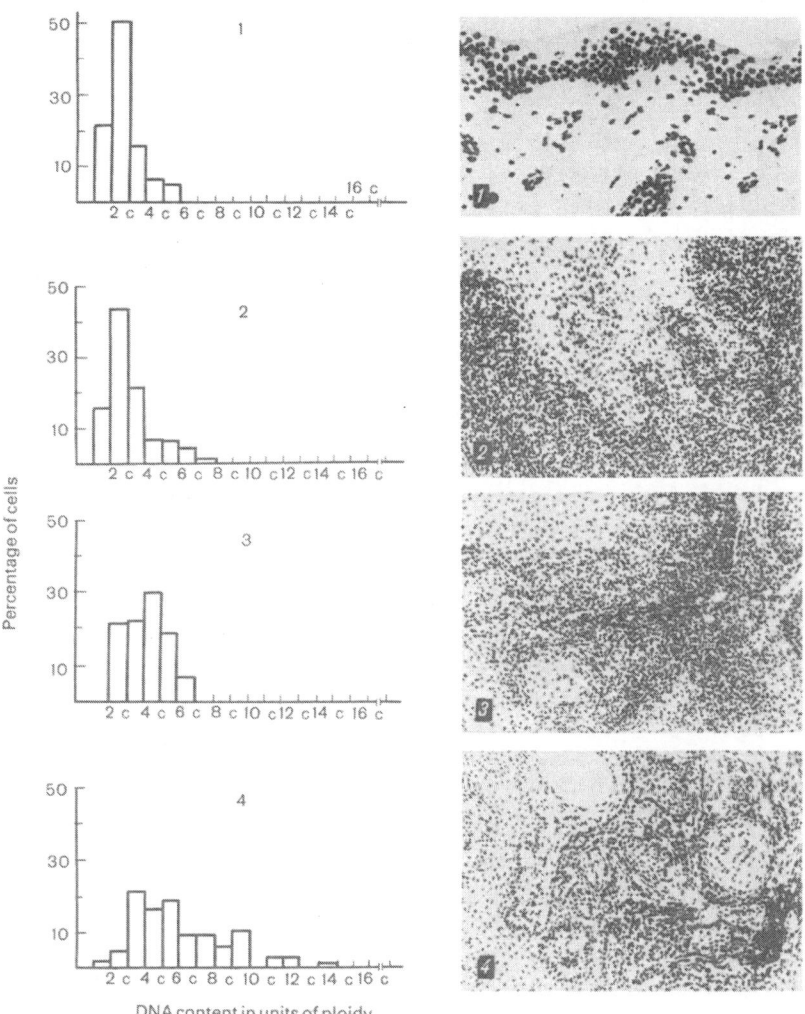

Fig. 31.  Histograms showing the distribution pattern of DNA in
          epidermal cell nuclei from patients.  (1) Normal epidermis;
          (2) pseudocarcinomatous hyperplasia; (3) precancerous
          acanthosis; (4) squamous cell carcinoma.


$\mu m^2$ occurred in only 20.4% of the cells, and those of 15 to 25 $\mu m^2$ in
as many as 71.2%; the remaining 8.4% of nuclei ranged in area 25 to
45 $\mu m^2$ and showed reduced optical densities of 0.09-0.17 unit.  The
cells constituting the stemline (59.7 ± 2.9%) had paradiploid DNA
values.  The percentage of paratetraploid cells was higher, as was,
to a greater degree, that of paraoctoploid cells.  The DNA accumulation index was only slightly higher than in the control.

Thus, the lesions showing pseudocarcinomatous hyperplasia differed but slightly from normal epidermis with regard to DNA content
in epidermal cell nuclei. The main difference was that nuclei with
DNA values in the tetraploid and octoploid ranges (paratetraploid and
paraoctoploid DNA values) were more frequent in the pseudocarcinomatous hyperplasia group. In this group the distribution patterns of
cells in terms of DNA content were very similar in all cases, irrespective of the degree to which the hyperplasia was expressed and of
the dermatosis (lichen verrucosus, warty tuberculosis, or so on) in
which it had arisen. In other words, the alterations in DNA content
were not specific for the particular dermatoses. The observed increase in the proportion of nuclei with paratetraploid and paraoctoploid DNA values may be attributed to enhanced mitotic activity of
the epidermal cells and to the fact that these were examined in
different periods of the mitotic cycle (S or $G_2$).

In the precancerous acanthosis group, nuclear optical density
was more variable (0.1 to 0.32 arbitrary unit) but the nuclear area
had a mean value of $22.2 \pm 0.4$ $\mu m^2$ and did not differ significantly
from that in the pseudocarcinomatous hyperplasia group (p>0.05), with
the incidence of nuclei 15 to 25 $\mu m^2$ in area being almost the same
(74%) as in the hyperplasia group (71.2%). The proportion of nuclei
with an area of 25 $\mu m^2$ or more was, however, much higher (18% against
8.4%). Cells with paradiploid DNA values were much less frequent and
those with paratetra- or paraoctoploid DNA values were much more
frequent (see Table 8). However, cells with hyperoctoploid DNA
values were never detected. The DNA accumulation index was increased
considerably (to 3.6), and this, together with the results presented
above, is an indication of increasing heterogeneity of the tissue
involved.

In the squamous cell carcinoma group, the range of nuclear
optical density variation was wider than in precancerous acanthosis
(0.07 to 0.31 arbitrary unit). Only 7.8% of the nuclei had an area
less than 15 $\mu m^2$, while the percentage of larger nuclei (15 to 40
$\mu m^2$) was as high as 86.6%, and giant nuclei with an area of 55 $\mu m^2$ or
more were observed. Cytospectrophotometry showed considerable differences in nuclear DNA content from the pseudocarcinomatous hyperplasia
and precancerous acanthosis. Thus, no particular stemlines were in
evidence; paradiploid DNA values were displayed by only $6.6 \pm 2.0\%$ of
the nuclei; and, although the percentage of paratetraploid elements
was somewhat lower than in the precancerous acanthosis group, the
percentage of cells with paraoctoploid DNA values was much higher,
and there appeared many cells with hyperoctoploid DNA values. The
DNA accumulation index rose to 5.5.

It may be concluded from the above that pseudocarcinomatous
hyperplasia and squamous cell carcinoma, while presenting similar
histologic and, not infrequently, clinical appearances, differ from
each other in the degree of heterogeneity of the cell populations.
And this conclusion has been borne out by our experiments on rabbits.

## 5.2  DNA CONTENT IN RABBITS

Comparative microspectrophotometric studies of DNA content in epidermal cell nuclei were carried out in 34 skin biopsy specimens from rabbit ears.  Twelve of these were from sites of reactive pseudocarcinomatous hyperplasia induced by injection of scarlet red in oil, 6 from sites of DMBA-induced obligatory precancerous acanthosis, and 7 from those of DMBA-induced squamous cell carcinoma; the remaining 9 specimens were controls.  A total of 2550 nuclei (2040 in epidermal cells and 510 in lymphocytes) was examined using the procedure described in the preceding section, except that cyto-photometry and karyometry were performed separately for basal cells and suprabasal cells.

The interphase nuclei of morphologically unchanged epidermis had an optical density of 0.2 to 0.4 arbitrary unit and did not vary greatly in area, with 91.3% of the nuclei having areas of 6 to 15 $\mu m^2$ (nearly half of them were less than $10\mu m^2$).  The microspectrophoto-metry demonstrated the basal and suprabasal layers to have prominent stemlines of cells with diploid or paradiploid DNA values; these cells accounted for 79.3 ± 1.9% of the cell population studied (Figure 32 and Table 9).  The percentage of paradiploid suprabasal cells was somewhat higher than that of paradiploid basal cell.  Paratetradiploid cells accounted for 19.0 ± 1.8% and paraoctoploid ones, for as little as 1.7 ± 0.6% of all cells, and these were present in the basal layer only.  The difference in DNA accumulation index between basal and suprabasal cells was small (see Table 9).

In the pseudocarcinomatous hyperplasia group, the percentage of nuclei up to 15 $\mu m^2$ in area was lower than in the control, whereas the percentage of nuclei with areas between 15 and 35 $\mu m^2$ was much higher.  Such nuclei had reduced optical density (0.1-0.25 arbit-rary unit).  The modal class was formed by paradiploid cells which were present in nearly equal proportions in the basal and suprabasal layers.  Nuclei with paratetra- and paraoctoploid DNA values were much more frequent than in the control.  No hyperoctoploid cells were detected.  The DNA accumulation index was only slightly greater than in the control (see Table 9).

In the areas of precancerous acanthosis within DMBA-induced papillomas and keratoacanthomas and within regions adjoining the sites of invasive epidermal growth, the nuclear area was greater than in the pseudocarcinomatous hyperplasias.  The proportion of nuclei up to 15 $\mu m^2$ in area averaged 40.7% and that of nuclei 15 to 40 $\mu m^2$ in area, 59.3%, with nuclei having an area between 25 and 40 $\mu m^2$ com-prising 10.3% of all the nuclei examined.  Nuclear optical density varied within wider limits (0.09 to 0.23 arbitrary unit).  The pro-portion of cells with paradiploid DNA values was lower than in the pseudocarcinomatous hyperplasia group, with such cells being con-siderably less frequent among basal than among suprabasal cells.

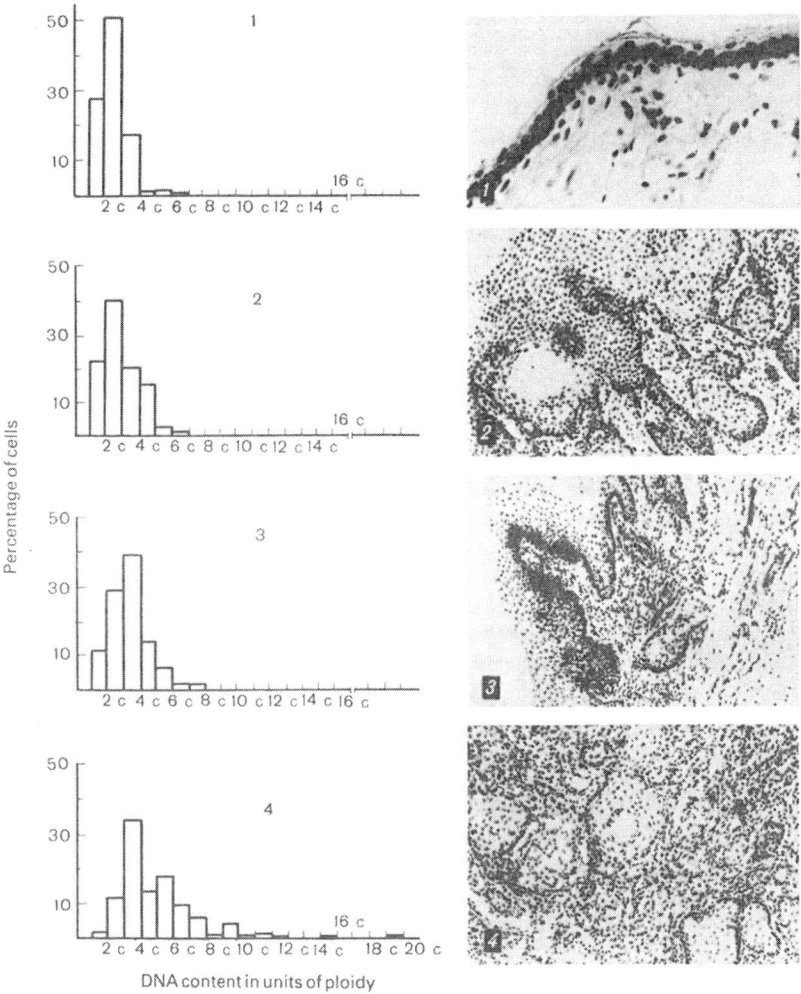

Fig. 32.  Histograms showing the distribution pattern of DNA in
          epidermal cell nuclei from rabbit ears.  (1) Normal
          epidermis; (2) pseudocarcinomatous hyperplasia; (3)
          precancerous acanthosis; (4) squamous cell carcinoma.


Nuclei with paratetra- and paraoctoploid DNA values were more frequent, particularly in the basal layer cells.  As in the pseudocarcinomatous hyperplasia group, no nuclei with a ploidy of over 8C were
detected.  The DNA accumulation index was somewhat higher than in the
hyperplasia group.

     Finally, in the invasive squamous cell carcinoma group, the
range of optical density variation in nuclei was wider than in the

Table 9. Percentage Distribution of Rabbit Epidermal Cells by DNA Content (As Expressed in Units of Ploidy).

| Condition | Cells | Percentage of Cells | | | | DNA accumulation index |
|---|---|---|---|---|---|---|
| | | Paradiploid (2C) | Paratetraploid (4C) | Paraoctoploid (8C) | Hyperoctoploid (>8C) | |
| Pseudocarcinomatous hyperplasia | Basal | 62.4 ± 3.3 | 32.8 ± 3.2 | 4.8 ± 1.4 | – | 2.4 |
| | Suprabasal | 60.7 ± 4.8 | 38.7 ± 3.9 | 0.6 ± 0.4 | – | 2.1 |
| | Total | 61.6 ± 2.5 | 35.3 ± 2.3 | 3.1 ± 0.8 | – | 2.3 |
| Precancerous acanthosis | Basal | 26.0 ± 3.5 | 60.0 ± 4.0 | 14.0 ± 2.8 | – | 3.3 |
| | Suprabasal | 53.3 ± 4.0 | 44.7 ± 4.0 | 2.0 ± 1.1 | – | 2.3 |
| | Total | 39.6 ± 2.8 | 52.4 ± 3.1 | 8.0 ± 1.5 | – | 2.8 |
| Squamous cell carcinoma | Basal | 0.8 ± 0.6 | 35.0 ± 3.0 | 51.3 ± 3.2 | 12.9 ± 2.1 | 5.3 |
| | Suprabasal | 25.4 ± 2.8 | 59.2 ± 3.1 | 15.0 ± 2.3 | 0.4 ± 0.1 | 3.3 |
| | Total | 13.2 ± 2.1 | 47.1 ± 1.1 | 33.0 ± 3.0 | 6.7 ± 1.6 | 4.3 |
| Normal epidermis | Basal | 80.0 ± 2.4 | 17.0 ± 2.2 | 3.0 ± 1.0 | – | 1.9 |
| | Suprabasal | 88.4 ± 2.3 | 11.6 ± 2.3 | – | – | 1.6 |
| | Total | 79.3 ± 1.9 | 19.0 ± 1.8 | 1.7 ± 0.6 | – | 1.9 |

other groups (0.05–0.4 arbitrary unit).  Only 15.6% of the nuclei had
an area less than 15 $\mu m^2$, the remaining nuclei having areas 15 to 60
$\mu m^2$ or even more.  Nuclei with paradiploid DNA values accounted for
only 13.2 ± 2.1% of all nuclei examined (for as little as 0.8 ± 0.6%
in basal cells), the proportion of nuclei with paratetraploid DNA
values was somewhat lower than in the precancerous acanthosis group,
but that of nuclei with paraoctoploid DNA values was much higher,
particularly in the basal cells (see Table 9).  There appeared cells
with hyperoctoploid DNA values, mainly in the basal layer.  THe index
of DNA accumulation was nearly twice that in the reactive hyperplasia
and precancerous acanthosis groups.

Thus, the changes in the DNA content of epidermal cell nuclei in
rabbits were essentially similar to those recorded for human
patients.


## 5.3  CONCLUSION

The results of our quantitative studies of DNA in epidermal cell
nuclei from human patients and rabbits with pseudocarcinomatous
hyperplasia, precancerous acanthosis, and squamous cells carcinoma
may be summarized as follows.

In pseudocarcinomatous epidermal hyperplasia, both in patients
in which it arises in various dermatoses and in rabbits in which it
arises as an inflammatory response to intradermal injection of
scarlet red, DNA synthesis is increased but the modal class is
formed, as in normal epidermis, by paradiploid cells.

Obligatory precancerous acanthosis is characterized by increased
genetic heterogeneity of the involved tissue, as is indicated by
a large increase in the frequency of cells with paraoctoploid DNA
values and a large decrease in that of paradiploid cells as
compared with pseudocarcinomatous hyperplasia.

Genetic heterogeneity of the lesional tissue is still greater in
areas of squamous cell carcinoma, both in human subjects and in
rabbits, as is indicated by a greatly reduced frequency of paradiploid cells and the appearance of hyperoctoploids.

The present cytophotometric studies have thus shown that cancerous and pseudocancerous epidermal hyperplasias, which present as they
do similar clinical and histologic appearances, differ substantially
in the distribution pattern of epidermal cell nuclei in terms of DNA
content.  A high incidence of diploid or paradiploid cells and a low
incidence of aneuploid cells should suggest that the hyperplasia in
question is benign.  By contrast, if the hyperplasia is pursuing a
malignant course, the cell population becomes extremely heterogeneous, as is reflected by alterations in DNA content.

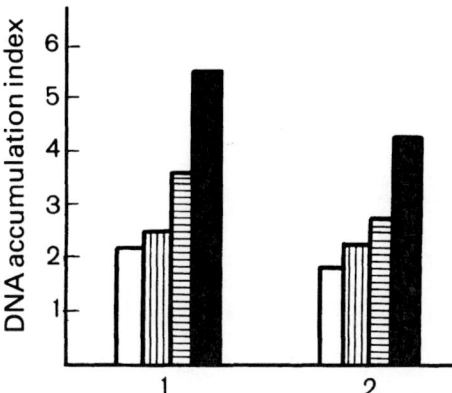

Fig. 33.  Values of the DNA accumulation index in reactively
          hyperplastic and malignant transformed epidermis.  (1)
          Humans; (2) rabbits.  ☐ = normal epidermis; ▥ =
          pseudocarcinomatous hyperplasia; ▤ = precancerous
          acanthosis; ■ = cancer.

     Estimates of DNA content in terms of the DNA accumulation index
proposed by Avtandilov (Avtandilov, 1973) have shown that this index
is close to normal in pseudocarcinomatous hyperplasia, is increased
in precancerous acanthosis, and is greatly increased in invasive
carcinoma (Figure 33).

     It may be concluded from the foregoing that cytophotometric
measurement of nuclear DNA content in proliferating epidermis can
provide a reasonably objective indication of the biologic nature of
the proliferation.  The important practical implication of this is
that cytophotometric determination of DNA content may be used as part
of the diagnostic work-up to differentiate pseudocarcinomatous hyperplasia from squamous cell carcinoma.  It should be noted, though,
that microspectrophotometry, although a fairly accurate method,
yields only indirect evidence regarding the numerical variation of
chromosomes and cannot of course provide information about qualitative changes in them (Pogosyants and Zakharov, 1965).

     However, the process of malignant transformation is well known
to be assoicated with qualitative chromosomal alterations (e.g.
Makino, 1957; Hauschka, 1961; Pogosyants, 1969; Atkin and Baker,
1966; Zakharov, 1970).  Hence of particular importance in the study
of mechanisms by which pseudocarcinomatous hyperplasia and malignant
transformation come about, are cytogenetic analysis (study of chromosomes and of sex chromatin) and cytophysiologic characterization of
epidermal growth patterns in vitro.  These aspects are dealt with in
the next chapter.

# 6
# Cytophysiologic and Cytogenetic Characteristics of Epidermal Cells in Pseudocarcinomatous Hyperplasia and in Squamous Cell Carcinoma

The progress achieved by cytophysiologic and cytogenetic research in oncology has been largely due to the application of comprehensive analyses in which various methods are used to study, in particular, the growth patterns of cultured cells and the chromosomes and sex chromatin in interphase nuclei of such cells. Although these aspects are interrelated, each of them has an independent value of its own, and it is desirable to consider them separately. Accordingly, the three sections which follow are concerned, respectively, with growth patterns of epidermal cells in vitro, karyotypic characteristics of cultured cells, and sex chromatin in squamous cell carcinoma and in pseudocarcinomatous hyperplasia, both in humans and in experimental animals.

## 6.1 GROWTH PATTERNS OF PRIMARY SKIN CULTURES

It is common knowledge that the method of tissue culture has been well developed and put to extensive use in biology, oncology, and cytogenetics (e.g. Khrushchev, 1931; Timofeevskii, 1934, 1947, 1971; Khlopin, 1940, 1947; Ford and Hamerton, 1956; Tjio and Puck, 1958; Hardnen, 1960; Bochkov and Nemtsov, 1962; Blok, 1966; Dobrynin, 1968; Korfsmeier, 1968; Grinberg, 1969; Belen'kii, 1970; Egorkina, 1970; Levine, 1972; Vasil'ev, 1973). As pointed out by Timofeevskii (1971), who was one of those responsible for introduction of tissue culture techniques in the USSR, "the tissue culture method ... can provide valuable information about biologic characteristics of the cell, mechanisms of action of various factors at the cellular level, and carcinogenic processes, and it can be used in the cytogenetic analysis of cell populations from various tissue and organs, in the differential diagnosis of tumors and in the elucidation of their histogenesis." A large contribution to the study of tissue growth in culture was made by Khlopin (1940, 1947) who was the first to show that a tissue grown outside the body retains its genetically determined characters. This applies not only to embryonal and normal adult animal and human tissues, but to tumor tissues as well. In cytophysiologic studies of cultured tissues, including neoplastic tissue, one is primarily interested to know the time when cells begin to grow out from the explant, the pattern of that growth, to which tissues the growing cell populations belong, the relationship between the populations of epithelial-like and fibroblast-like cells, and the features of cell differentiation.

Although skin is readily accessible to biopsy and the material required for tissue culture is easy to procure, the information about growth characteristics of normal and pathologically altered human and animal skins in culture is scarce in dermatologic literature. There are only a few publications concerned with growth patterns in culture of normal human skin (e.g. Khlopin, 1940; Hardnen, 1960; Burdette, 1962; Blok, 1966; Karasek, 1967; Korfsmeier, 1968; Pruniéras, 1975; Pricl et al., 1980), of human skin involved with lichen planus, Darier's disease, psoriasis, or lupus erythematosus (Belen'kii, 1970; Egorkina, 1970; Karasek, 1972), and of neoplastic skin from humans (Cobl et al., 1961, Söltz–Szötz, 1963; Walker et al., 1964; Schindler, 1965; Korfsmeier, 1967, 1968) and experimental animals (Abercombie and Ambrose, 1962; Mercer, 1962; Issa et al., 1968).

The paucity of literature can probably be explained by the fact that in tissue culture it is difficult to secure the growth of epithelioid cells alone. Ordinarily, fibroblast-like cells also proliferate to supplant epithelioid cells upon further incubation (Karasek, 1967; Korfsmeier, 1968). This has been attributed to technical faults in the procedures used to prepare epidermal explants and to the tendency of fibroblasts for more active growth in culture (Vasil'ev, 1961, 1965). Egorkina (1970), in her observations of growing normal skin explants, noted the predominant growth of epithelial-like cells in some cases, of fibroblast-like cells in others, and of both of these types in still others, and she emphasized that in the cases of such mixed growth, fibroblastic cells "pave the way, not unlike pathfinders, for a sheet of epithelioid cells which follows them ....." A similar observation was made by Walker et al. (1964) for cutaneous basal-cell carcinoma.

It has been observed (e.g. Walker et al., 1964) that fibroblast-like cells not only show active growth, but are also capable of stimulating, together with connective tissue, the growth of other cellular elements in the culture. Karasek (1972), in studying the effects of dermal factors on cell proliferation rates, noted that proliferation was particularly rapid on collagen which is a component part of the dermis; another factor observed to stimulate epithelial cell growth were protein-bound acidic mucopolysaccharides.

Usually, the explants of normal tissue begin to grow out
epithelioid cells as soon as within the first 24 h of incubation.  In
one study on in vitro growth patterns of normal skins from 15 human
donors, all explants were found to start growing out epithelial-like
cells after 24 h of incubation, and with the course of time the
boundary between cells in the culture was obliterated, the contours
of the cell nuclei became blurred, the cells decreased in volume,
underwent vacuolation, and acquired a fine-grained structure (Blok,
1966); in other words, processes were taking place in the epidermal
culture similar to those of differentiation and keratinization of
epidermal cells.  Korfsmeier (1968), in studying the growth patterns
of cultured normal skin, noted that intercellular connecting strands
and bridges were forming during epithelioid cell growth and that the
monolayer sheet of epithelioid cells gradually came to resemble the
stratum spinosum of the epidermis; when the monolayer sheet attained
a considerable size, its further growth slowed down or ceased, and by
that time fibroblast-like cells, if present, were seen to have grown
through the full thickness of the sheet.  It has been observed that
in a culture of biopsied normal skin, epidermal cells grow like a
membrane whereas fibroblastic cells extend in a radial pattern to rim
the sheet of epithelial cells (Hentzer and Kobayashi, 1975).

The multiplication of cultured normal cells is controlled by the
local density of the cells: the greater the density, the slower the
multiplication rate because of a prolongation of the $G_1$ phase of the
mitotic cycle (Söltz-Szöts, 1963; Brodskii et al., 1971; Vasil'ev,
1973).

Another constant feature of multiplying cultured cells, in
particular fibroblasts, is their ability to attach to a suitable
solid substratum.  Only after they have achieved attachment to the
substratum do the cells settle down and start proliferating (Levine,
1972; Macieira-Coelho, 1967; Vasil'ev, 1973; Vasil'ev and Gel'fand,
1973).

What are the growth characteristics of cultured epidermis
biopsied from sites of pseudocarcinomatous hyperplasia and of
squamous cell carcinoma of the skin?  Evidence in the literature
indicates, first of all, that tumor cells have no or greatly diminished capacity for attachment to substratum and can proliferate in
culture without first attaching to the glass or other backing
(Brodskii et al., 1971; Vasil'ev, 1973; and others).  In their experiments with cultured tumor fibroblasts from mice, Vasil'ev and
Gel'fand (1973) found that the tumors cells, which were only loosely
adherent to the glass, were displaced by normal cells, but continued
to proliferate rapidly on the surface of the normal cell monolayer.
Another distinctive growth feature of cultured tumor cells is that
the rate of their proliferation does not depend on the cell population density.  Because they are no longer subject to contact
inhibition, tumor cells, even when in close contact with highly

differentiated cells, proceed to multiply rapidly and to overlie
these cells. However, as found by Söltz-Szöts(1963) in a study of
cultured cutaneous epithelioma and melanoma cells, if the explant
placed in a culture medium contains connective tissue cells in
addition to tumor cells, the former will grow through the tumor cell
monolayer. Similar observations were reported by Korfsmeier (1968)
in a study of growth patterns of cultured skin from sites of squamous
cell carcinoma: epithelioid tumor cells began separating from the
explant as soon as within the first 24 h of culture to form a monolayer later, but subsequently fibroblast-like cells were often seen
to grow through the epithelioid cell monolayer. It has often been
observed that the explants of squamous cell and basal cell carcinomas
begin to grow out epithelioid cells earlier than do the explants of
normal tissue (Söltz-Szöts, 1963; Walker et al., 1964; Korfsmeier,
1968).

The foregoing brief review shows that the in vitro growth of
tumor cells differs from that of normal cells in several respects.
However, because of the small number of relevant studies, it is not
yet possible to draw any definite conclusions about the cytophysiologic characteristics displayed by primary cultures of skin from
squamous cell carcinomas. As regards pseudocarcinomatous epidermal
hyperplasia, we have not found any studies at all concerned with the
in vitro behavior of epidermal cells from sites of such hyperplasia.

Our comparative investigations of cultured human and rabbit
skins involved by atypical yet benign epidermal hyperplasia and by
squamous cell carcinoma have revealed a number of cytophysiologic
differences in growth patterns between these two conditions.

In these studies, use was made of the plasma clot method developed in detail by Avrorov and Timofeevskii (1914), Khlopin (1940),
and Timofeevskii and his associates (Timofeevskii, 1934, 1947;
Timofeevskii and Dobrynin, 1967). The average time of cultivation
required to obtain adequate cell populations in the primary plasma
cultures of lesional skin was 23-25 days for human skin and 42-72
days for rabbit skin. The cultures were observed for growth every 2
or 3 days in a light microscope at low magnification. The criteria
by which culture growth was characterized were time of onset of cell
migration from the explant, histogenetic features of the migrating
cells, and developmental pattern of the monolayer.

## 6.1.1  Human Skin Cultures

We studied primary plasma cultures of skin biopsied from 40
patients, including 16 women and 24 men, ranging in age from 21 to
78 years. Twenty of the patients had various dermatoses in which a
reactive pseudocarcinomatous (often pronounced) hyperplasia had
developed (3 of these patients had lichen ruber verrucosus, 6 had

trophic ulcers, 4 had chronic ulcerative pyoderma, 2 had prurigo
nodularis, and the remaining 5 had warty tuberculosis, cutaneous
leishmaniasis, lichen planus, psoriasis in its warty form, or
Darier's dyskeratosis). Eight patients had benign skin tumors
(3 had keratoacanthoma, 2 senile keratoma, 2 cutaneous horn, and 1
seborrheic wart). The remaining 12 patients (3 women and 9 men) had
keratinizing squamous cell carcinoma of the skin; in 6 cases this was
preceded by a dermatosis (unhealing ulcers in 2 cases, Buschke-
Loewenstein's condyloma in 2, keratoacanthoma in 1, and Bowen's
disease in 1).

From the 28 patients with dermatoses or benign skin tumors, a
total of 290 explants were studied, 24 of which (8.2%) gave no outgrowth during the observation periods which ranged from 26 to 44
days. Of the remaining 266 explants, more than a half (55.5%) were
growing out predominantly epithelial-like cells and 10.9%, fibroblast-like cells throughout the incubation period, while the remaining 33.6% showed a mixed type of growth.

With 163 explants (61.3%), outgrowth of cells and their
migration began at days 3-5, and with the remaining 103 explants,
at days 6-10 postexplantation.

As already mentioned, most explants grew out mainly epithelioid
cells; these were progressively increasing in number around the
explants and at a considerable distance from them where they formed
small islands (Figure 34). In such cultures, extensive continuous
fields of epithelioid cells were not observed until days 20-30 of
cultivation (Figure 35). In the cultures with the mixed type of
growth, fibroblast-like cells were seen to grow initially and both
these and epithelioid cells subsequently, with fibroblast-like cells
appearing to grow ahead of epithelioid cells to provide a substratum
for them on the glass over which epithelioid cells then proceeded to
migrate and multiply. To secure good growth of epithelioid cells, it
is essential to treat properly the tissue to be explanted, taking
special care to separate the epidermis with basement membranes from
the dermis; otherwise, the monolayer may show a predominance of
fibroblast-like cells, as was the case with 10.9% of our explants.
Contrary to the observations by Belen'kii (1970), the cultured hyperplastic epidermis did not show any specific structures pathognomonic
of the particular dermatoses. This was probably due to the fact
that, unlike Belen'kii, we did not run subcultures because our experiments were designed for other purposes than those of that author.

In the squamous cell carcinoma group (12 patients), a total of
129 specimens were cultured. Of these, 62 (48%) began to exhibit
growth at 24-48 h and the rest at days 3-5 of culture. Thus, contrary to the situation with explants from sites of pseudocarcinomatous hyperplasia, in no case did growth start at a later time.
Predominant growth of epithelioid cells was observed in 95 (73.6%) of

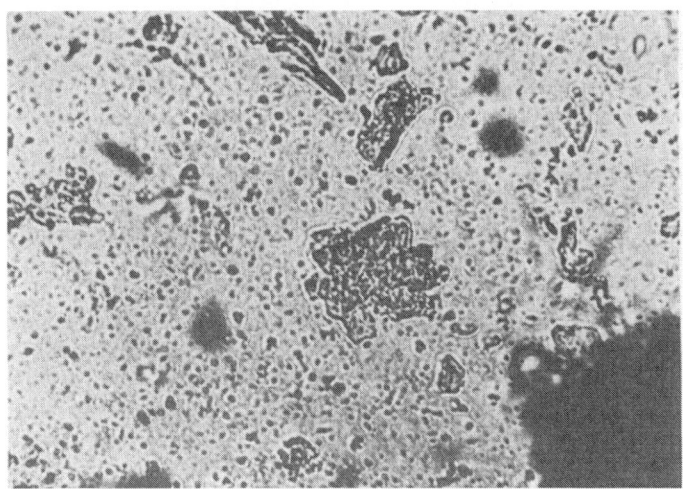

Fig. 34. Unstained 5-day-old live culture of lesional skin from a patient with chronic ulcerative pyoderma, showing small islands formed by epithelial-like cells during early period of growth.

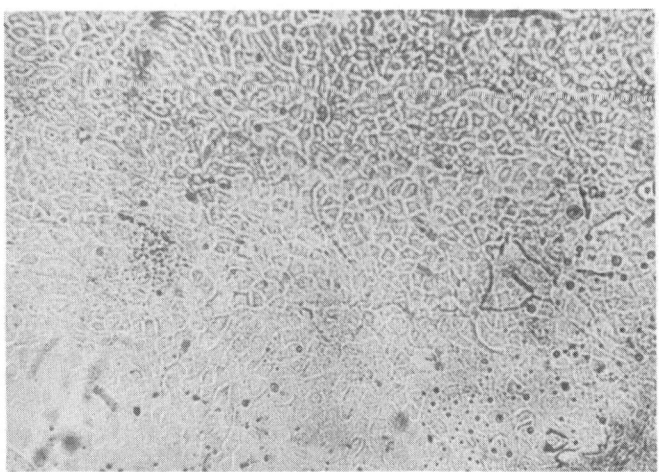

Fig. 35. Unstained 25-day-old live culture of lesional skin from a patient with trophic ulcer of the shin, showing a continuous field of epithelial-like cells.

the explants, of epithelioid and fibroblastlike cells in 24 (18.6%), and of fibroblast-like cells in 10 (7.8%). Active migration of cells was noted in all the explants without exception.

A characteristic feature of the epidermal tissue cultures in this group was the rapid growth of explants from the beginning. Cells migrating from the explant were seen in about half of the cultures as soon as after 24 to 48 h of incubation, and by days 7-10 a sheet of cells (25-30 rows) growing out directly from the explant was observed in these cases (Figure 36). By days 20-25, a dense monolayer of polymorphic cells (Figure 37) had developed in almost all the cultures. Where connective tissue elements (fibroblast-like cells) appeared in the culture, these elements were seen to be pushed aside by a sheet of epithelioid cells upon further cultivation.

In summary, the primary cultures of human skin from sites of pseudocarcinomatous hyperplasia were characterized by late start of migration of epithelioid cells from the explant, by formation of cell islands, and by slow expansion of the monolayer, whereas such cultures from sites of squamous cell carcinoma showed an early start of growth, with a monolayer sheet of cells growing out directly from the explant and rapidly expanding.

6.1.2  Rabbit Skin Cultures

We followed the growth of primary cultures of 32 skin biopsy specimens from ears of 18 rabbits with pseudocarcinomatous hyperplasia induced by scarlet red and 14 rabbits with squamous cell carcinoma induced by DMBA.

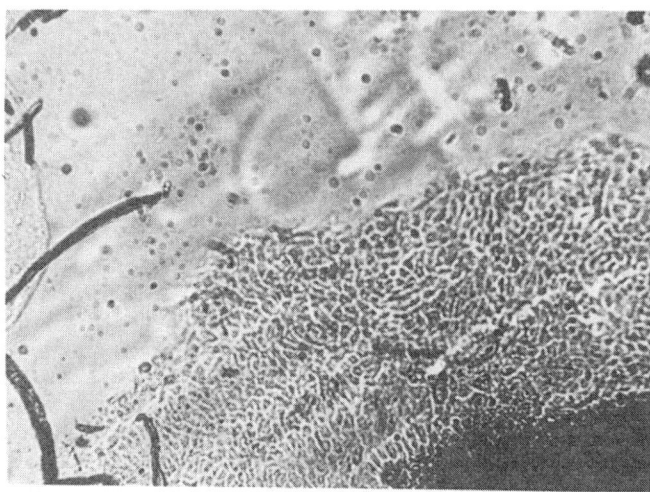

Fig. 36.  Unstained 7-day-old live culture of lesional skin from a patient with keratinizing squamous cell carcinoma, showing a sheet of epithelioid cells growing out from the explant.

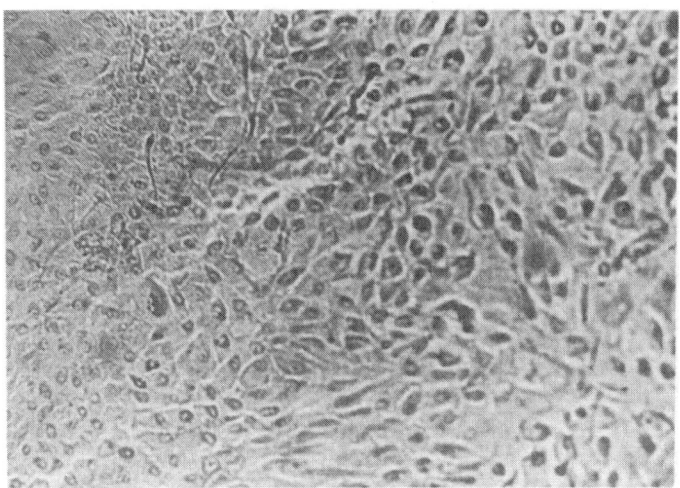

Fig. 37.  Unstained 27-day-old live culture of lesional skin from a
patient with keratinizing squamous cell carcinoma, showing
a dense monolayer of polygonal epithelioid cells which
display pronounced polymorphism.

    In the pseudocarcinomatous hyperplasia group, where 179 explants
were cultured, 65 explants (36.3%) failed to produce growth during
the observation periods which ranged from 45 to 75 days.  Of the 114
explants that showed outgrowth, predominant proliferation of epithelioid cells was seen in 38% of cases, mixed growth in 43.6%, and
growth of "fibroblastic" cells in 18.4%.

    Generally, growth started much later than it did in the group of
human pseudocarcinomatous hyperplasia considered above, with only
9.5% of the explants showing migration of cells at days 4-7 of incubation and with the remaining explants showing no active migration
until days 8-15.  Such a late onset of growth was probably due to the
presence of scarlet red oil in the cultures despite careful preparation of the material before its placement into the culture medium.
Where the explants were growing out epithelioid cells, the initial
growth was characterized by the propagation of these cells around the
explant as well as at a considerable distance from it with formation
of cell islands (Figure 38).  Continuous fields of closely packed
epithelioid cells (Figure 39) did not appear until days 45-70 post
explantation.

    Where the explants exhibited mixed growth, the initial growth
was characterized by advancement of a sheet of fibroblast-like cells
over whose surface epithelial-like cells were seen to migrate subsequently.

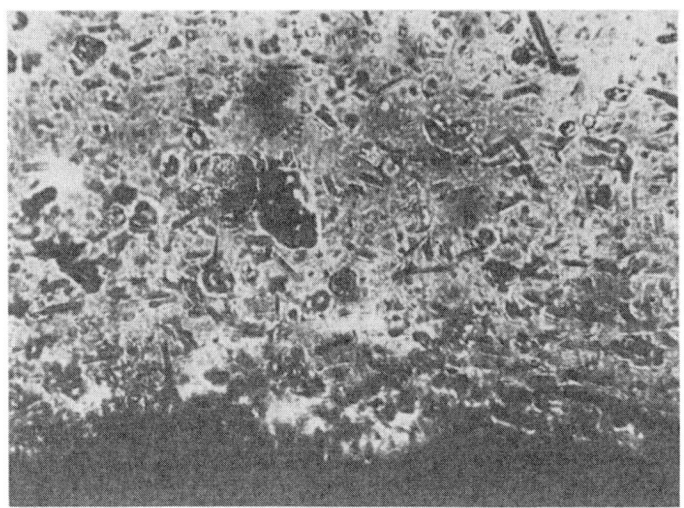

Fig. 38.  Unstained 10-day-old live culture of lesional skin from a
          rabbit ear with pseudocarcinomatous epidermal hyperplasia.

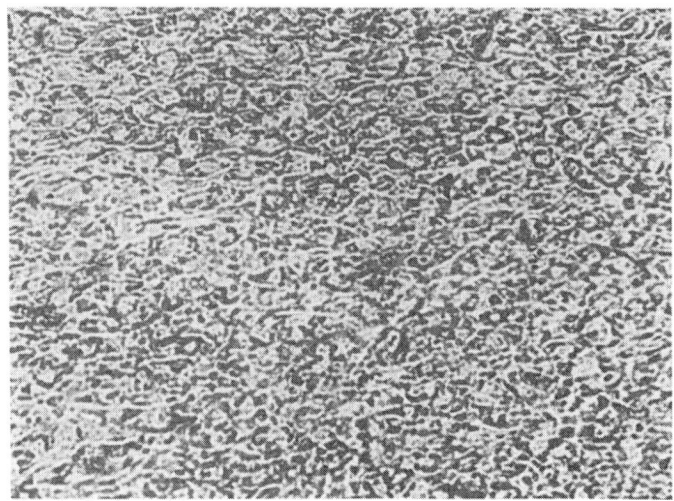

Fig. 39.  Unstained 56-day-old live culture of lesional skin from a
          rabbit ear with pseudocarcinomatous epidermal hyperplasia.


       In the squamous cell carcinoma group, where 164 explants were
cultured, 65 explants (36.6%) failed to show any outgrowth throughout
the observation periods of 42 to 79 days.  Of the remaining 99
explants, more than a half (54.4%) were growing out epithelioid
cells.

Generally, the explants of malignant epidermis showed a more rapid onset of growth than did those of reactively hyperplastic epidermis.  Of the 99 explants that displayed growth, about 75% started growing out cells within the first week of cultivation (31% within the first 3 days).  As with the human epidermis explants, a sheet of epithelial cells was seen growing directly from the explant (Figure 40) with subsequent formation of a continuous monolayer (by days 42-72).  Cellular polymorphism and impaired cell adhesion were noted (Figure 41).

Thus, the differences in growth pattern between the primary cultures of rabbit skin from sites of reactive hyperplasia and those from sites of squamous cell carcinoma were similar to such differences seen with human skin.  In reactive hyperplasia, the involved rabbit skin likewise showed a late migration of epithelial cells from the explant, the formation of cell islands, and a slow expansion of the monolayer.  By contrast, the cultures of malignant epidermis were characterized by a much earlier onset of growth, with a monolayer sheet of cells growing out directly from the explant and expanding rapidly.

6.2  CHROMOSOMAL ANALYSIS OF CELLS FROM PRIMARY SKIN CULTURES

It has been established in numerous studies that human and animal malignant tumors of various sites display the phenomenon of chromosomal variability and that it is this variability which is responsible for the variability in the karyotypes observed within

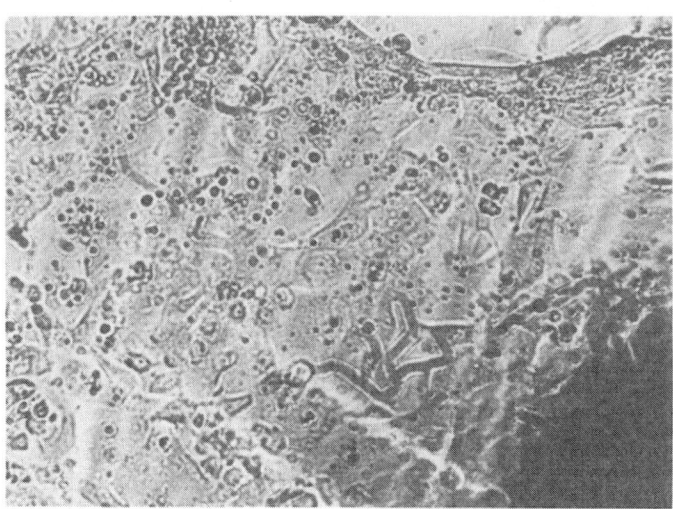

Fig. 40.  Unstained 7-day-old live culture of lesional skin from a rabbit ear with squamous cell carcinoma.

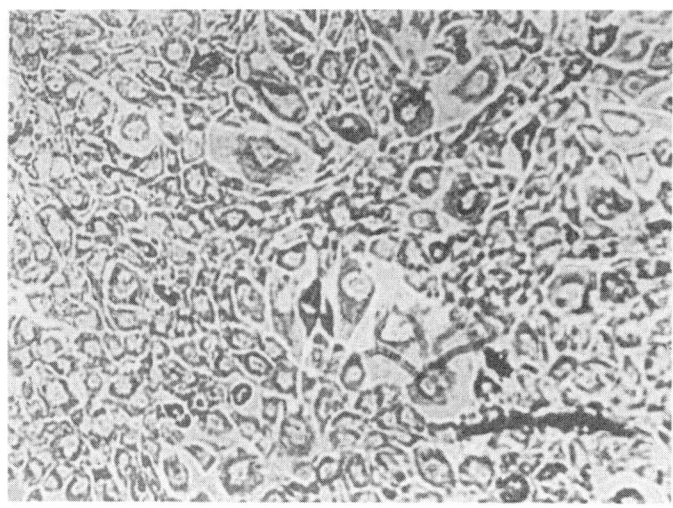

Fig. 41.  Unstained 67-day-old live culture of lesional skin from a
rabbit ear with squamous cell carcinoma.


cancer cell lines (e.g. Levan, 1956; Makino, 1957; Hauschka, 1963;
Pogosyants and Zakharov, 1963; Pogosyants, 1969, 1973; Zakharov,
1970; Genes, 1971; Lelikova, 1972; Dehuhard et al., 1975).

     The karyotypes of cancer cells differ from those of normal cells
in both the number and structure of the chromosomes.  Instead of the
diploid chromosome number of 46 (2n), the karyotypes of different
tumors or even of a single tumor demonstrate great variability
(heterogeneity) of chromosome numbers which range from hypoploid
through hyperploid to polyploid.  Despite the karyotypic variability
of cell populations, it is possible to find, within a malignant
tumor, a modal number or class of cells, that is , cells with a given
chromosome number which occurs most frequently in the cell population
(Hauschka, 1953; Makino, 1957).  A stemline concept in cancer has
been developed, according to which selection of one type of cell over
others results in progression and maintenance of the cancerous state
(Makino 1957; Hauschka, 1961).  In firm, solid tumors, the modal
class is not prominent, however; it constitutes only from 10 to 40%
of the cell population (Yamada et al., 1966; Sandberg et al., 1967;
Sandberg et al., 1970; and others).  Under various influences, or
spontaneously, cells with a different chromosome set may become
predominant, that is, one stemline may be replaced by another with
the course of time (Hauschka, 1961).

     In cytogenetics, the term "aneuploidy" is used to designate
numerical chromosome variation, that is, any deviation from an exact
multiple of the haploid number of chromosomes, whether fewer (hypoploidy) or more (hyperploidy).

In a normal somatic cell population, cells with hyperploid chromosome numbers are generally believed to be less common among aneuploids than cells with hypoploid numbers. The more frequent occurrence of hypoploids is considered by some to result from arti- facts or from methodologic faults in the assessment of karyotypes (Bochkov et al., 1966; Moorhead, 1967). Hyperploidy usually arises because of chromosome nondisjunction and hypoploidy because of non- disjunction or loss of chromosomes (Bochkov et al., 1966). Poly- ploidy, that is the state of having a chromosome number that is a multiple of the normal diploid number, is attributed to mitotic abnormalities, in particular abnormal cytokinesis (Brodskii, 1963) but it may also occur as a result of endomitosis or endoreduplication (Pogosyants and Zakharov, 1965).

Aneuploidy is regarded as a common characteristic of tumor cells (Field, 1972). In malignant tumors of various localizations and histogenesis, aneuploidy is most often due to hyperploidy (Sandberg et al., 1963; Vincent et al., 1964; Pogosyants and Zakharov, 1965; Sandberg, 1966; Miles, 1967; Pogosyants and Zakharov, 1969, 1973; Genes, 1971), but there are also reports of hypodiploid malignant neoplasms. Pogosyants et al. (1972), for example, having examined 1358 cells from 22 ovarian tumors, found 12 of the tumors to be hypodiploid. In malignant epithelium the modal number of chromosomes may be difficult to identify (Ishihara et al., 1963; Miles, 1967), or else more than one modal number may be present (e.g. Koller, 1947; Makino et al., 1959, 1964; Kirkland et al., 1967).

Of special importance for understanding the role of chromosomal heterogeneity in malignancy is chromosomal analysis of benign tumors and precancerous lesions. It has been demonstrated that the modal cells remain diploid in benign human and animal tumors of various localizations (e.g. Palmer, 1959, Hauschka, 1961; McMicheal et al., 1963; Socolov et al., 1964; Jackson, 1967; Toews et al., 1968). As regards chromosomal alterations during carcinogenesis, evidence in the literature is controversial . Whereas some authors have found no substantial changes in chromosome number in precancerous tissues (Stich et al., 1960; Janeja and Stich, 1965; Lamb, 1967; Toews et al, 1968), others have reported pronounced aneuploidy (Makino et al., 1959, Kirkland, 1966; Katajama and Jones, 1967; Granberg, 1971). Of great interest is the evolution of chromosomal alterations from the early phases of malignancy all the way to invasive and metastasizing tumors. Although it is extremely difficult to follow this evolution in man, there are reports of studies on chromosomal changes during various stages of malignant transformation (e.g. Kirkland, 1966; Atkin and Baker, 1969; Jaffurs et al., 1970; Granberg, 1971; Katajama et al., 1972; Dehuhard et al., 1975). These studies warrant the conclusion that heteroploidy appears and progressively increases as the epithelium undergoes histopathologic changes from dysplasia to invasive carcinoma.

Generally, evidence in the literature indicates that epithelial malignant transformation in various parts of the body is accompanied by changes in chromosome number, but that these alterations are highly variable and are not specific for particular malignant tumors.

Tumors of the skin have received little cytogenetic study in comparison with solid tumors of other organs, apparently because of the technical difficulties involved in securing suitable metaphase plates from epidermal cells. There are only occasional reports in the literature of chromosomal changes in premalignant and malignant cutaneous lesions. Thus, Palmer (1959) studied in rabbits the chromosomes of early Shope papillomas and transplantable carcinomas derived from papillomas and found the benign papillomas to be essentially diploid (2n = 44) with a low frequency of hyperdiploid cells. The transplantable carcinomas had varying chromosome counts (from 50 to 88), but no consistent abnormalities were noted. Beyreuther (1960) examined five benign rabbit papillomas and five early primary carcinomas derived from such papillomas and discovered that the benign tumors had normal chromosome counts, but that each of the primary carcinomas had a different hyperdiploid chromosome complement. McMichael et al. (1963), in chromosome studies of 25 primary rabbit tumors induced by the Shope virus, detected no specific chromosomal changes that could be associated with particular stages of tumor development, but found that at late stages the tumors had a variety of chromosome counts in the diploid and hyperploid ranges; they pointed out that similar cutaneous tumors may show many karyotypically diverse stemlines and modes of chromosomes and concluded that alterations in the karyotype were not causally related to the initiation of the tumors or to their conversion to malignancy. Mark (1965) found a diploid stemline of cells in all 13 rabbit papillomas caused by the Rous virus. Manocha (1969) likewise reported the diploid chromosome number to prevail in cells from mouse papillomas induced by chemical carcinogens; heteroploid chromosome numbers were seen to appear increasingly as the papillomas underwent malignant transformation.

The above findings from animal experimentation suggest that malignant transformation of the epidermis, as that of epithelia elsewhere in the body, is often accompanied by changes on the part of chromosomes. And similar results have been obtained for human tumors. Makino et al. (1959) detected cells with chromosome numbers ranging from 54 to 74 in patients with precancerous dermatoses. Ehlers (1968) found, by the method of DNA cytophotometry, a considerable degree of aneuploidy in epidermal cells from sites of squamous cell cancer, but only the diploid modal chromosome number in basal cell carcinoma. It is noteworthy that variability of chromosome numbers is observable already in obligatory precancerous dermatoses (Ehlers, 1971). Hauschka (1961) reported no alterations in chromosomes of epidermal cells in warts.

In the available literature, we have been unable to find any reports of studies on chromosome alterations in sites of pseudo-carcinomatous hyperplasia which, as has been repeatedly mentioned above, closely simulates keratinizing squamous cell carcinoma of the skin. Moreover, the available reported evidence regarding cytogenetic changes in epidermal cells in foci of squamous cell cancer is inconclusive. Comparative studies on chromosomal changes in atypical, but benign epidermal hyperplasia and in squamous cell carcinoma of the skin may be expected to make possible a more objective evaluation of those abnormalities in the chromosome apparatus which arise during malignant transformation. The plasma clot method of culture which we employed in such studies, allows one to secure a sufficiently large population of epithelioid cells necessary to prepare metaphase plates and to perform chromosome analysis.

Our comparative studies, which were started in 1967, have shown that the proliferation of epidermal cells in sites of squamous cell carcinoma is accompanied by a much greater numerical variation in chromosomes than in those of pseudocarcinomatous epidermal hyperplasia arising in various dermatoses (e.g. Belen'kii and Berenbein, 1967; Belen'kii et al., 1968; Berenbein and Egorkina, 1974; Berenbein, 1977). These studies have led us to suggest that chromosomal analysis may be of value in diagnostic differentiation between an atypical, but benign epidermal hyperplasia and a squamous cell carcinoma in cases where other methods of investigation (clinical, histologic, etc.) have failed to provide an unequivocal diagnosis.


6.2.1  Human Skin Cultures

Chromosomal Changes in Pseudocarcinomatous Hyperplasia

We performed cytogenetic analyses of cultured skin from 18 patients with various dermatoses or benign cutaneous tumors in which pseudocarcinomatous hyperplasia (often pronounced) had developed. Chronic pyoderma ulcerosum vegetans was present in 3 of these patients, trophic ulcers of the lower leg in 2, lichen ruber verrucosus in 1, the warty form of psoriasis in 1, prurigo nodularis in 1, cutaneous leishmaniasis in 1, Darier's disease in 1, circumscribed chronic balanoposthitis in 1, keratoacanthoma in 2, senile keratoma in 2, seborrheic wart in 1, cutaneous horn in 1, and angioleiomyosarcoma in 1.

Metaphase plates were prepared according to the procedure described by Ford and Hamerton (1956). Only undamaged metaphases with well separated chromosomes meeting the requirements of suitability for chromosomal analysis were used. In preparing the idiograms, the distribution of chromosomes on the photomicrographs was considered in relation to the results of their examination under the microscope. The chromosomes were arranged to the various karyo-

type groups according to the Denver system as modified by Patau
(1960) (groups A, B, C, D, E, F, and G).  No pairing of chromosomes
within these groups was made.  From 50 to 100 or more metaphases were
analyzed in each case.  The results are summarized in Figure 42 where
the histograms are presented in the order of increasing chromosomal
changes.

The mode of cells containing 46 chromosomes was sharp in all
cases.  A total of 1130 metaphase plates were analyzed.  The percentage of diploid cells ranged from 70% to 40% for a mean value of
50.5%, and among the aneuploid cells (49.5%) the average proportion
of hyperploids metaphases was slightly higher than that of hypoploids
(28.8% against 20.5%).

Although the dermatoses displayed clinical and histopathologic
features characteristic of each of them, the numerical chromosome
variation in the vast majority of cases was such as to suggest a
benign hyperplastic process.  Here is one case report.

Patient I., a woman aged 49, presented with a clinical
diagnosis of keratoacanthoma.  Histopathologic examination
revealed a picture of pronounced epidermal hyperplasia with
cellular disarray, nuclear polymorphism, destruction of the
basement membrane, and other features suggestive of malignancy.

A cytogenetic study of 70 metaphase plates (see Figure
42, 3) showed a distribution of chromosome numbers from the
hypoploid to triploid range, a paradiploid modal number of
cells, and a stemline of cells containing 46 chromosomes
(57% of all metaphases).  On a structural analysis of 9
metaphase plates, the chromosome counts differed from the
theoretically expected values in all karyotypic groups, but
the differences were insignificant, except in group B where
the chromosome count was significantly increased (p<0.005)

In this case, the absence of marked hyperploidy in the karyotype, the paradiploid modal class, and the stemline of cells containing 46 chromosomes along with the absence of marker chromosomes all
indicated that the hyperplasia was pseudocarcinomatous, and this was
confirmed by the follow-up studies: no pathologic changes were noted
on the skin when the patient was examined 5 years after excision of
the tumor.

In another case, the chromosomal analysis had a prognostic
value.

Patient K., a man aged 58, was admitted to our department complaining of an eruption over the left popliteal
fossa.  The eruption had appeared about 10 years before to

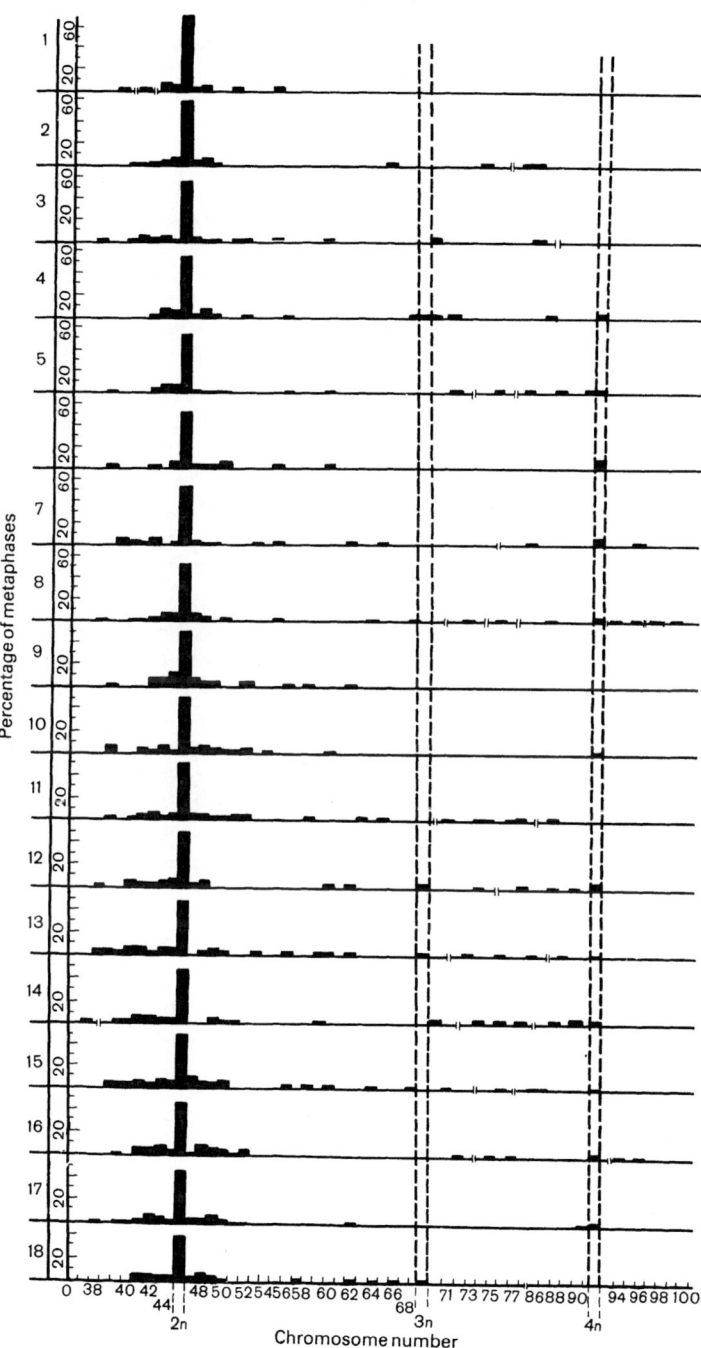

Fig. 42. Histograms showing the distribution of metaphase plates by chromosome number in 18 patients with various dermatoses accompanied by pseudocarcinomatous epidermal hyperplasia.

regress and recur periodically ever since. He was unable
to say anything definite as to the cause of his condition.
He had been treated externally with various antibiotic-
containing lotions and ointments, but with only temporary
relief.

On examination, a circumscribed lesion composed of
confluent nodes of soft consistency and cyanotic appearance
was seen in the left popliteal fossa, overlaid by vegetations and sanguinopurulent crusts from which pus could
be expressed. The regional lymph nodes were not palpable,
The presumptive clinical diagnosis was ulcerative vegetating pyoderma.

Histologic examination of the skin biopsied from the
lesion presented a picture of pseudocarcinomatous hyperplasia. Epidermal ridges had penetrated deep into the
dermis and in places had separated out to appear as epithelial nests. There was pronounced hyper- and parakeratosis. The cells were arranged disorderly in some areas.
The dermis contained an infiltrate of lymphocytes and
histiocytes with some plasma cells whose elements had
invaded the epidermis in places. The histologic diagnosis
was vegetating pyoderma with pronounced pseudocarcinomatous
hyperplasia.

The cytogenetic analysis of 70 metaphases (see Figure
42, 18) showed a paradiploid modal class with a stemline of
cells containing 46 chromosomes (40% of all cells); 60% of
the cells were aneuploid (21.4% were hypoploids and 38.6%
were hyperploids).

In this karyotype, the percentage of diploid cells was lower
(40%) and that of hyperploid cells (38.6%) was higher than in any
other of the analyzed cases, while the percentage of hypoploid cells
(21.5%) was close to the average value for this group. No marker
chromosomes were detected. In three metaphases, however, deletions
in the long arms of group C chromosomes were noted.

An analysis of chromosome distribution by karyotypic groups
carried out in 6 metaphases showed the mean chromosome counts to
differ from the theoretically expected values in all groups; the
differences were, however, insignificant (p>0.05), except for group G
where the chromosome numbers were significantly decreased (<0.01).

Thus, the cells of cultured skin from this patient were characterized by a low percentage of diploid cells constituting the stemline, a high percentage of hyperploid cells among aneuploids, and
chromosome arm deletions in Group C. All this, coupled with clinicopathologic findings, aroused the suspicion that the hyperplastic

process in the epidermis was progressing toward malignancy.  Two years afterwards, this patient sought assistance in another clinic where keratinizing squamous cell carcinoma was diagnosed after a biopsy, and a course of roentgen therapy was carried out.  When the patient was re-examined 6 years later, a radiation ulcer with peripheral atrophic scars was seen at the site of the lesion.  The ulcer was removed and a plastic operation was done to repair the defect.

To summarize, the alterations in chromosomes observed in pseudo-carcinomatous epidermal hyperplasia were not specific for this hyperplasia or for the dermatosis in which it arose.  However, the chromosome counts did reflect the benign biologic nature of the hyperplasia, and this was confirmed by follow-up studies of the patients over periods of 2 to 6 years.  There was only one case where the karyotype studies aroused suspicion of malignancy, and the malignant nature of the process was confirmed later.  It may be added that chromosome counts in moderate pseudocarcinoma hyperplasia did not differ substantially from those in cases where the hyperplasia was very pronounced, which suggests that karyotypic analysis reflects, not the degree of reactive epidermal hyperplasia, but rather its biologic nature, that is, benignity.

Of considerable interest is the question of how altered chromosome numbers are distributed among the karotypic groups, that is, whether and how many chromosomes are supernumerary or missing in the particular groups.  As far as pseudocarcinomatous epidermal hyperplasia is concerned, we have not encountered any reports shedding light on this question.  Table 10 summarizes the results of our analyses of the distribution of chromosomes by karotypic groups for 120 cells of cultured tissues from sites of pseudocarcinomatous hyperplasia, and it can be seen that the chromosome counts are distributed nonuniformly both among the different karotypic groups of the same patients and within the same karotypic groups among the different patients.  The overall mean deviations indicate that the observed chromosome numbers were greater in groups B, C, F, and G and smaller in groups A, D, and E, than the theoretically expected values.  These differences, however, were statistically significant only in groups B and F.

From a practical point of view, it is useful to compare chromosomal changes in the karotypic groups in pseudocarcinomatous hyperplasia with those in squamous cell carcinoma.

## Chromosomal Changes in Squamous Cell Carcinoma of the Skin

We performed cytogenetic analyses of cultured skin from 7 biopsies taken in 6 male patients aged 52 to 64 years.  The lesion was located in the lower extremity or trunk in 3 of them, on the penis in 2, and on the lower lip in 1.  In all the patients, keratin-

Table 10. Summary of Deviations of Chromosome Counts in Karyotypic Groups from the Theoretically Expected Chromosome Numbers in Cultured Skin Cells from Patients with Pseudo-carcinomatous Hyperplasia.

| Case No. | No. of cells counted | Mean No. of chromosomes per cell | Mean deviations of chromosome counts from expected values in various karyotypic groups | | | | | | |
|---|---|---|---|---|---|---|---|---|---|
| | | | $XA_1-A_2$ | $XB_1-B_2$ | $XC_1-C_2$ | $XD_1-D_2$ | $XE_1-E_2$ | $XF_1-F_2$ | $XG_1-G_2$ |
| 2 | 19 | 51.8 | +0.1 | +0.5 | -0.1 | -0.2 | +0.2 | +0.1 | -0.3 |
| 3 | 9 | 45.4 | +0.1 | +0.2 | +0.3 | -0.1 | -0.1 | +0.1 | -0.2 |
| 5 | 8 | 71.8 | -0.1 | -0.1 | -0.1 | -0.3 | -0.5 | +0.3 | +0.5 |
| 8 | 12 | 47.2 | +0.3 | +0.4 | -0.5 | -0.2 | +0.1 | 0.0 | +0.5 |
| 10 | 4 | 46.7 | 0.0 | +0.2 | +0.1 | -0.3 | +0.5 | +0.2 | -0.3 |
| 11 | 17 | 54.6 | -0.8 | -0.1 | +1.7 | +0.1 | -0.3 | +0.1 | -0.2 |
| 14 | 91 | 45.7 | +0.1 | +0.2 | +0.2 | +0.3 | -0.4 | -0.2 | +0.2 |
| 15 | 28 | 49.7 | -0.3 | -0.1 | -0.4 | +0.2 | -0.2 | +0.2 | +1.0 |
| 17 | 8 | 57.5 | -0.2 | -0.1 | +0.4 | -0.4 | +0.4 | +0.2 | -0.1 |
| 18 | 6 | 47.0 | -0.1 | 0.0 | +0.2 | +0.2 | +0.2 | +0.1 | -0.4 |
| Overall mean deviation | | | -0.09 | +0.11 | +0.18 | -0.01 | -0.1 | +0.11 | +0.07 |
| Level of significance ($p$) | | | >0.05 | <0.01 | >0.05 | >0.05 | >0.05 | <0.01 | >0.05 |

Designations: X = means; $A_1$, $B_1$, etc. = observed chromosome numbers (chromosome counts) in karyotypic groups; $A_2$, $B_2$, etc. = expected values; $A_1-A_2$, $B_1-B_2$, etc. = difference between observed and expected values. The significance of differences was assessed by Wilcoxon's test.

izing squamous cell carcinoma of the skin had been diagnosed both
clinically and histopathologically.

The results are summarized in the histograms of Figure 43 which
are arranged in the order of increasing chromosomal changes.  A total
of 680 metaphase plates were analyzed.  The percentage of diploid
metaphases in sites of squamous carcinoma was considerably reduced
(see Figure 43) to give a mean value of 23.4%.  The aneuploid metaphases, which accounted for as much as 76.6% of all metaphases,
showed a wide variation in chromosome number (from 41 to 108), with
the percentage of hyperploid metaphases being much higher than that
of hypoploids (65.3% and 11.3%).

In all instances, the proportion of diploid metaphases was lower
than even the lowest level of such metaphases found in the pseudocarcinomatous hyperplasia group.  In 5 of the 6 cases, the percentage
of aneuploid metaphases was much higher than the highest level of
such metaphases in pseudocarcinomatous hyperplasia.  It was only in
the patient with a highly differentiated squamous cell carcinoma

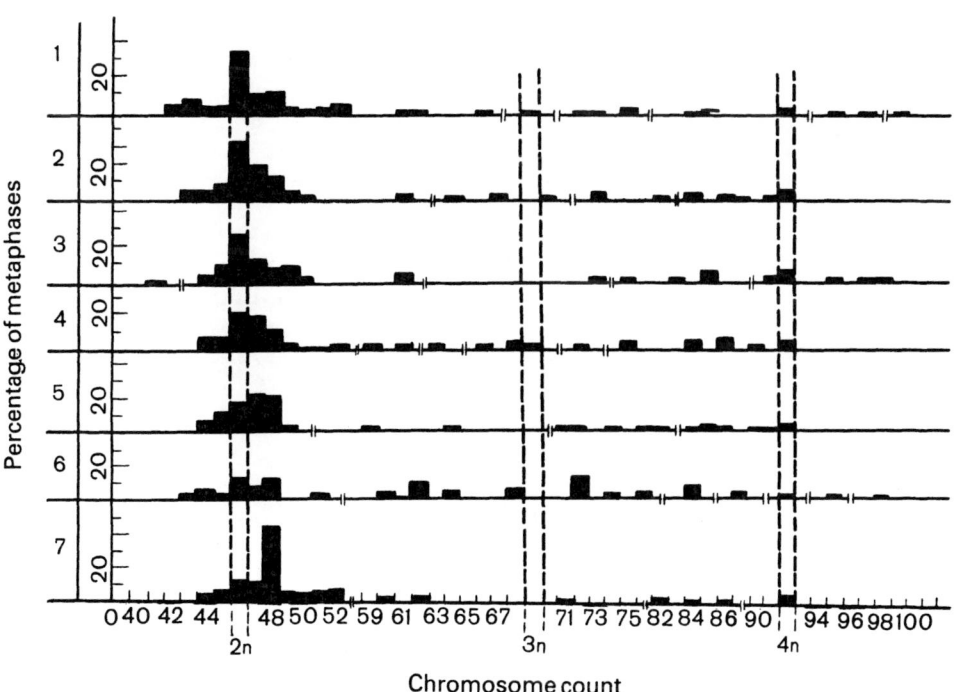

Fig. 43.  Histograms showing the distribution of metaphase plates by
          chromosome number in 7 patients with squamous cell
          carcinoma of the skin.

which had supervened on a keratoacanthoma that the percentage of
aneuploid metaphases (62.5%) was nearly the same as that (60%) in the
patient with pyoderma ulcerosum vegetans with pronounced pseudocarcinomatous hyperplasia described above.  But, as already
mentioned, this latter patient was found to have developed cancer
subsequently.

Thus, the squamous cell carcinoma group was characterized by a
low percentage of diploid metaphases (10 to 37.5%) and a high percentage of aneuploid ones (62.5% to 90.2%), most of which were hyperploid (50 to 85% of all metaphases).  Here is a case report.

Patient Sh., a 50-year-old man, was referred to our
clinic for consultation because of an ulcer on the lower
lip with no tendency to heal.  The ulcer developed from a
fissure which had appeared about 4 years before and had
healed and recurred periodically.  The ulcer was excised
but reappeared in the same site 6 months thereafter.  Over
the past year or so, it had been growing in size and became
painful to touch.

On examination, an oval ulcer about 1.5 cm in diameter
with a firm roundish border was seen on the vermilion
border of the lower lip and encroaching on the mucosa.  The
floor of the ulcer was covered by a sanguinous discharge
which had dried up at the ulcer margin to form a crust
(Figure 44).  The regional lymph nodes were not palpable.
The presumptive diagnosis was squamous cell carcinoma of
the lower lip.

Histologic examination of the margin of the ulcer
revealed a moderately acanthotic surface epithelium with
para- and hyperkeratosis.  The middle and lower layers of
the dermis contained sheets of epithelial cells showing

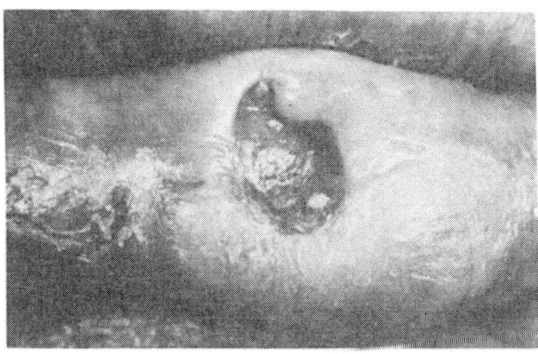

Fig. 44.  Keratinizing squamous cell carcinoma of the lower lip.

marked architectural disorganization, polymorphism, and
individual cell keratinization.

A cytogenetic analysis of 100 metaphases from the
cultured epithelium of the margin of the ulcer (see Figure
43, 4), revealed a modal number of 46 chromosomes (20% of
the metaphases) with a wide distribution of chromosomes
around the mode (from 44 to 102). Hypodiploid metaphases
accounted for 10% and hyperdiploid ones for 70% of all
metaphases. A noteworthy feature was a large percentage
(18%) of cells with 47 chromosomes. An analysis of 100
metaphases from the deeper portions of the ulcer showed
higher percentages of cells containing 47 and 48 chromosomes (22% and 20% respectively).

These findings suggest that different portions of a given tumor
may contain clones of cells with similar chromosome numbers and that
constant selection of such clones can assure progression of the
tumor. In the case just described, the metaphases were generally
characterized by hyperploid chromosome numbers (Figure 45). However,
a structural analysis of 35 metaphases showed that the chromosome
counts were significantly lower (p<0.01) in some karyotypic groups
(groups A, B, and E) and significantly higher (p<0.01) in the others
(groups C, D, F, and G) than the theoretically expected numbers.

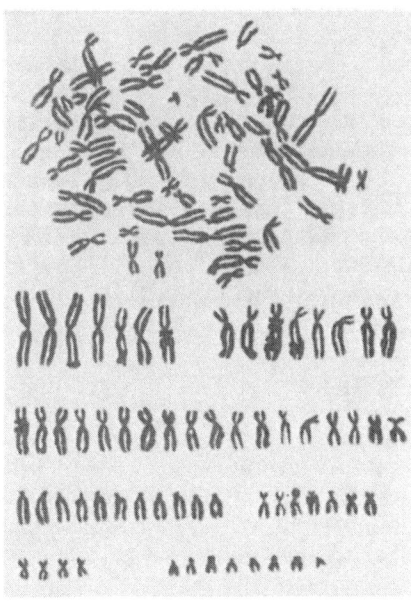

Fig. 45.  Metaphase and arrangement of its hyperploid karyotype (63
          chromosomes) from the carcinoma shown in Fig. 44. (Azure
          and oesin stain.)

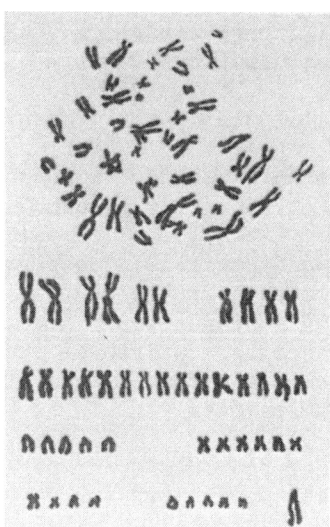

Fig. 46.  Metaphase and arrangement of its karyotype showing a marker
          chromosome from the squamous cell carcinoma of the penis in
          patient K.


In one of the tumors, the proportion of diploid cells was as low
as 10% and the modal number was constituted by metaphases containing
48 chromosomes (see Figure 43, 7); in 9 metaphases (9%), marker
chromosomes resembling group D chromosomes in morphology were found
(Figure 46).

The data on changes in  chromosome numbers in the various karyotypic groups, based on an analysis of 107 metaphases, indicate (Table
11) that in squamous cell carcinoma of the skin these changes are
similar to those in malignant tumors of other sites.  The most frequent changes in cutaneous carcinoma were significantly decreased
chromosome counts in groups A and B (p<0.01) and significantly
increased counts in groups C and D (p<0.01).


6.2.2  Rabbit Skin Cultures

It has been shown that the diploid chromosome number in normal
somatic rabbit cells is 44 (Issa et al., 1968).  We distributed the
chromosomes by karyotypic groups according to the classification
proposed by Issa et al (1968) who divided the rabbit karyotype into
11 groups in the combined basis of the arm ratio and relative length
of the chromosomes, as follows:

groups I-IV (the first four pairs) comprising large metacentric
chromosomes; group V (pairs 5-8), nearly acrocentric chromosomes;
group VI (9-13 + X), nearly metacentric chromosomes; group VII

Table 11. Summary of Deviations of Chromosome Counts in Karyotypic Groups from the Theoretically Expected Chromosome Numbers in Cultured Skin Cells from Patients with Squamous Cell Carcinoma.

| Case No. | No. of cells counted | Mean No. of chromosomes per cell | Mean deviations of chromosome counts from expected values in various karyotypic groups | | | | | | |
|---|---|---|---|---|---|---|---|---|---|
| | | | $XA_1-A_2$ | $XB_1-B_2$ | $XC_1-C_2$ | $XD_1-D_2$ | $XE_1-E_2$ | $XF_1-F_2$ | $XG_1-G_2$ |
| 1 | 19 | 50.4 | -0.5 | -0.3 | +0.2 | +0.7 | +0.3 | 0.0 | 0.0 |
| 2 | 12 | 63.5 | -1.1 | 0.0 | +2.0 | +0.1 | 0.0 | +0.5 | +1.3 |
| 3 | 15 | 67.0 | -2.7 | -1.1 | +0.4 | +3.2 | +1.5 | -0.2 | -1.1 |
| 4 | 35 | 60.7 | -0.8 | -0.1 | +0.3 | +0.9 | -0.6 | +0.2 | +0.2 |
| 5 | 8 | 62.0 | -2.0 | -0.5 | +0.4 | +0.3 | +0.2 | +2.1 | +1.1 |
| 6 | 18 | 47.6 | 0.0 | -0.1 | +0.7 | +0.1 | -0.1 | -0.1 | -0.1 |
| Overall mean deviation | | | -1.18 | -0.35 | +0.68 | +0.9 | +0.2 | +0.4 | +0.23 |
| Level of significance ($p$) | | | $<0.01$ | $<0.01$ | $<0.01$ | $<0.01$ | $>0.05$ | $>0.05$ | $>0.05$ |

Designations: $X$ = means; $A_1$, $B_1$, etc. = observed chromosome numbers (chromosome counts) in karyotypic groups; $A_2$, $B_2$, etc. = expected values; $A_1-A_2$, $B_1-B_2$, etc. = difference between observed and expected values. The significance of differences was assessed by Wilcoxon's test.

(14-15) and group VIII (16), small metacentric chromosomes; group IX
(17-18), telocentric chromosomes; group X (19), small metacentric
chromosomes; and group X1 (20-21 + Y), small acrocentric chromosomes.
Figure 47 depicts rabbit metaphase plates and karyotypes for one male
and one female cell. We did not identify chromosomes within the
groups because our purpose was solely to compare numerical changes of
chromosomes in cells from morphologically unaltered and pathologically changed rabbit ear epidermis.

Chromosome analyses were performed in 667 metaphases, including
58 prepared from cells of histologically unchanged epidermis, 70 from
cells of epidermis showing pseudocarcinomatous inflammatory hyperplasia, and 539 from cells of epidermis from sites of obligatory
precancerous tumors (papillomas, keratoacanthomas) and of squamous
cell carcinomas derived from these tumors. The distributions of
chromosome counts in these groups of cells are shown in the histograms of Figure 48. It can be seen that in the morphologically
unchanged epidermis, most cells (81%) were represented by diploid
metaphases with 44 chromosomes. Among the aneuploid metaphases
(19%), the percentage of hypoploids was somewhat higher than that of
hyperploids (10.4 and 8.6). No marker chromosomes were found.

In the cases of pseudocarcinomatous hyperplasia, there was a
prominent paradiploid modal class of cells with a stemline containing
44 chromosomes. The percentage of aneuploid metaphases was approxi-

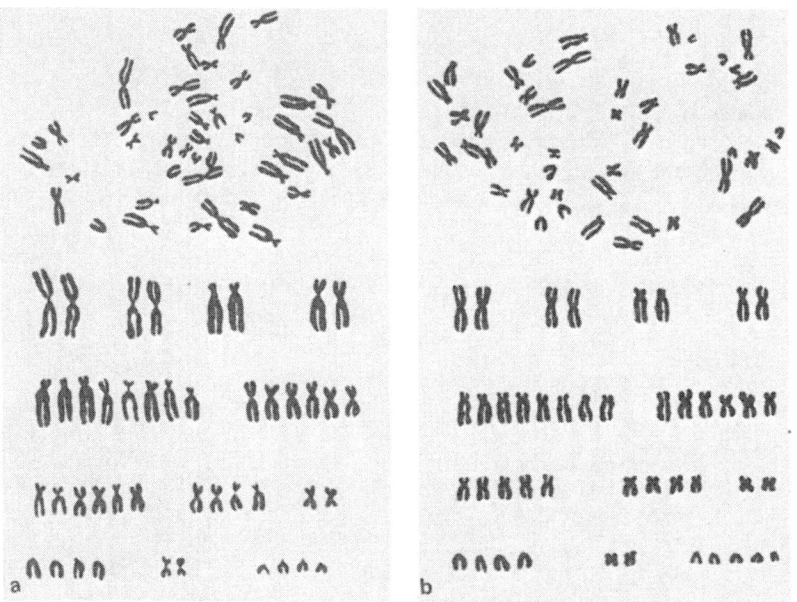

Fig. 47.    Unaltered metaphases and karyotypes of cells from cultured
normal rabbit skin.    (a) Female; (b) male.    (Azure and
eosin stain.)

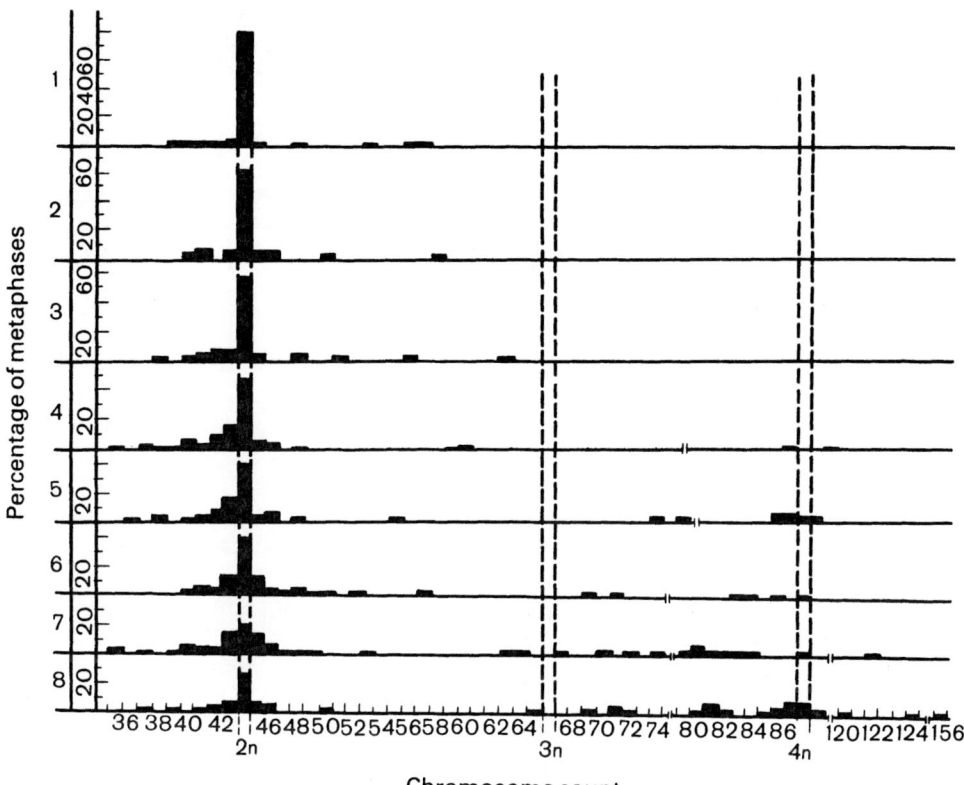

Fig. 48.  Histograms showing the distribution of chromosome counts in
          rabbit ear epidermis.  (1) Normal epidermis; (2) and (3)
          pseudocarcinomatous hyperplasia; (4), (5), and (6)
          obligatory precancerous tumors; (7) and (8) keratinizing
          squamous cell carcinoma.

mately the same in all cases, but the ratio of hypo- to hyperploid
metaphases varied from one case to another.  Thus, whereas in case 2
the proportion of hyperploids was somewhat higher than that of hypoploids (21.4% and 17.6%), the reverse was true in case 3 (23.6% and
16.6%).  Chromosome counts in the hypoploid metaphases ranged from 38
to 43, and such decreased counts occurred in various karyotypic
groups.

     Thus, the pseudocarcinomatous hyperplasia involved some re-
duction in the level of diploid cells and an increase in the level of
aneuploid cells.  However, there was always a well-defined diploid
stemline and no consistent changes could be discerned for aneuploid
cells.

In the cases of obligatory precancerous tumors and squamous cell
carcinomas, the percentage of diploid metaphases was lower (37 to
47.6%) and that of aneuploid ones was higher (52.4 to 62.4%) than in
the previous groups.  The stemline of cells containing 44 chromosomes
was, however, prominent.  Among the aneuploid metaphases, hypoploids
predominated over hyperploids (29.3 to 38.5% and 13 to 33% of all
metaphases).  In most hypoploid metaphases, chromosome counts ranged
from 40 to 43.  In some cases, chromosomes with broken arms were
noted (Figure 49).  Hyper- and polyploid metaphases were frequent
(Figure 50).

## 6.3  SEX CHROMATIN IN EPIDERMAL CELL NUCLEI

The problem of sex chromatin has been attracting the attention
of investigators since 1949 when Barr and Bertram discovered a
nucleolar satellite body in nerve cells of adult cats.  This body was
smaller than a nucleolus in size and was usually nucleolus-associ-
ated, but in some cases no such association was seen and the chromatin body was situated at the nuclear membrane or in the nucleoplasm.
Since these bodies were detected in females of various animal
species, including man, but only in a small percentage of nuclei from
male individuals, the terms "sex chromatin" and "sex chromatin body"
(or "Barr body") have come to be used instead of "neucleolar satellite".

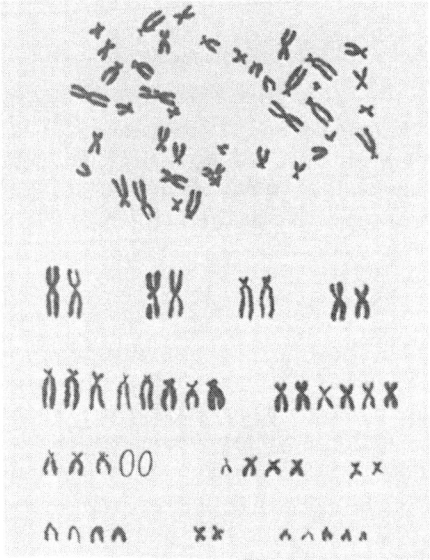

Fig. 49.  Hypoploid metaphase and arrangement of its karyotype from
          rabbit ear epidermis affected by an obligatory precancerous
          tumor (keratoacanthoma).  There are 42 chromosomes, with
          breakage of an arm of one chromosome of the second pair.
          (Azure and eosin stain.)

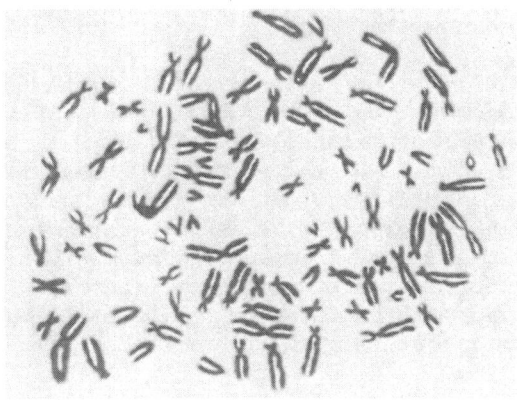

Fig. 50.  Hyperploid metaphase from rabbit ear epidermis during
          development of squamous cell carcinoma.  There are 87
          chromosomes.  (Azure and eosin stain.)


     Barr and Bertram (1949), Moore and Barr (1954), and other
authors believed that the "nucleolar satellite" is formed by fusion
of the heterochromatic portions of the two X-chromosomes and, con-
sequently, is a female structure.  However, further studies led to
the conclusion that the sex chromatin body represents a single X-
chromosome in a coiled state (Ohno et al., 1959).  This conclusion
was based on the finding that one of the X-chromosomes stains more
deeply early during mitosis.  The modern concepts about the biologic
nature of the sex chromatin are reflected in Lyon's (1961) hypothesis
postulating essentially that in female cell nuclei one of the two
X-chromosomes is heteropycnotic in prophase and is represented in the
form of genetically inactive sex chromatin in interphase.

     Moore et al. (1953) and Holzer and Marberger (1957) reported sex
chromatin to be contained in 45 to 90% of nuclei of tissues from
women and in 0 to 20% of nuclei from men.  Gautier (1961) concluded
for his studies of fibroblasts in tissue culture that sex chromatin
is absent in the normal nuclei of somatic cells from healthy male
humans, being present only in chromosomal disorders characterized by
an increased number of X-chromosomes.  According to Moore and Barr
(1954), the percentage of sex chromatin-positive nuclei in women
varies from tissue to tissue and is 25% on the average.

     Sex chromatin may occupy three positions in the nucleus: (1) at
the inner surface of the nuclear envelope, (2) at the nucleolus, or
(3) in the nucleoplasm (Klinger, 1966; Grinberg, 1969).  Most commonly, it occurs closely applied to the inner nuclear membrane (e.g.
Grinberg, 1969; Belen'kii, 1970; Kryazheva, 1971).  If it occurs at
the nucleolus or within the nucleoplasm, sex chromatin may be diffi-

cult to identify because it is then indistinguishable from other
DNA-containing chromocenters.

An inverse correlation has been noted to exist between the
frequency of sex chromatin-positive nuclei in a tissue and the
mitotic activity of that tissue. Golovin and Zus' (1981) have concluded from their studies on cytophotometric measurement of DNA
content and mitotic activity and sex chromatin determinations in cell
nuclei of the same histologic specimens that changes in the number of
sex chromatin-positive nuclei in tumor tissue signify, not the disappearance of the X-chromosome or its incorporation into the interphase nuclei as is often believed to be the case, but rather alterations in the proliferative activity of the cells.

James (1964) found from autoradiographic and cytophotometric
studies in tissue culture that chromatin-negative nuclei dominated in
the middle and last parts of the S phase of the cell cycle, when very
few chromatin-positive nuclei were present. He observed two morphologically different types of chromatin body: a small type which
occurred in the $G_1$ phase, and a larger type which occurred late in
the S phase and in the $G_2$ phase.

Large nuclei with a low incidence of sex chromatin despite a
high degree of ploidy, are usually present within malignant tissues
(Kallenberger et al., 1968; Ganina and Loboda, 1969; Ganina, 1970).
The number of chromatin-positive nuclei in tumors has been reported
to decrease in proportion to the increase in the number of large
nuclei (Meier-Ruge and Kallenberger, 1967). There is abundant evidence to show that the development of malignant tumors in various
sites of the body is accompanied in most cases by a reduction in the
frequency of sex chromatin-containing nuclei in women (e.g. Lenz,
1963; Atkin, 1964; Mardakhiashvili and Shats, 1969; Sluzhinskaya et
al., 1969; Belen'kii, 1970; Baruffi et al., 1971; Naleskina, 1971;
Siracky, 1971; Odinokova et al., 1973; Ganina et al., 1976).

There are indications that the tumor tissue and buccal epithelium of men with malignant neoplasm contain a high percentage of
sex chromatin-positive cells (e.g. Avtsyn and Shibaeva, 1969;
Sluzhinskaya et al., 1969; Egorkina et al., 1972; Odinokava et al.,
1973; Voitenko, 1976).

The observations that sex chromatin-positive nuclei are consistently decreased in number in women with malignant tumors have provided a justification for sex chromatin determination in the differential diagnosis of malignancy.

As early as 1957, Moore and Barr reported the percentage of
nuclei containing sex chromatin in lesional skin to be, on the average, lower in women with squamous cell carcinoma than in those with
basal cell carcinoma (54% against 64%), with variations from 2% to

84% in individual cases of squamous cell carcinoma; no differences in sex chromatin frequency were observed in men. By contrast, Rodermund (1957), in a study of 13 squamous cell carcinomas, 4 basal cell carcinomas, 3 melanomas, and 3 keratoacanthomas in women, detected no differences in sex chromatin incidence among these tumors or between these and areas of normal skin, which led that author to conclude that the sex of a tumor corresponds to that of the tumor bearer. The same conclusion was reached by Tavares (1955) in sex-chromatin studies of 110 malignant tumors of various localizations in women (including 27 squamous cell carcinomas) in which 60 to 80% of nuclei (average, 72%) were found to possess sex chromatin; no differences in sex chromatin were found between tumor cells and histiocytes of the tumor stroma.

However, in a later study Tavares (1957) found that two squamous cell carcinomas out of the five studied, did not correspond to the female sex of their bearers, but that histiocytes in the tumor stroma were invariably chromatin-positive. Tavares noted that undifferentiated tumors always contained fewer nuclei with sex chromatin than did differentiated tumors. Heite and Rüssmann (1960) found reduced frequencies of sex chromatin-containing nuclei in sites of squamous cell carcinoma (21.5%, on the average, in 20 patients) as compared to keratoacanthoma (30.9% in 21), basal cell carcinoma (30% in 15), and senile keratoma (35.2% in 15 patients). Since the difference in sex chromatin between squamous cell carcinoma and keratoacanthoma was statistically significant, they considered that sex chromatin studies might be of value in diagnostic differentiation between these conditions. Lenz (1963) compared the number of nuclei with sex chromatin in histologic specimens of malignant and benign tumors of the skin and of surrounding connective tissue and noted that sex chromatin frequency was significantly reduced at sites of squamous cell carcinoma in women, but that in men the number of chromatin-positive nuclei was equally low in malignant tumors, benign tumors, and surrounding connective tissue elements, with the exception of basal cell carcinomas in which the percentage of nuclei with sex chromatin was high (up to 60%). The above author likewise concluded that sex chromatin determination may be a valuable adjunct in the diagnosis of malignant neoplasms.

Decreased numbers of nuclei with sex chromatin in malignant melanomas as compared to pigmented nevi and epidermal areas adjacent to the tumor have been reported by Ganina (1970), Naleskina (1971), and a number of other authors, who have all emphasized that these decreases are accompanied by increased nuclear volume and DNA content. Basal cell carcinomas, which are known to run a benign course, have been reported to have the diploid chromosome complement and high percentages of sex chromatin-positive nuclei (Manocha, 1969).

Evidence in the literature therefore suggests that changes in the incidence of sex chromatin-containing nuclei of tumor cells

reflect the functional state of the chromosomal apparatus and the
degree of malignancy. We however, have not been able to find any
reports of comparative studies on sex chromatin in nuclei of cells
from sites of pseudocarcinomatous hyperplasia and squamous cell
carcinoma, although such studies may contribute to a more objective
evaluation of the role which changes in the genetic apparatus of
epidermal cells may play in the development of pseudocarcinomatous
hyperplasia and squamous cell carcinoma. Our comparative studies in
this area, which were initiated in 1968 (Belen'kii et al., 1968) have
shown that proliferating epidermal cells in sites of pseudocarcinomatous hyperplasia differ in the incidence of sex chromatin-containing
nuclei from those in sites of squamous cell carcinoma.

### 6.3.1  Sex Chromatin Studies in Patients

Sex chromatin was studied in 62 skin biopsy specimens from 56
patients (27 women and 29 men) with various dermatoses or benign
epithelial skin tumors in which pseudocarcinomatous epidermal hyperplasia (often pronounced) had arisen, and in 37 skin biopsy specimens
from 24 patients (10 women and 14 men) with keratinizing squamous
cell carcinoma. Although the patients ranged in age from 18 to 82
years, the differences in age were not taken into account in the
analysis of the biopsied material, since the percentage of nuclei
with sex chromatin had been shown to vary only insignificantly from
one age group to another (Kayumov and Dmitrieva, 1973).

Sex chromatin was studied in paraffin-embedded histologic skin
sections not more than 7 μm in thickness fixed with 10% neutral
formalin and stained with hematoxylin and eosin. Only interphase
nuclei with even membranes and delicate chromatin structures were
analyzed.

Areas of acanthosis, those of invasive proliferations, and those
of morphologically unaltered epidermis adjacent to the lesions (controls) were studied separately. In each area selected for examination, 200 to 500 cells were analyzed and the mean number of nuclei
with sex chromatin was then calculated. Since basal cells are germi-
native and many of them as in mitosis, only suprabasal cells were
used.

In the control (9 biopsy specimens), where a total of 4500
nuclei were counted for women and 4000 for men, the mean percentage
of chromatin-containing nuclei was 25.6 ± 0.65& (range: 18 to 34%) in
the females and 3.27 ± 0.64% (range: 0 to 18%) in the males.

The results obtained for pathologically changed epidermis are
summarized in Table 12. The mean percentage of nuclei with sex
chromatin in areas of moderate acanthosis in women with various
dermatoses (a total of 11 disease entities, including chronic ulcer-

ative pyoderma, trophic ulcers of the lower leg, lichen ruber verrucosus, keratoacanthoma, etc.) was 24.1 ± 0.7%. This is lower than in the control, but the difference in insignificant (p>0.05). The zones of invasive proliferations of the pseudocarcinomatous hyperplasia type in the same histologic specimens were characterized by a significantly (p<0.01) decreased percentage of nuclei containing sex chromatin (21.2 ± 0.56) as compared to the areas of moderate acanthosis. This decrease in sites of pseudocarcinomatous hyperplasia is probably attributable to increased mitotic activity of the tissue.

In the male patients with dermatoses (a total of 15 disease entities), the percentage of chromatin-positive nuclei in areas of moderate acanthosis likewise differed insignificantly from the control (p>0.05), but was significantly lower than in areas of pseudocarcinomatous hyperplasia (p<0.01) in which the incidence of sex chromatin-positive nuclei remained, however, within normal limits of variation (0 to 10%). No changes in sex chromatin frequency specific for particular dermatoses were noted.

The foci of obligatory precancerous acanthosis and of invasive squamous cell carcinoma were characterized by more marked changes in sex chromatin. In the women, the percentage of Barr-positive nuclei in sites of precancerous acanthosis was significantly lower than in those of inflammatory acanthosis (p<0.01). The invasive cancerous proliferations were particularly low in chromatin-positive nuclei and often did not correspond to the sex of the host in this respect. The mean percentage of chromatin-positive nuclei in these areas was significantly lower (p<0.01) than in those of precancerous acanthosis and pseudocarcinomatous hyperplasia. Figure 51 shows an area of tumorous proliferations where chromatin-containing nuclei are not apparent and an area of precancerous acanthosis in the same histo-logic preparation where clumps of sex chromatin can be seen in the nuclei.

In the male patients, the mean percentage of sex chromatin-positive nuclei was significantly higher both in areas of precancerous acanthosis and in invasive cancerous proliferations.

These differences in the percentage of nuclei with sex chromatin between squamous cell carcinoma and pseudocarcinomatous hyperplasia reflect the biologic essence of epidermal proliferation in each of these differential diagnostic purposes.


## 6.3.2  Sex Chromatin Studies in Rabbits

Our sex chromatin studies in rabbits with reactive pseudocarci-nomatous hyperplasia and rabbits with obligatory precancerous tumors progressing to squamous cell carcinoma have produced results similar to those reported in the preceding section for human patients.

Table 12. Percentage Sex Chromatin-containing Nuclei in Sites of Pseudocarcinomatous Hyperplasia (PCH) and of Squamous Cell Carcinoma in Human Patients.

| Sex | Condition | No. of histo-logic specimens examined | Acanthosis adjacent to areas of invasion | | Areas of invasive epidermal growth | |
|---|---|---|---|---|---|---|
| | | | No. of cells examined | Percentage of sex chromatin-containing nuclei (M±m) | No. of cells examined | Percentage of sex chromatin-containing nuclei (M±m) |
| Women | Miscellaneous dermatoses accompanied by PCH | 32 | 5000 | 24.1 ± 0.7 | 5000 | 21.2 ± 0.56 |
| | Squamous cell carcinoma | 18 | 3600 | 18.8 ± 0.8 | 4900 | 10.7 ± 0.64 |
| Men | Miscellaneous dermatoses accompanied by PCH | 30 | 4800 | 4.1 ± 0.4 | 4400 | 5.6 ± 0.36 |
| | Squamous cell carcinoma | 19 | 5700 | 6.1 ± 0.5 | 5900 | 11.8 ± 0.78 |

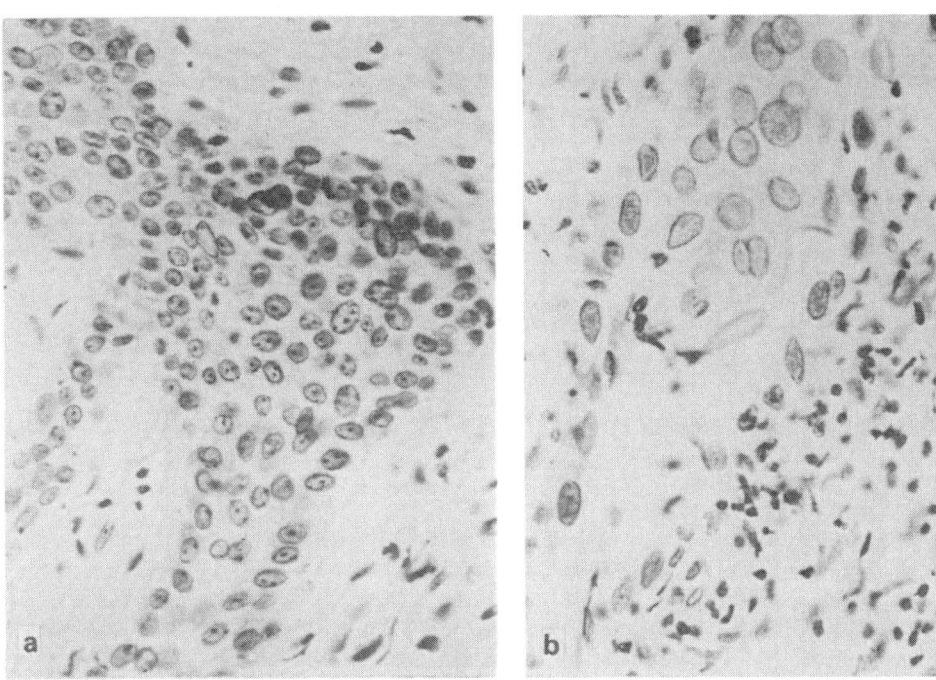

Fig. 51.  Sex chromatin in epidermal cell nuclei from a patient with
          squamous cell carcinoma of the skin.  (a) Area of
          acanthosis showing clumps of sex chromatin in cell nuclei;
          (b) proliferations of tumor cells, with sex chromatin being
          indetectable in cell nuclei.  ((a) 500 X; (b) 1100 X;
          Feulgen stain).

In the control group, where a total of 6900 female and 4000 male
cell nuclei from morphologically unchanged ear epidermis were
counted, the mean percentage of chromatin-positive nuclei was 30.3 ±
0.75 (range: 18 to 44) in the females and 3.4 ± 0.43 (range: 0 to 14)
in the males.

It can be seen from Table 13 that in the female rabbits with
pseudocarcinomatous hyperplasia the mean percentage of chromatin-
positive nuclei was somewhat higher in inflammatory acanthosis than
in invasive epidermal growth and that in squamous cell carcinoma this
percentage in females was much lower than in areas of pseudocarcinomatous hyperplasia and of obligatory precancerous acanthosis.
Figure 52 shows cell nuclei in an area of tumorous proliferation low
in sex chromatin and in an area of precancerous acanthosis in the
same histologic specimen where many clumps of sex chromatin are
present.

Table 13. Percentage Sex Chromatin-containing Nuclei in Sites of Epidermal Pseudocarcinomatous Hyperplasia and of Malignant Transformed Epidermis in Rabbits.

| Sex | Condition | No. of histologic specimens examined | Acanthosis adjacent to areas of invasion | | Areas of invasive epidermal growth | |
|---|---|---|---|---|---|---|
| | | | No. of cells examined | Percentage of sex chromatin-containing nuclei (M±m) | No. of cells examined | Percentage of sex chromatin-containing nuclei (M±m) |
| Females | Reactive pseudocarcinomatous hyperplasia | 29 | 8300 | 25.0 ± 0.48 | 8700 | 21.0 ± 0.5 |
| | Obligatory precancerous tumors and squamous cell carcinoma | 17 | 4800 | 20.6 ± 0.62 | 52.00 | 10.7 ± 0.64 |
| Males | Reactive pseudocarcinomatous hyperplasia | 6 | 1400 | 4.6 ± 0.7 | 1800 | 3.2 ± 0.4 |
| | Obligatory precancerous tumors and squamous cell carcinoma | 17 | 4000 | 7.0 ± 0.56 | 5300 | 12.4 ± 0.7 |

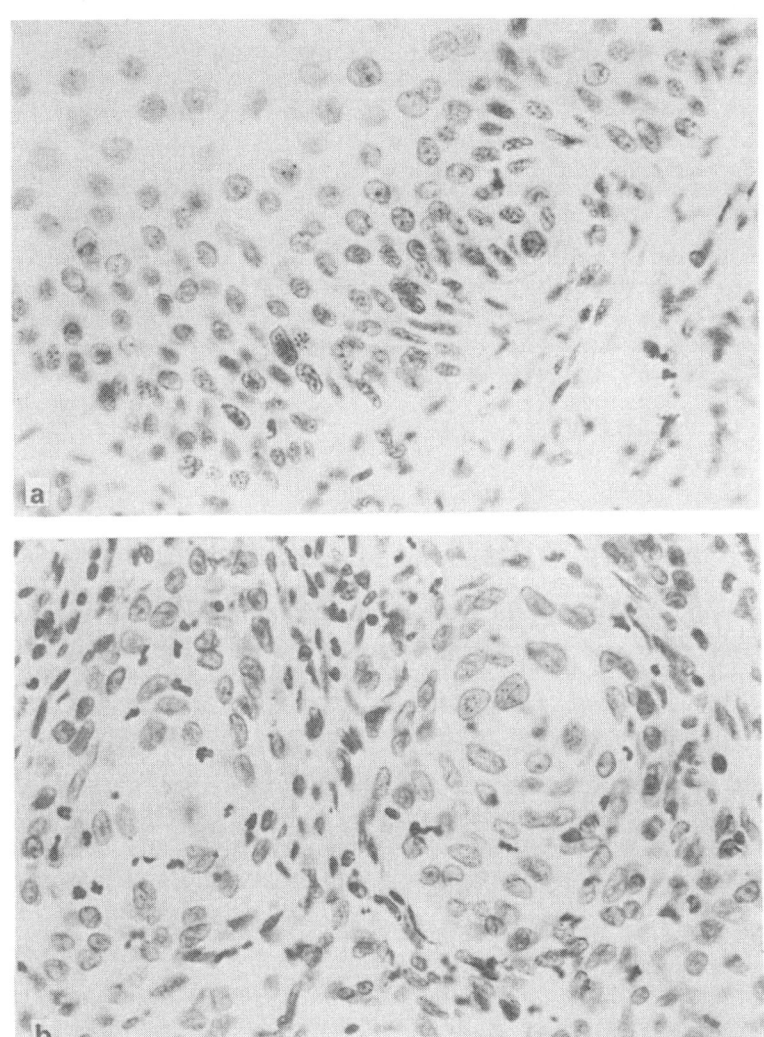

Fig. 52.   Sex chromatin in epidermal cell nuclei from rabbit ear
           affected by squamous cell carcinoma.   (a) Area of
           acanthosis, showing clumps of sex chromatin in cell nuclei;
           (b) chromatin clumps are scarce in nuclei of proliferating
           tumor cells.   (500 X; Feulgen stain.)


     In male rabbits, the mean percentages of Barr-positive nuclei
were higher in areas of precancerous acanthosis and in invasive tumor
cell proliferations than in sites of reactive hyperplasia, without,
however, exceeding the normal limits of variation.

## 6.4  SUMMARY AND CONCLUSION

The foregoing cytophysiologic and cytogenetic studies of
lesional skin from patients and rabbits have indicated changes which
may occur in the genetic apparatus of epidermal cells at sites of
pseudocarcinomatous reactive hyperplasia as well as differences
between these changes and those arising in squamous cell carcinoma
of the skin.

Differences between inflammatory epidermal hyperplasia and
squamous cell carcinoma are evident already in the growth patterns of
primary skin cultures.  Epidermal cells from areas of pseudocarcinomatous hyperplasia are no longer subject to the stimulatory action
of the inflammatory infiltrate and so grow much slower in such cultures than do cancer cells.  Tumor cells, which are capable of autonomous growth without stimulatory action of connective tissue, grow in
culture much faster and form, within one week of cultivation, a
monolayer sheet of cells which grows out directly from the explant.

The chromosome analyses of cells from cultured skin have shown
that the range of quantitative chromosomal changes in such cells is
wider in pseudocarcinomatous hyperplasia than in normal epidermis.
However, both in man and in rabbits, pseudocarcinomatous hyperplasia
is characterized by a prominent diploid stemline of cells and by
approximately the same percentages of hypo- and hyperploid metaphases
among aneuploids.

As the human epidermis undergoes transformation to malignancy,
the percentage of diploid metaphases decreases and that of aneuploid
metaphases rises, mainly because of an increase in the number of
hyperploids.  Our studies have demonstrated that a low percentage of
diploid cells (40% or less) combined with a high percentage of hyperploid cells (50% or more) is suggestive of incipient malignant transformation of the epidermis.  In sites of well-differentiated squamous
cell carcinomas, the modal class of cells remained paradiploid,
and aneuploidy was pronounced only when the tumor was far advanced.
Similar chromosomal changes occurred in rabbits in the process of
chemical carcinogenesis.

A structural analysis of chromosomal alterations in the karyotypic groups has shown that a consistent feature of pseudocarcinomatous hyperplasia is an increased chromosome count in group B, and of
squamous cell carcinoma, decreased counts in groups A and B and
increased counts in groups C and D.  The changes in chromosome
numbers within the karyotype seen in pseudocarcinomatous hyperplasia
and squamous cell carcinoma thus appear to reflect the overall trend
in mitotic pathology in each of these processes.

As regards the sex chromatin, the frequency of chromatin-
positive nuclei provides a clear indication of the biologic nature

of epidermal hyperplasia in females, since the percentage of nuclei with sex chromatin has been found to be consistently reduced in tumor cell proliferations. One should agree with those (Therkelssen and Lamm, 1966; Kallenberger et al., 1968; Mardakhiashvili and Shats, 1969; Ganina et al., 1976; Golovin and Zus', 1981) who attribute the reduction in the number of Barr-positive nuclei seen in cancerous tumors of various sites in women to a high mitotic activity of the tissue and to increased nuclear volume. This view is supported by the results of our studies which indicate that mitotic activity, pathologic mitoses, and nuclear ploidy all increase in squamous cell carcinoma of the skin. As for the observed increase in the number of sex chromatin-positive nuclei in sites of squamous cell carcinoma in men, it is difficult to explain this phenomenon because the origin of sex chromatin in men still remains a matter of controversy. If one accepts the hypothesis that the sex chromatin in men, as in women, derives from X-heterochromatin (Voitenko, 1976), then an increase in sex chromatin in men can probably be attributed to the overall increase of chromosome number in the karyotype in cancer. As shown above, the hyperploid cells within a cutaneous squamous cell carcinoma display a significantly increased number of chromosomes in group C to which the sex X-chromosome is known to belong. Although we have not identified chromosomes by pairs, it may be assumed that an inactive X chromosome may occur in the interphase nucleus among the supernumerary group C chromosomes.

In our view, the results of studies such as those described in this chapter, considered in relation to clinicopathologic findings, can permit a more valid and correct assessment of the hyperplastic process in the epidermis and thus may be of considerable practical value in diagnostic differentiation between pseudocarcinomatous epidermal hyperplasia and squamous cell carcinoma of the skin.

# 7
# Regulation of Epidermal Proliferation

Unraveling the mechanisms by which cells proliferate represents one of the greatest challenges for biomedical research today. It is the proliferation of epithelial cells and of epidermal cells in particular that is the major determinant of hyperplastic and neoplastic processes all the way from reactive to precancerous hyperplasia through cancerous lesions in situ to invasive squamous cell carcinoma.

In dermatology, epidermal cell proliferation is of special significance because most dermatoses, regardless of their etiology and pathogenesis, can be associated, at some stage of their evolution, with disorders of cellular reproduction and differentiation such as acanthosis, hyperkeratosis, parakeratosis, hypergranulosis, and dyskeratosis. Voorhees et al. (1976) have proposed the term "proliferative skin disease" to cover all skin ailments characterized by abnormal proliferation of keratinocytes. Specifically, they include in this group psoriasis, eczema, ichthyosis, and cancer. They state that "although these proliferative entities probably have multiple etiologies, the universality of common physiologic mechanisms implies that the molecular basis of cellular proliferation has mechanisms common to all cells."

It is not yet clear how precisely the epidermal cell population is being continuously renewed so that cell production equals the constant physiologic loss of cells. Although it has not been established what specific mechanisms operate to maintain this steady state which is essential for the preservation of normal epidermal structure and for the performance by the epidermis of its various functions, the advances made by biochemistry, molecular biology, genetics, and cytology have provided important clues to an understanding of these mechanisms.

134

A substantial contribution in this respect has been made by the cell cycle concept, which was first proposed by Howard and Pelc in 1953 and which is based on the fact that proliferating eukaryotic cells synthesize DNA at a specific time. The cell cycle is now known to consist of four periods, or phases. Following mitosis (M phase), the cell enters the interphase period ($G_1$ phase) which continues until DNA synthesis begins (S phase). The interval between the completion of DNA synthesis until the beginning of the next mitosis represents the $G_2$ phase. The ordered sequence of events as defined by the cell cycle constitutes a "proliferative program" (Voorhees et al., 1976). At the termination of mitosis, there are two progeny cells, and these cells may continue to cycle, enter a resting phase ($G_0$), or leave the cycle and enter upon the path of functional development, that is, of differentiation (Baserga, 1971). The normal epidermis balances the rates of proliferation and differentiation so that a steady state is maintained (Voorhees et al., 1976). The balance may be upset by emotional stress, hormonal or immune stimuli, mechanical damage, or so on, resulting in an increased size of the proliferating cell population (Watson et al., 1972).

According to Voorhees et al. (1976), a normal physiologic analogue of proliferative skin disorders is the process of wound healing, in which the organism responds to injury by a directed proliferation whereby proliferation begins to dominate over differentiation. The increase in the rate of proliferation is accompanied by an increase in the cellular content of glycogen; by migration of the epithelial cells into the area of the wound; and, in some cases (as in psoriasis), by diminished rate of epidermal differentiation (Watson et al., 1972).

In normal epidermis, members of the cell community are closely interrelated functionally. It has been shown, for example, that the upper cells of the epidermis are in communication with cells of the basal layer (Rothberg et al., 1976): removal of the topmost layer of the epidermal stratum corneum by stripping resulted in acceleration of the cell cycle in basal cells (which were ten to twenty cell layers away from the site of stripping), as was indicated by increased tritiated thymidine incorporation which showed two peaks occurring between 12 and 24 h and 48 and 54 h after the stripping. The above authors have concluded from this that in response to injury a signal is generated in the epidermal surface to initiate a chain of events that culminate in the production of new basal cells. A similar conclusion has been made by Bertsch et al. (1976) who found that mechanical stimulation of dorsal mouse skin by massage or by removal of the stratum corneum led to "mutually comparable increases in DNA labeling and mitotic activity."

While it is now certain that a mitogenic signal can be initiated in epidermal cells, the nature of this signal remains unknown. Evidence has been obtained that mitogenic signals can be transmitted

from cell to cell. Rowe and Dixon (1972, 1975), in studying the
distribution pattern of mitotic figures in human skin biopsy specimens, found that mitoses occur both isolated and closely clustered in
groups or nests of two or three cells. Studies using labeled thymidine indicated a significant degree of mitotic synchronization among
the cells in such a nest. Rowe and Dixon have concluded from their
in vitro studies that mitotic stimuli pass from cell to cell via
cytoplasmic bridges and that the clustering observed in human epidermis can also be probably accounted for by the spreading of mitotic
signals from mitotic cells. A statistical analysis showed that the
clustering was highly significant in excess of what could be explained by chance (Rowe and Dixon, 1972).

In 1957 Weiss and Kavanau postulated, on the basis of a cyber-
netic model, that a given tissue regulates cellular proliberation by
a feedback mechanism whereby the tissue responds to a loss of cells
(as in skin injury) by increasing cell proliferation and maintaining
it at an accelerated pace until the defect is repaired. They
suggested essentially that in a normal tissue the cells themselves
elaborate an inhibitor which restrains their division to maintain
cellular proliferation at a level required by the tissue.

In 1960 Bullough and Laurence invoked the concept of a locally
produced humoral substance that exerts an inhibitory influence on
mitosis in the tissue concerned, and they proposed the name "chalone"
for the substance. The theory of chalones as intracellularly produced and intracellularly acting substances that control cellular
proliferation by negative feedback inhibition has gained wide currency in the last decade or so, and it is noteworthy that all the
more important findings regarding the properties and action mechanism
of the chalones have come from studies of epidermal tissues. This
theory can explain why normal epidermis retains its size, thickness,
and constant rates of proliferation and differentiation as well as
why it shows enhanced proliferation in response to injury whereby the
defect, if not too large, can be repaired in a matter of days. As
pointed out by Bullough (1967), when chalone-producing cells are lost
by wounding, the total concentration of chalone in the wound area is
reduced to weaken its inhibitory influence so that a burst of mitotic
activity ensues.

Epidermal chalone is believed to be a basic glycoprotein with
molecular weight of 30,000 to 40,000 and requiring the presence of
epinephrine for its action (Weinstein, 1979).

Chalones are tissue-specific rather than species-specific.
Thus, as shown in many studies, the aqueous extracts of epidermal
chalone from cod and from pig, mouse, and other mammals are all
equally effective mitotic inhibitors in epidermal cells but have no
inhibitory effect on cells of liver or other tissues (e.g. Bullough
and Laurence, 1960; Bullough, 1967).

It has been shown in the past decade that the division of epidermal cells in controlled by two tissue-specific chalone-type inhibitors, one of which inhibits epidermal cells in the $G_2$ phase thus preventing them from entering mitosis (the epidermal $G_2$ inhibitor), while the other inhibits the transit of cells from the $G_1$ phase into the S phase (the epidermal $G_1$ inhibitor) (Marks, 1971; Vamaguchi et al., 1974; Elgjo, 1975; Bertsch et al., 1976).  It has been shown that the $G_1$ inhibitor occurs in the more differentiated epidermal layers (Elgjo et al., 1972) and that the $G_2$ inhibitor is present predominantly in the basal layer (Elgjo et al., 1971).  These latter authors have concluded that since the inhibition in phase $G_1$ of the cell cycle is more important in terms of cell proliferation, the substance responsible for this inhibition should be considered as the true epidermal chalone.  It has been suggested that chalone acts as a repressor in inhibiting the set of genes required for mitosis to be accomplished and also that chalone may be directly associated with the cell membrane (Süss et al., 1973).

Of considerable theoretic and practical interest is the research into the roles of chalones in epidermal hyperplasia and neoplasia. It has been demonstrated that whereas in normal mouse epidermis, the synthesis of DNA can be greatly inhibited by intraperitoneal injection of a chalone-containing skin extract, no inhibition occurs, over a period of time, if the epidermis has been pretreated with a substance that stimulates cell proliferation (Marks, 1973).  To explain this phenomenon, the above author has suggested that either the mitogen interferes with a hypothetical chalone-receptor mechanism or the cells pass into a state in which they are unresponsive to the inhibitor.

Bertsch et al. (1976) have described what they call a "hyperplastic transformation" which is shown by mouse skin in response to mechanical removal (stripping) of the epidermal stratum corneum - a phenomenon characterized by a transient abolition of the responsiveness to epidermal $G_1$ inhibitor (chalone).  They have found that, unlike stripping, ordinary skin massage neither interferes with this responsiveness nor induces hyperplastic transformation, and they explain these observations by assuming that the epidermal stem cell population is heterogeneous and consists of $G_1$ chalone-sensitive and $G_1$ chalone-insensitive cells.

It has been proposed that in the process of neoplastic transformation the cells may diminish or discontinue the production of chalone so that its restraining action is abolished and the cells can enter mitosis without hindrance or that, alternatively, the cells may lose the capacity of responding to the inhibitory action of chalone and may begin to proliferate autonomously (Süss et al., 1973).  The processes involved here appear to be irreversible, whereas the cells of a reactively hyperplastic epidermis regain chalone sensitivity after the stimulus that has invoked the hyperplasia is withdrawn (Marks, 1973).

The hypothesis of Holley (1972) that cells do not need special
messages to stimulate or inhibit their division deserves special
mention.  According to it, proliferation is possible as long as the
cell is continued to be supplied by low-molecular mass nutrients
(calcium, zinc, glucose, certain amino acids), but when the influx of
these trophic factors is drastically reduced, the cell is no longer
able to divide.  This hypothesis ascribes a large role to cell membrane permeability on which the nutrients depend for their penetration into the cell's interior and also to the hormones and other
humoral substances that control the permeability.  It has been shown
that tumor cells have increased membrane permeability permitting the
accumulation of trophic factors and therefore the unrestrained reproduction of the cells (Shapot, 1975).

In recent years, a central role in the regulation of cellular
proliferation has been assigned to the cyclic nucleotides, substances
of protein nature responsible for the recognition of hormonal signals
acting on the cell membrane and for their transmission into the cell.
Although the nature of the proliferative signals themselves remains
unknown, there is evidence to implicate the cyclic nucleotides in
their initiation and transmission.  Since Sutherland and his co-
workers discovered in 1957 the presence in animal tissues of cyclic
3',5'-adenosine monophosphate (cyclic AMP, or cAMP), this intracellularly located nucleotide has been shown to be the most important
intermediate in hormonal action on cells of the target organs.

Cyclic AMP is known to be produced in the cell from ATP by
adenyl cyclase which is activated by hormonal action (Rao, 1971).
Like AMP, adenyl cyclase has been found in all mammalian cells with
the exception of human erythrocytes.  This enzyme is firmly bound to
or is a constituent of, the plasma membrane.  Chemically, it is a
lipoprotein composed of two subunits, one of which carries a receptor
site facing the extracellular space and the other, a catalytic site
located on the inner surface of the membrane (Sutherland et al.,
1965; Robison et al., 1968).  The enzyme activity is stimulated by
magnesium, fluorides, and prostaglandins (Sutherland et al., 1962;
Butcher and Baird, 1968) and is inhibited by calcium (Drummond and
Duncan, 1970).

The hormones acting primarily on adenyl cyclase to transfer it
from the inactive to an active state are known as first messengers.
The activated cyclase attacks the intracellular ATP to produce cAMP.

Numerous recent studies have been devoted to elucidating the
role of cAMP in the intimate mechanisms by which cellular activities
are regulated.  Since the pioneering work by Greengard et al. (1969)
and Cheung (1972), a large body of evidence has been amassed to
demonstrate that cATP acts as an intermediate (second messenger) for
the action of hormones on cells in target organs.  Cyclic AMP is now
known to be a regulatory substance involved in the regulatory control

of DNA synthesis and mitosis, malignant transformation, and other
cellular processes.

Severin (1975) has stated that "... because of the complex
cascade of reactions elicited by the adenyl cyclase system, the
cyclic nucleotides produce a great diversity of biologic effects:
cAMP inhibits cell division, retards malignant growth, alters enzyme
activities thereby modifying the direction of metabolic processes,
facilitates synaptic transmission of impulses, alters membrane permeability, stimulates synthesis of adaptive enzymes, etc." The cyclase system has a particularly important role to play in the regulation of cell division. The mechanisms of the enzymatic reactions
involved are highly complex.

In 1969 Iversen suggested that cAMP can mediate the regulation
of epidermal proliferation. In 1972 Williams noted the level of cAMP
to be altered in epithelial wound healing, observing that epidermal
glycogen accumulation, enhanced proliferative rate, and cellular
migration were decreased or nonexistent following injection into an
area near the wound either of dibutyryl cAMP or agents which raise
cellular levels of cAMP, such as epinephrine or theophylline. In
1975 Elgjo reported cAMP to the involved in the regulation of the
rate of transit of epidermal cells from the $G_1$ to the S phase.
Pastan and Johnson (1974) and Pastan et al. (1975) found that malignant fibroblasts contained lower levels of cAMP and that following
the addition of exogenous cAMP the fibroblasts tended to revert
toward normal. They noted that the proliferation of lymphosarcoma
cells in response to mitogens was suppressed by cAMP. It has been
hypothesized that the maintenance of the block of the $G_1$ phase of the
cell cycle is related to the ratio of cAMP to cyclic guanosine monophosphate (cGMP) in such a way that a high level of cAMP serves to
modulate the nonproliferating state (Goldberg et al., 1974). On the
other hand, proliferation is favored by increased cGMP levels. In
particular, Chambers et al. (1974) have shown that cGMP can act as a
weak mitogenic agent for lymphocytes.

It has been reported that a stable level of cAMP is not important for proliferative processes since these may increase only in
response to changes in the level of the nucleotide (Halprin, 1975).
It is now beyond doubt that lowering the level of cAMP leads to
increased mitotic activity. All types of actively proliferating
cells including tumor cells, have been shown to have much lower cAMP
levels than their nonproliferating counterparts (Abell and Monachan,
1975). What is particularly important is that the level of cAMP is
variable during the cell cycle and that the intracellular concentration of cAMP is regulated by cGMP. Although the location of cGMP
in the cell has not been determined, it is well established that this
nucleotide can stimulate cell proliferation by acting on phosphodiesterase, an enzyme which modulates the level of cAMP. The concentration of cGMP in animal and human tissues is very low (10-50 times

less than that of cAMP), and yet this nucleotide plays a highly important role in the regulation of cell dividion. Whether cGMP, like cAMP, is a second messenger is debatable. Hadden et al. (1972) have suggested that cGMP acts as an intermediate in transmitting the mitogenic signal from the cell membrane to the nucleus to trigger a whole series of biochemical reactions which eventually cause the cell to undergo division. As regards cAMP, the above authors assign to it an auxiliary role in the regulation of normal mitotic activity.

A major regulatory factor is also considered to be phosphodiesterase. A correlation has been found to exist between phosphodiesterase activity and cAMP level (Prasad and Sheppard, 1972; Wao and Manery, 1973), and this correlation has been used as a basis for the development of therapeutic approaches to control excessive cell proliferation.

Important factors in the maintenance of cAMP and cGMP metabolism are the prostaglandins (PG). It has been reported that $PGE_1$ and $PGE_2$ can modulate the level of cAMP and PGF, the level of cGMP (Whitefield, 1972; Aso et al., 1976; Adachi et al., 1977). It is believed that prostaglandins E are localized in the epidermis and that their release from epidermal cells may influence the adjacent cells by stimulating their proliferative activity (Aso et al., 1975, 1976). The level of cAMP was found to increase considerably following the addition of prostaglandin $E_1$ in a concentration as low as $10^{11}$M (Aso et al., 1976).

It is believed by most investigators that basic to the molecular mechanism of cAMP action is the ability of this nucleotide to bind to specific tissue protein kinases (e.g. Langan, 1968; Walton and Gill, 1973).

Birnbaum et al. (1976) have shown for mouse ear skin that an inhibitory adrenergic influence that sustains mitotic rate at a normally low level can be prevented by pretreatment of mice with reserpine. Reserpine depletes the endogenous catecholamines, produces a state of enhanced mitotic activity, and makes the epidermal cells particularly susceptible to mitotic inhibition by agents that raise the levels of cAMP.

Cyclic AMP has been reported to inhibit a number of physiologically active substances (Birnbaum et al., 1976), which supports the view that cAMP regulates the $G_2$ phase of the epidermal cell cycle. According to ELgjo (1975), the $G_2$ inhibitor requires a particular level of cAMP to be active.

It has been reported that epidermal chalone can interact with adenyl cyclase to stimulate it to produce a fairly high level of cATP (Duell et al., 1975), which implies that the chalone also plays an important role in the maintenance of the cAMP/cGMP ratio within the range required to ensure epidermal homeostasis.

It should be stressed that the various processes referred to above are interdependent and closely interrelated, and that any disturbance in some one link of this highly complex chain can modify the entire cascade of biochemical events involving adenyl cyclase and cAMP. Alterations in this cascade are considered to be an important factor in bringing about abnormal proliferation of epidermal cells (e.g. Yoshikawa et al., 1975; Bauer, 1977).

The cyclic nucleotides are now generally recognized to be involved in the proliferation of malignant cells (e.g. Pastan, 1975). No less important role is assigned to the nucleotides in the proliferative processes occurring in cutaneous diseases such as psoriasis accompanied by reactive epidermal hyperplasia. Voorhees et al. (1976) believe that an elevated ratio of cGMP to cAMP may be central to the initiation and/or maintenance of abnormal epidermal characteristics in psoriasis-affected skin, so that normal epidermal proliferation can possibly be restored by use of phosphodiesterase inhibitors.

As pointed out by Severin (1981), the evidence available so far regarding the involvement of the adenyl cyclase system in mechanisms of proliferation reflects the initial stage of research into the possibility of regulating normal, retarded, and accelerated cell division in the process of regeneration.

In addition to the proliferation-inhibiting system, there exist factors that stimulate mitotic activity; one of these is the epidermal growth factor (EGF) described by Cohen (1972). This factor has been chemically purified as a polypeptide with a molecular weight of 6,000 to 7,000 (Weinstein, 1979). EGF exerts its specific action under conditions of reduced concentrations of chalone, epinephrine, prostaglandin, and cAMP and elevated concentrations of histamine or other physiologically active substances.

It is difficult to enumerate all the diverse mechanisms involved in epidermal proliferation. Many of these mechanisms have been studied inadequately, if at all. It is beyond doubt, however, that neurohumoral and biochemical alterations have major roles to play in the proliferative processes and that the further elucidation of the complex mechanisms responsible for the proliferation of cells in general and of epidermal cells in particular will largely depend on the progress achieved in the fields of biochemistry, molecular biology, genetics, and cytology.

# 8
# Skin Diseases with Obligatory Development of Pseudocarcinomatous Hyperplasia

This chapter is concerned with those cutaneous diseases which display pseudomalignant epidermal hyperplasia as their almost invariable and often essential feature (obligatory pseudocarcinoses). They include keratoacanthoma, papillomatosis cutis carcinoides of Gottron, and giant condyloma acuminatum of Buschke and Loewenstein.

## 8.1 KERATOACANTHOMA

Keratoacanthoma is a relatively uncommon benign epithelial neoplasm characterized by rapid growth and spontaneous regression. It has been described under a multiplicity of names including, among others, vegetating sebaceous cyst, pseudoepithelioma, and epithelioid verrucome (Gougerot, 1917); kysté sebacé atypique (Dupont, 1930; Huriez et al, 1957); molluscum sebaceum (McCormac and Scarff, 1936); tumorlike keratosis (Poth, 1939); diverticule épidermique à paroi végétante (Dupont, 1952); molluscum pseudocarcinomatosum (Hamperl and Kalkoff, 1954); pseudoepitheliomatous hyperplasia (Weidman, 1955); benign acanthoma (Finnerud, 1955); keratopapilloacanthoma (Gardat and Baseux, 1955); idiopathic cutaneous pseudoepitheliomatous hyperplasia (Grinspan and Abulafia, 1955); and horny molluscum (Glazunov and Blinova, 1960).

It has been generally held that the first clear-cut description of the tumor was given by Dupont in 1930, but there are indications in the literature that conditions similar to keratoacanthoma had been described much earlier. Thus, according to Burge and Winkelmann (1969), a variant of multiple keratoacanthoma was described in several members of a family by Hatchinson as early as 1889. Apatenko (1973) considers that the first to report cases of keratoacanthoma

was apparently Lassar in 1893 when he described several patients who
had had what was then thought to be squamous cell carcinoma and who
had been cured by treatment with arsenicals.  There is also a view
that the first description of keratoacanthoma was provided by
Gougerot in 1917 under the title "verrucome".  More recently, a
number of reports were published of solitary skin tumors which
mimicked a squamous cell carcinoma both clinically and histologically, but which disappeared in response to intravenous injections of neoarsphenamine without any external therapy (Gougerot,
1917; Gougerot et al., 1929; Raymond et al., 1931).  In 1930, at a
meeting of the Belgian Dermatological Society, Dupont presented a
patient with a tumor on the face which, judging from the clinical
picture described by Dupont, was a typical keratoacanthoma.

    In 1936, McCormac and Scarff reported on 10 patients with cutane-
ous tumors which, while generally resembling squamous cell carcinoma,
differed from it in several clinical and histologic features.  They
designated these tumors "molluscum sebaceum", a name which had gained
wide currency before the term "keratoacanthoma" firmly established
itself.

    The wide acceptance of the word keratoacanthoma, which was
coined by Freudenthal and first used by Dauling in 1940 (Rook and
Whimster, 1979), was promoted by Rook and Whimster (1950) who
reported 29 cases of benign epithelial tumors which showed clinical
and histologic similarities to cutaneous squamous cell carcinomas,
but which, unlike these, underwent resolution spontaneously or under
symptomatic treatment.

    By 1970, well over a thousand cases of keratoacanthoma had been
reported in the literature (Mashkilleison, 1970).  By far most of the
available publications concern individual observations, probably
because keratoacanthoma is a relatively uncommon tumor, although its
true incidence must be much higher than is thought because it is
often erroneously diagnosed as squamous cell carcinoma.  In the
Soviet literature the most complete reviews appear to have been
published by Torsuev (1959), Glazunov and Blinova (1960), and
Glazunov (1962).

    Keratoacanthoma accounts for 3 to 5% of all malignant cutaneous
neoplasms (Rook and Whimster, 1959).  The frequency ratio of keratoacanthoma to squamous cell carcinoma among Caucasians has been
reported to be approximately 1:3 irrespective of climatic differences
(Sanderson, 1968).

    Keratoacanthoma tends to occur more frequently in the male
(e.g. Blinova, 1959; Torsuev, 1959; Montgomery, 1967; Apatenko, 1973;
Sanderson, 1968).  According to Silberberg et al. (1962) and
Sanderson (1968), it affects men three times as frequently as women.
Torsuev (1959) found, from a review of nearly 300 keratoacanthoma

cases, that men had accounted for 55.3% of the cases and that the
mean age of the patients at onset of the disease was 61 ½ years.
Blinova (1959) reported the age of onset to range from 15 to 80 years
in the cases reviewed by her, with the tumor occurring most frequently between the ages of 40 and 70.  Silberberg et al. (1962)
reported a mean age of 52 years.  Sanderson (1968) remarks that
keratoacanthoma is most common in middle-aged persons and that, in
contrast to squamous cell carcinoma, the incidence does not increase
with age.  Keratoacanthoma has also been seen in children and even
infants.

Among 21 of our patients with keratoacanthoma, 9 were men and 12
women, ranging in age from 32 to 70 years (mean age = 55.6).  In the
women, the age at onset was between 61 and 70 years in 6, between 51
to 60 in 3, and between 31 and 40 in 2.  By contrast, only 3 of the 9
men were aged over 50 at onset of the disease.

The sites of predilection are exposed areas of the skin, notably
the scalp and face (e.g. Torsuev, 1959; Venkei and Sugar, 1965;
Isaeva et al., 1966,; Mashkilleison, 1970, Apatenko, 1973; Il'in,
1974; Sanderson, 1968).  According to Il'in (1974), the tumor arises
on the scalp or face in 80-85% and on the hands or arms, in 10-15% of
cases.  On the face, the favored sites are the cheeks, temples, and
nose (Il'in, 1974).  Occasionally, a solitary keratoacanthoma
develops on the vermilion border of the lip.  Mashkilleison (1970)
reported the vermilion border to have been the site of keratoacanthoma in only 70 out of over 1000 cases reported in the literature.  Silberberg et al. (1962) found the lower lip to be affected in
nearly 90% of such cases.

Among our patients, the distribution of keratoacanthomas by site
was as follows:  the face, 17 patients (cheeks in 6, nose in 5,
mandible in 3, eyelids in 2, lower lip in 1); the neck in 1; the
extremities in 2; and the trunk in 1.  Thus, in keeping with the
reports by other investigators, the tumor was located on exposed skin
areas in most of our patients.  There are also reports of atypically
located keratoacanthomas in the nail bed region (Shapiro and Baraf,
1970), conjunctiva (Freeman et al., 1961; Bellamy et al., 1963), oral
mucosa (solitary or multiple tumors) (e.g. Helshan and Buchunan,
1960; Winkelmann and Brown, 1968; Scafield et al., 1974), perineal
region (Il'in, 1974), and mucosal surface of the prepuce (Lejman and
Starzycki, 1977).  These observations of atypically sited keratoacanthomas are of considerable importance both for the histopathologic differential diagnosis of these lesions and for understanding
their histogenesis.

A vast majority of keratoacanthomas are solitary, but reports of
multiple tumors also appear in the literature from time to time (e.g.
Nehl and Ghadially, 1966; Winkelmann and Brown, 1968; Thambiah, 1969;
Vollum, 1976; Green et al., 1977; Schnitzler et al., 1977).

Clinical manifestations. In the typical case, a mature keratoacanthoma is a solitary grayish-pink or skin colored round or oval
tumor of firm consistency which is not fused with the subjacent
tissue. The center of the tumor consists of a dense grayish horny
mass which is depressed or elevated relative to the surface of the
rest of the tumor and is surrounded with a rolled rim covered by
tightly stretched epidermis, The size of this epithelial elevation
depends on the area occupied by the horny mass, and may be larger in
a developing lesion (Figure 53a) than in an established one (53b).
In some cases, the keratinous crater is ill defined (Figure 54) and
appears to consist of partially fused keratinous plugs; in such cases
the roundish shape of the keratoacanthoma is preserved. Usually
keratoacanthomas are 10 to 20 mm in diameter, although giant tumors
are occasionally observed; Del Rossi et al. (1977) have described a
keratoacanthoma as large as 22 x 19 cm.

There are three phases in the development of keratoacanthoma.
The first phase is one of growth which lasts 3-4 weeks, but is particularly fast during the first 8-10 days after onset of the tumor
(Torsuev, 1959). This attains its maximum size approximately in a
month after which growth stops and the static phase begins which
lasts 2-3 weeks to be succeeded by one of involution. In this last
phase, the keratoacanthoma progressively flattens, the horny mass
detaches, and the border of the lesion becomes indistinct in places
(Figure 55); finally the tumor regresses completely leaving behind a
puckered or pitted scar.

Kopf (1968) distinguished the following atypical clinical forms
or types of keratoacanthomas: (1) periungual and subungual; (2)
multiple; (3) eruptive (as many as several hundred tumors may be
present); (4) giant; (5) multinodular (synonyms: centrifugal or
aggregated) - a form which results from coalescence of several
lesions, grows slowly, and often lack a central crater; (6) verrucous (the tumor surface is covered with a hyperkeratotic mass);
(7) vegetating (the tumor surface is made up of polypoid excrescences
capped by horny material; and (8) persistent (the tumor persists up to
8 months or longer). Hundeiker (1978) has pointed out that the typical "crateriform" keratoacanthoma occurs in approximately 90% of
cases, while in the remaining cases atypical forms are seen, such as
flat keratoacanthomas, keratoacanthoma marginatum centrifugum, the
aggregated form (several closely spaced tumors), or multiple keratoacanthomas arising in succession.

The question of how long keratoacanthomas develop and persist is
of great interest, for the criterion of time has often been relied
upon in attempts to differentiate a keratoacanthoma from a squamous
cell carcinoma (Montgomery, 1967; Burge and Winkelmann, 1969;
Sanderson, 1968). It must be acknowledged that this question is
still debatable.. Usually, a keratoacanthoma takes 2 to 3 months to
develop and regress, but instances of slowly developing and long-

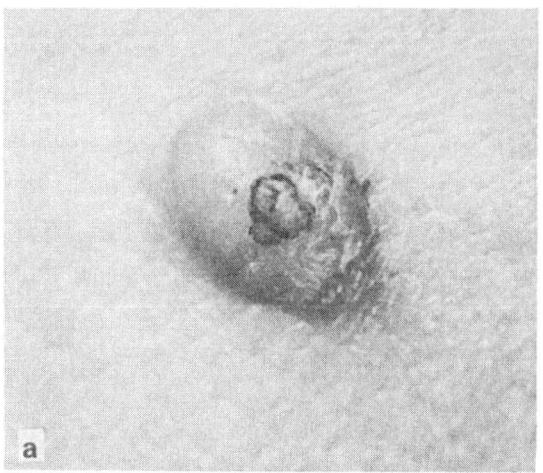

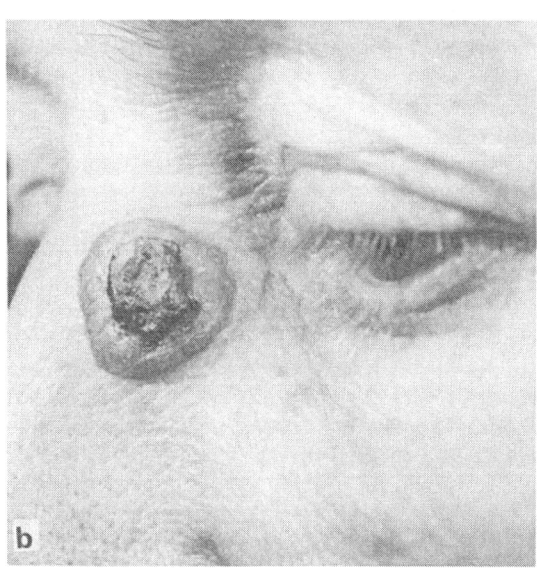

Fig. 53. Keratoacanthoma.  (a) Five-week-old tumor on the cheek;
(b) fully developed tumor of 2½ months' duration on the
nose.

lasting keratoacanthoma have been reported.  For example, Rook and
Whimster (1979) and Huriez et al. (1957) described cases where
keratoacanthoma underwent resolution as late as 4 to 6 months after
onset, and Vollum (1976) saw a woman with dozens of keratoacanthomas
that had persisted for 2½ years.  Shanin (1969) stated that in young
persons certain keratoacanthomas located on the back or in the anal
region may run a course protracted for years, fail to resolve spontaneously, and show a poor response even to roentgen therapy; should

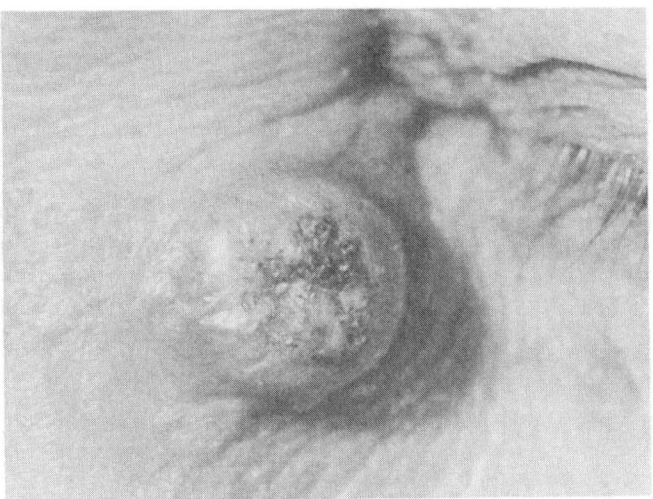

Fig. 54.   Keratoacanthoma of 7 weeks' duration with an ill-defined
horny crater.

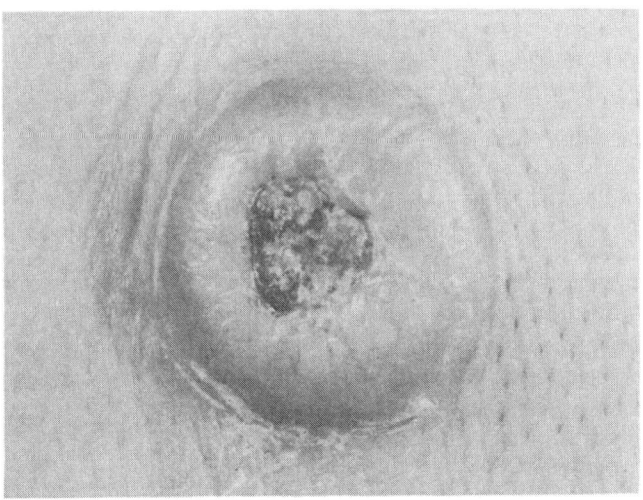

Fig. 55.   Keratoacanthoma undergoing involution 3 months after onset.

the tumor take such an atypical course, the diagnosis of keratoacanthoma may well be questioned.

In our patients, the age of the lesion at the time of examination was approximately 1 month in 1 patient, 1-2 months in 2, 2-3
in 4, 3-4 in 2, 4-6 in 7, 6-7 in 3, and about 12 months in 2.   Thus,

in only a third of the patients had the tumors been evolving for
periods characteristic of the "classical" keratoacanthoma, that is
for 3 months or so.  In 5 of the remaining 14 patients, they had been
present for 5 to 12 months and could be assigned to the atypical
persistent type according to Kopf's (1968) classification.  These
findings may suggest that keratoacanthomas of relatively long duration are not so uncommon as is thought.

Histologic appearance.  The histologic structure of keratoacanthoma has been well described in detail in many publications
(e.g. Grzhebin and Tseraidis, 1969; Montgomery, 1967; Apatenko, 1973;
Vikhert et al., 1973; Golovin, 1975; Lever and Schaumberg-Lever,
1975; Sanderson and Mackie, 1979).

This is a sharply demarcated elevated tumor showing considerable
hyperkeratosis and pseudocarcinomatous epidermal hyperplasia.  A
section passing through the center of the tumor reveals an invagin-
ation of the acanthotic epidermis which forms a crater filled with
horny material predominantly of orthokeratotic structure.  At the
margin of the crater the epidermis thins and extends like "lips"
which overhang the crater and strive, as it were, to embrace the
horny mass in the manner of a collarette.  The overall histologic
picture resembles a horn-filled cup (Figure 56a).  The epidermis at
the base of the cup extends irregularly down into the dermis to the
level of the sweat glands in places or even, according to Glazunov
and Blinova (1960), into the muscle. The sheets of stratified epithelium produce irregular outgrowths from which aggregates of cells
have budded off to form epithelial nests separated from the
acanthotic epidermis (Figure 56b).  Basal cells within the zone of
epidermal outgrowths are arranged disorderly or are indescernible in
places.  The cytoplasms of spinous cells stain unevenly.  In the
center of the epidermal strands, one observes horny material surrounded by concentrically arranged spinous cells with partially
preserved, elongated nuclei.  There is marked cellular disarray and
nuclear polymorphism.  Cells with giant hyperchromic or homogeneous
nuclei that resemble dyskeratotic elements are present (Figure 56c).
The tumor stroma and the upper portions of the dermis show a diffuse
infiltrate composed of lymphocytes and histiocytes admixed with
plasma cells and polymorphonuclear leukocytes.  Cells of the infiltrate surround the epidermal proliferations in a tight manner, but
only the occasional cells penetrate into these.  Although individual
keratoacanthomas may have specific histologic characteristics, the
basic feature is, as already mentioned, a pseudocarcinomatous hyperplasia which is difficult, or at times even impossible (Rook and
Whimster, 1950), to distinguish from a well-differentiated squamous
cell carcinoma.

The question of how keratoacanthoma relates to squamous cell
carcinoma is central to determining the identity of the tumor.  The
frequency of keratoacanthoma relative to that of squamous cell
carcinoma has been variously reported to range from 1:4 to 1:2
(Scarpa, 1971).

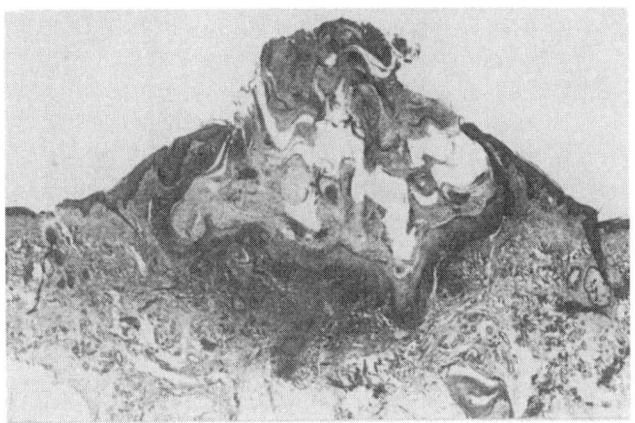

Fig. 56a.  Keratoacanthoma on cheek skin.  General view, showing a
horny cup with overhanging epithelial "lips" (13 X).

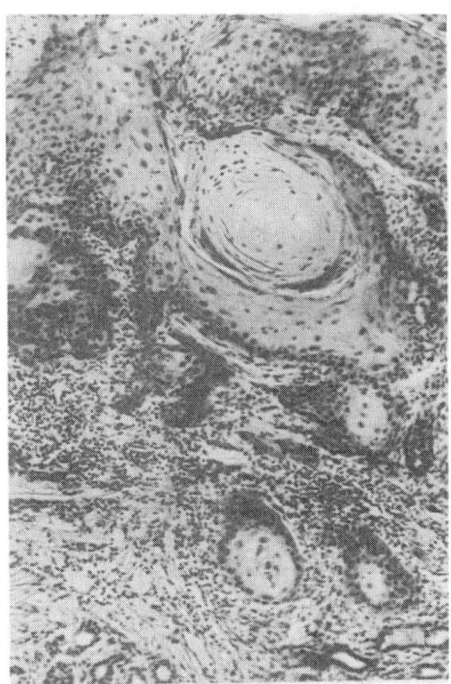

Fig. 56b.  Keratoacanthoma on cheek skin.  Epidermal proliferations
deep in the dermis (75 X).

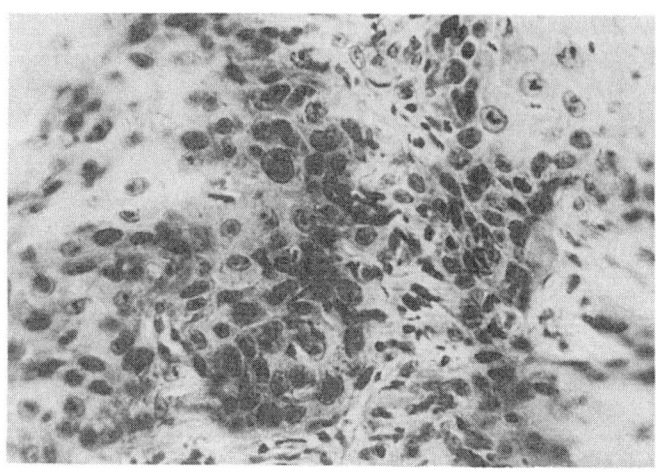

Fig. 56c.  Keratoacanthoma on cheek skin.  Same specimen at higher
           (250 X) magnification, showing cellular disorganization
           and nuclear polymorphism within epidermal proliferations.
           (Hematoxylin and eosin.)


        Rook and Gronin (1962) found from a review of 404 kerato-
acanthoma cases that the tumor had recurred in 5% of the cases and
noted that malignant transformation of keratoacanthoma always remains
a possibility.  Scarpa (1971), for example, observed such transformation in 5 cases out of 8.  Accordingly, a number of authors place
keratoacanthoma in the group of precancerous cutaneous conditions
(e.g. Grzhebin and Tseraidis 1960; Pinkus and Mehregan, 1969; Shanin,
1969; Zegarelli, 1975) and some even go as far as to identify keratoacanthoma with squamous cell carcinoma.  Lowry et al (1972), for
instance, regard them as essentially identical conditions, stating
that the course and spontaneous resolution of a keratoacanthoma
depend on the general state of the body and of its defences.  Muer et
al. (1967), Bakker and Tjou (1971), and Poleksis (1974) consider
keratoacanthoma and squamous cell carcinoma as being closely related
conditions on the ground that some patients with keratoacanthoma have
primary squamous cell carcinoma of internal organs.  It appears, though
that in such cases the keratoacanthoma is a cutaneous manifestation of
the underlying internal malignant disease.

        There are reports of metatases occurring in regional lymph nodes
several years after excision or irradiation of a typical keratoacanthoma (e.g. Belisario, 1954; Anderson, 1957).  Such reports,
however, testify to the difficulties involved in diagnostic differentiation between keratoacanthoma and squamous cell carcinoma, rather
than to a causal relationship between the two.

The histogenesis of keratoacanthoma is still a matter for debate. There are three points of view regarding its origin. Some authors (e.g. McCormac and Scarff, 1936; Venkei and Sugar, 1965; Kalkoff et al., 1968; Connors and Ackerman, 1976) believe that ordinarily this neoplasm springs from the pilosebaceous follicles. Others (e.g. Rook and Whimster, 1950; Santha Cruz and Clausen, 1977) hold the view that it arises from the excretory ducts of sweat glands. Thus, Santa Cruz and Clausen (1977) found sweat gland ducts to be hyperplastic in all 20 keratoacanthomas which they studied. Still others (e.g. Blinova, 1959; Glazunov and Blinova, 1960; Apatenko, 1973) are of the opinion that keratoacanthoma takes its origin in the surface epithelium. This view, which is believed by Apatenko (1973) to be the most valid and widespread, is supported by the occurrence of keratoacanthomas on the oral mucosa, the vermilion border of the lip, and the mucosal surface of the prepuce, that is, in areas devoid of both pilosebaceous follicles and sweat glands.

Etiology and pathogenesis. The causes of keratoacanthoma have not yet been fully elucidated. Many authors have presented evidence strongly suggestive of viral origin (Fouracres and Whittick, 1953; Hamperl and Kalkoff, 1954; Glazunov, 1962; Ereaux et al., 1955; Glazunov and Blinova, 1960; Gay Prieto et al., 1964). As noted by Sanderson (1968), the viral concept is supported by the fact that keratoacanthoma has been observed to arise in skin autografts in patients with multiple keratoacanthomas. Structures resembling virus particles have been reported present in histologic sections of keratoacanthoma (Glazunov, 1962), including those examined under the electron microscope (Ereaux et al., 1955; Gay Prieto et al., 1964), although no one has ever succeeded in isolating a keratoacanthoma virus and infecting experimental animals with it. It is thought by many that keratoacanthomas are caused by various agents that irritate the skin, such as solar radiation (Randazzo and Tichera, 1963; Sanderson, 1968); mechanical or thermal trauma (Montgomery, 1967; Kopf, 1968): and tar, pitch, mineral oils, or other chemical irritants (Rook and Whimster, 1950; Whiteley, 1957; Ghadially et al., 1963). Montgomery (1967) emphasized the possible involvement of immune and genetic factors in the production of keratoacanthoma. Gay Prieto et al (1964) reported other family members to be affected in 0.5% of keratoacanthoma cases. Rook and Maffatt (1962) consider that cases of unilaterally distributed multiple keratoacanthomas should be classed among nevoid conditions. Keratoacanthomas may arise on a dermatosis such as lupus vulgaris, lupus erythematosus, neurodermatitis, toxicodermas, psoriasis, ichthyosis, etc. (Randazzo, 1966; Kopf, 1968; Miedzinski et al., 1973). In view of this, the possibility of a causal relationship existing between keratoacanthoma and the dermatitis in which it arises has been under discussion, as has been the possible stimulatory effect on the production of keratoacanthoma of various medicines, in particular tuberculostatic drugs (Randazzo, 1966).

Among our patients, the tumor was found to have followed a mechanical trauma in 8 cases, prolonged exposure to sunlight in 3, and insect bites in 2, while in 1 case it arose in disseminated lupus erythematosus.

Differential diagnosis. The primary differential diagnostic consideration is well-differentiated squamous cell carcinoma. It must be noted, however, that the existing clinical and especially histopathologic diagnostic criteria for distinguishing between these two different neoplasms cannot always be relied upon and, indeed, it is believed by some (e.g. Rook and Whimster, 1950; Belisario, 1954; Maggiera, 1968; Zegarelli, 1975) that in some cases it is quite impossible to distinguish a keratoacanthoma from a squamous cell carcinoma. A review of the literature and our personal experience indicate that the differential diagnosis must involve comprehensive assessment and correlation of clinical and histopathologic features. These may be subdivided into absolute and relative. The absolute clinical features of keratoacanthoma include development of the tumor on unaltered skin, presence of a central horn-filled crater, absence of ulceration and of regional lymph node enlargement even a long time after onset of the tumor, and spontaneous regression of the lesion. A relative clinical feature is growth rate. This is usually slow with keratoacanthomas and rapid with squamous carcinomas, although the reverse may be true occasionally (Montgomery, 1967; Maggiera, 1968; Pinkus and Mehregan, 1969).

The absolute histopathologic features of keratoacanthoma may be taken to include presence of a collarette and of "lips" overhanging the horn-filled crater, predominantly ortokeratotic structure of the horny material, absence of cellular anaplasia, and exocytosis. It is held by a number of authors (e.g. Raichev et al., 1964; Randazzo, 1966; Sanderson, 1968; Pinkus and Mehregan, 1969) that in kerato-acanthoma, in contrast to squamous cell carcinoma, the epidermal strands do not extend beyond the sweat gland level, the nucleo-cytoplasmic ratios are normal, there is no dyskeratosis, the number of mitoses is small, and the basement membrane is intact. Our own experience suggests, however, that these are only relative diagnostic criteria at best. For example, during the growth phase mitotic activity in keratoacanthoma may be the same as, or even higher than, in squamous cell carcinoma, and only the number and types of patho-logic mitoses may be different. Also, in keratoacanthoma, epidermal strands may extend beyond the sweat gland level, at times even into the subcutaneous fat (Montgomery, 1967; Glazunov, 1962), and the basement membrane may be indetectable in places. As observed by Montgomery (1967), nests of epithelial cells deep within the dermis and basement membrane destruction are not uncommon in kerato-acanthoma, but, unlike in squamous cell carcinoma, cells of the infiltrate invade the epithelial aggregates.

Many authors (e.g. Rook and Whimster, 1950; Grzhebin and Tseraidis, 1960; Apatenko, 1973; Lever and Schaumburg-Lever, 1975; Pinkus and Mehregan, 1976) have emphasized that in keratoacanthoma, epithelial cells display individual cell keratinization so that horn pearls are often found in deep portions of the tumor, but that, in contrast to a well-differentiated squamous cell carcinoma, many of the pearls are parakeratotic in structure.  It has been considered by some that a feature of considerable diagnostic importance is the development, during the regressive phase of keratoacanthoma, of granulation tissue with giant cells which is subsequently replaced by fibrosis (e.g. Glazunov and Blinova, 1960; Raichev et al., 1964).

A correlation of the clinical and histopathologic findings is of course necessary if the correct diagnosis is to be arrived at, and teamwork between the clinician and pathologist is important in difficult cases.  One may well agree with Sanderson (1968) in that if the clinician and pathologist have failed to come to an agreement, the final judgement rests with the clinician.

Keratoacanthoma should be separated also from verruca vulgaris, giant mulluscum contagiosum, senile keratoma, cutaneous horn, Kyrle's disease, and multiple self-healing squamous cell carcinoma of Ferguson-Smith.

The distinctive features of verruca vulgaris are the predominant localization to the hands (fingers) and feet; the frequent presence of multiple lesions; the absence of a keratinous crater; the papillomatous epidermal growth; and the presence of vacuolated cells.

Giant molluscum contagiosum appears as a round shiny structure with central umbilication, often accompanied by multiple eruptions; there is no keratinous crater, and histologic examination reveals Feulgen-positive intracytoplasmic inclusion bodies ("molluscum bodies").

Senile keratoma, unlike keratoacanthoma, is a slowly developing lesion characterized by the absence of epithelial elevation or horn-filled crater and by histologic changes in the epidermis resembling Bowen's disease.

The verrucous form of keratoacanthoma is sometimes difficult to distinguish from cutaneous horn, but a cutaneous horn develops very slowly, does not display a pronounced epidermal elevation, and reveals an erosive and ulcerative surface when removed forcibly. Histologically, cutaneous horns are characterized by irregular thickening of the granular layer and sometimes by cellular polymorphism resembling that seen in senile keratoma, and by severe hyperkeratosis; no marked acanthosis and no "horny cup" are present.

Hundeiker (1975) has reported from his experience that the clinical diagnosis of keratoacanthoma is confirmed histologically in 75% of cases, but that in 20% of cases histologic examination reveals squamous cell carcinoma. In a subsequent paper, Hundeiker (1978) has observed that keratoacanthoma is misdiagnosed as cancer in approximately 30% of cases and as nodular basalioma in 12%. These observations serve to emphasize the need for close collaboration between clinicians and pathologists in the diagnosis of keratoacanthoma.

Kyrle's disease (hyperkeratosis follicularis et perifollicularis in cutem penetrans) has as its distinguishing features a multiplicity of lesions which are located on clothed areas of the skin, and a follicular hyperkeratosis which extends down into the dermis.

Multiple keratoacanthoma is not easy to distinguish from a multiple self-healing squamous cell carcinoma of Ferguson-Smith, but the latter tends to run in families and to occur before the age of 40 years. However, some authors (e.g. Grzybowski, 1950; Fouracres and Wittick, 1953; Sanderson, 1968; Schnitzler et al., 1977) do not see any essential difference between these two conditions and are inclined to regard Ferguson-Smith's self-healing carcinoma as a variant of multiple keratoacanthoma.

## 8.2  PAPILLOMATOSIS CUTIS CARCINOIDES OF GOTTRON

In 1932, Gottron reported a case of tumorlike and papillomatous epidermal growths on the lower legs characterized histologically by invasive epidermal proliferation and hyperkeratosis without any other signs of malignancy. Although the lesions had persisted for as long as 15 years, the regional lymph nodes displayed only reactive changes and there were no mestastases. Gottron called this condition "papillomatosis cutis". A few years later he described a similar condition in a 40-year-old man in whom cauliflowerlike growths had arisen in a lichen on the sole of the foot to encroach on the dorsolateral aspect of the foot; the regional lymph nodes were enlarged, but no metastases were apparent, even though the disease had persisted for about 17 years. In 1950, Nikolowski and Eisenlohr described yet another patient with clinical and histopathologic features similar to those observed in the two cases referred to above. In view of the close external similarity of the lesions in squamous cell carcinoma to those in papillomatosis cutis, the above authors expanded the latter title by adding to it the word carcinoides and also the name "Gottron" to do credit to the man who was first to describe this condition. Subsequently, the term papillomatosis cutis carcinoides of Gottron became firmly established in the dermatologic literature.

Papillomatosis cutis carcinoides of Gottron is a rare disease, only about 30 cases having been reported up to 1976 (Ribodli and Del Pozzo, 1976). However, the actual frequency is likely to be higher, for some cases of what was a true papillomatosis cutis carcinoides were probably diagnosed as squamous cell carcinoma because these two conditions are so similar both clinically and histologically.

Although the absence of a comprehensive review of cases of papillomatosis cutis carcinoides of Gottron precludes any definite judgement as to the age and sex predilection, it appears that men beyond the age of 40 years are affected most frequently. Thus, among the 5 cases seen by us and 18 others described in the available literature (Gottron, 1932, 1954; Miescher, 1950; Nikolowski and Eisenlohr, 1950; Rathjens, 1953; Adams et al., 1956; Schuppiner and Steinke, 1960; Wodniansky, 1960; Döring, 1961; Khristin et al., 1963; Schimpf and Seller, 1963; Venkei and Sugar, 1965; Fomin et al., 1971; Roboldi and Del Pozzo, 1976) 15 were men and only 8 women, ranging in age from 40 to 85 years.

Clinical manifestations. The lesions persist for years or decades, do not undergo necrosis or ulceration, show no metastases, and, in the early reports, are described as being distributed symmetrically and confined to the lower extremities. More recent observations have shown, however, that they may be arranged asymmetrically and occur on the upper extremities, trunk, and even the oral mucosa (Rathjens, 1953; Grixoni, 1955; Adam et al., 1956; Scheicher-Gottron, 1958). The disease usually arises on a preexisting dermatosis of long standing (eczema, lichen planus, ichthyosis, lupus vulgaris, etc.) or in scars.

An established lesion presents as a flattened plaque the size of a child's palm or larger sharply delimited from the uninvolved skin and rising 1-1½ cm above its level. The surface of the plaque is covered with tumorlike structures of doughy consistency resembling raw meat in color, and with vegetations resembling a cauliflower. Between the villous excrescences and between the tumorous conglomerates there are furrows filled with a yellowish-whitish ointment-like horny mass. Not uncommonly the surfaces of papillomatous growths are covered with a malodorous dense sticky secretion, which has dried up in places to produce yellowish-gray crusts; in some cases erosions and superficial ulcerations may be present on a background of macerated vegetations.

In individual cases the clinical appearance may differ somewhat from the one described above; thus, a pronounced hyperkeratosis or exuberant granulations that bleed readily may be found in an occasional case.

Fomin et al. (1971) observed areas of calcification within the lesions of Gottron's papillomatosis and stated that calcification areas, if present, may be helpful in the differential diagnosis of this disease.

With the course of time, the clinical changes described above tend to obliterate completely those of the preexisting dermatosis, but residual manifestations of the latter, expressed to varying degrees (depending on the skin area involved), may occasionally persist at the periphery of the lesion.

Of the five cases seen in our clinic, papillomatosis cutis carcinoides had arisen in lichen planus hypertrophicus in two and in chronic eczema and varicose veins in the other three.

Histologic appearance. This is characterized mainly by a carcinomatous epidermal hyperplasia. Acanthotic epidermal ridges that are composed of spinous cells penetrate deep into the dermis and may appear as thin processes or be highly irregular in outline, and collections of epithelial cells that had separated out from the acanthotic epidermal proliferations may be seen. However, as pointed out by Gottron and Nikolowski (1960), there is no cellular atypia, and the basement membrane remains intact everywhere, and the epidermal processes show keratinization, tubular horny masses, and incompletely keratinized cells resembling "pearls". According to Gottron and Nikolowski, a characteristic feature is the presence of large amounts of glycogen in the proliferating keratinocytes. The stroma surrounding the epithelial proliferations displays a pronounced lymphohistiocytic infiltrate admixed with plasma cells. The histologic appearance may vary from one lesional area to another as the disease evolves (Schimpf and Seller, 1963). The small nodules seen early during its course present an appearance marked by acanthosis, circumscribed papillomatosis, and exudative inflammation in the dermis which shows a lymphohistiocytic infiltrate with many mast cells. Larger nodules (the size of a pea or kidney bean) are characterized by acanthosis, papillomatosis and an exudative reaction of obscure origin in the connective tissue. Still larger, hemispheric tumors (the size of a chestnut) show acanthosis, papillomatosis, and the presence of deeply seated horny material. It is only with large tumorous growths that the acanthosis presents an appearance of pseudocarcinomatous hyperplasia with hyperkeratosis and horny masses within the aggregations of keratinocytes lying deep in the dermis. The histologic appearance bears close resemblance to that of a well-differentiated squamous cell carcinoma, especially when considered in relation to the clinical features.

The histogenesis of papillomatosis cutis carcinoides is not fully understood, and its nature remains unknown. Gottron himself regards it as a separate disease entity unrelated to squamous cell carcinoma. Some authors (e.g. Gay Prieto and Cascos, 1951; Civatte, 1967) equate it with the chronic vegetating pyoderma of Azua. Others (Adam et al., 1956; Miescher, 1957; Schruppiner and Steinke, 1960) do not draw any distinction between it and a well-differentiated squamous carcinoma. For instance, Schruppiner and Steinke (1960) described a case of cutaneous squamous cell carcinoma that had pre-

viously been interpreted as papillomatosis cutis carcinoides on both
clinical and histopathologic grounds, while Gonin (cited in Khristin
et al., 1963) reported metastases and a fatal outcome in a patient
diagnosed 10 years before as having Gottron's papillomatosis.
Raichev and Andreev (1965) and Venkei and Sugar (1965) consider
papillomatosis cutis carcinoides as a precancerous condition intermediate between cancer and noncancer.  Wodniansky (1960) believes
that papillomatosis cutis carcinoides of Gottron, as well as chronic
vegetating pyoderma of Azua, is not a disease entity, but represents
a kind of pseudocarcinomatous hyperplasia that may develop on the
basis of various chronic inflammatory disorders of the skin.

Etiology and pathogenesis.  Particular importance in the causation of this condition has been attached to mechanical trauma, but
it is possible that a significant role is played by the chronic
inflammation that occurs in the preexistent dermatosis (Nikolowski
and Eisenlohr, 1950; Rathjens, 1958; Wodniansky, 1960) and by circulatory disturbances in the lower extremities leading to acrocyanosis,
as well as by the altered general reactivity of the body which, in
the final analysis, determines the proneness to papillomatous growths
and their persistence (Schimpf and Seller, 1963; Raichev and Andreev,
1965; Fischer, 1975).

Differential diagnosis.  Papillomatosis cutis carcinoides of
Gottron has to be distinguished mainly from highly differentiated
squamous cell carcinoma and from chronic vegetating pyoderma.

The clinical features of carcinoid papillomatosis that distinguish it from squamous carcinoma include the gradual, slow
evolution of the lesions in the form of plaques which develop tumorlike excrescences and vegetations on their surfaces; the absence of
ulcerations and of elevated borders; the doughy consistency of the
fungating growths on the lesional surface; and the persistence of the
lesions for a long time (even for decades) without any metastases
or alterations being seen in the regional lymph nodes.

Diagnostic problems may arise if carcinoid papillomatosis arises
in scars, since the development of epidermal hyperplasia at sites of
atrophic scars always arouses suspicion of malignancy.  In such
cases, histologic findings should be helpful.  Two important points
of difference from a differentiated squamous cell carcinoma are that
in carcinoid papillomatosis the acanthotic epidermal strands (1) are
invariably composed of well differentiated cells without signs of
anaplasia and (2) show the presence of tubular horny masses.  Gottron
and Nikolowski (1960), who have attached great significance to histochemical findings, have pointed out that a distinctive feature of
carcinoid papillomatosis is a high content of glycogen in the cells
of epidermal proliferations.  However, as indicated by Apatenko
(1973), although glycogen is absent from the cells of undifferentiated squamous cell carcinoma, it is always abundant in those of a

well-differentiated growth.  More important distinguishing characteristics appear to be the intactness of the basement membrane and
the presence of a perivascular infiltrate composed of lymphocytes,
histiocytes, and mast cells which invade the epidermal proliferations
in places.  Prolonged follow-up of the patient, with repeated
biopsies taken from different lesion areas, is necessary, however,
if malignancy is to be ruled out completely.

Usually, papillomatosis cutis carcinoides of Gottron differs
from chronic vegetating pyoderma of Azua by showing symmetrical
distribution of the lesions which are confined to the lower legs, are
flat, large, and run a protracted, but not progressive, course.  On
the other hand, it is difficult, if not impossible, to separate
chronic vegetating pyoderma (pseudoepithelioma of Azua) from carcinoid papillomatosis in cases where the lesions are located atypically, asymmetrically, or are solitary.  Histopathologic findings may
then be helpful, for although pseudocarcinomatous hyperplasia is
pronounced in both these conditions, chronic vegetating pyoderma,
unlike carcinoid papillomatosis, often exhibits the presence of
cavities and cysts containing leukocytes and cellular detritus and
also the widespread permeation of the epidermal proliferations by
cells of a massive infiltrate.  Should the diagnosis still remain in
doubt, the problem may be resolved by observing the response to
treatment: combined antiinflammatory, antibacterial, and nonspecific
therapy is effective in chronic pyoderma vegetans, but not in papillomatosis cutis carcinoides.

Lastly, papillomatosis cutis carcinoides of Gottron should be
differentiated also from tuberculosis cutis verrucosa and the deep
mycoses.  Here, demonstration of the causative organisms in effusions
or histologic specimens from the lesions should clinch the diagnosis.
Moreover, warty tuberculosis shows a fairly typical clinical picture,
a multiplicity of lesions, and marked hyperkeratosis.

## 8.3  GIANT CONDYLOMA ACUMINATUM OF BUSCHKE AND LOEWENSTEIN

The first report of giant condyloma acuminatum was provided by
Buschke in 1896, and in 1925 Buschke and Loewenstein described a
giant condyloma of the penis under the name "carcinoma-like condyloma
acuminatum", thus emphasizing its close clinical resemblance to
squamous cell carcinoma.  They wrote that while the clinical presen-
tation of the giant condyloma acuminatum was that of a carcinoma, its
histologic appearance was devoid of any sign suggestive of malignancy.

Giant condyloma acuminatum of Buschke and Loewenstein is a rare
disease.  Thus, Netto et al. (1976) found only just over 90 cases
described in the literature.  But the true frequency is difficult to
establish because many cases of what was actually giant condyloma

acuminatum have been diagnosed as epidermoid cancer and, conversely, true carcinomas are at times misdiagnosed as giant condylomas.

The usual site of giant condyloma acuminatum is the penis (Buschke and Loewenstein, 1925; Loewenstein, 1939; Machacek and Weakley, 1960; Seigel, 1962; Anderson, 1971; Lever and Schaumburg-Lever, 1975; Goldstein et al., 1977; Wilkinson, 1968) but it has also been reported to occur in other areas of the skin, including the perineal (Dawson et al., 1965; Magenburg et al., 1977) and anorectal (Knoblich and Failing, 1967) regions, the inguinal fold (Machacek and Weakley, 1960), the vulva (Judge, 1969), the abdomen and thigh (Bedi and Pandhi, 1977), the mucous membranes of the urinary bladder and urethra (Bissada et al., 1974), and the oral mucosa (Bazex et al., 1972; Reiffers et al., 1976). Most of the patients were men. In women the disease is exceedingly rare (e.g. Dawson et al., 1965; Bissada et al., 1974; Mayenburg et al., 1977).

Clinical manifestations. As a rule, giant condyloma acuminatum affects middle-aged men and arises on the coronary sulcus or on the inner surface of the prepuce. The onset is sudden, with the appearance of small wartlike nodules or papillomatous elements in several areas at a time, usually on unaltered skin. Netto et al. (1976) noted, however, a frequent association of giant condyloma acuminatum with phimosis.

The lesions rapidly enlarge and become confluent to form a large sessile tumor whose surface is composed of vegetations and villous structures with intervening well-defined fissures. As the tumor enlarges, the vegetations become more pronounced and their surface comes to be partly covered by horny scales and partly macerated, with a foul-smelling exudate accumulating in the interpapillary fissures. In a well established tumor, especially if it shows invasive growth, the fissures give rise to deep sinuses whose exudate becomes secondarily infected.

A characteristic clinical feature of giant condyloma acuminatum is its relentless progression, with destruction of the prepuce, invasion of the cavernous bodies, and compression of the urethra or formation of urethral fistulas (Bedi and Pandhi, 1977). South et al. (1977) described a giant condyloma in the perineal region that had grown out into the small pelvis leading to a fatal outcome in a young woman. Another clinical feature of the tumor is its marked tendency to recur, even after a wide excision (Machacek and Weakley, 1960; Judge, 1969; South et al., 1977). However, even in cases of invasive carcinomalike growth, the regional lymph nodes show reactive changes only, without any metatases being detectable. In some cases the growth is predominantly expansive, with the formation of a cauliflowerlike lesion by confluent wartlike structures and with the appearance of satellite condylomata acuminata at the tumor periphery.

Of the five patients seen in our clinic, the tumor was located
in the penis in 4 and at the left upper eyelid in 1.  In this latter
case, small condylomalike lesions were also present on the right
lower eyelid and in the armpits.  As we have not encountered any
mention of similar cases in the literature,  it is worthwhile to
describe this case in detail.

Patient V., a 24-year-old male driver, was referred to
our department from the Department of Ophthalmology of our
Institute (Moscow Regional Institute for Clinical Research)
to undergo surgery for a tumor on the left upper eyelid.
He said that over the past six months sties had been appearing and disappearing repeatedly on his upper eyelid and
that the last of these had arisen 4 months before to grow
rapidly and to involve the entire eyelid in a month.  He
had consulted an oculist, a surgeon, and an oncologist at
the place of his residence, and on histologic grounds his
condition had been diagnosed as "papillomatosis without
signs of malignant change."  He had received antibiotics,
autohemotransfusions, and topical applications of a
mercurial ointment, but without any benefit. On the contrary, the lesion on the upper eyelid had evolved into a
tumor that closed the eye completely.  By that time, papillomatous elements had appeared also on the right lower
eyelid and in the axillae.  He had a history of measles and
dysentery in childhood.  He said he had never had tuberculosis or venereal disease and that no member of his family
had ever been afflicted with a condition similar to his.

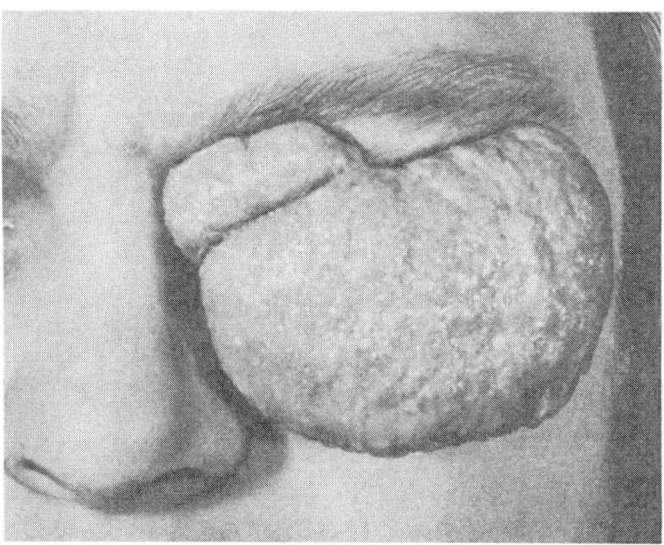

Fig. 57.  Giant condyloma acuminatum of Buschke and Loewenstein.

On physical examination, a massive tumor that had
closed the entire left eye was seen (Figure 57).  The tumor
was pink, firm to palpation and had a knobby surface composed of a multitude of smoothed-out villous formations
covered with a sticky seropurulent exudate.  The eyelid
skin at the base of the tumor was edematous and hyperemic.
In the region of the right lower eyelid there was a grayish
wartlike structure 0.5 x 1 cm in size covered by keratinizing papillomatous outgrowths.  Vision in the right eye
was normal.  The refractory media were transparent.  The
fundus oculi: the optic disk was pink, the borders well
defined, and the vessels normal.  In the axillae, dark pink
lesions with rather well defined but irregular borders and
containing multiple condylomatous structures were seen
(Figure 58).  Some of the lesions had fused to produce a
larger diffuse lesion showing deep folds and grooves, while
the other, smaller, lesions (about 0.5 cm in diameter) were
composed of individual elements arranged in groups and were
covered by thick malodorous exudates.  At the upper pole of
one such larger lesion there was a cone-shaped condyloma
with a macerated knobby surface measuring about 3 cm in
diameter at the base and some 2.5 cm in height.  The
exudates from the lesions in the left eye region and

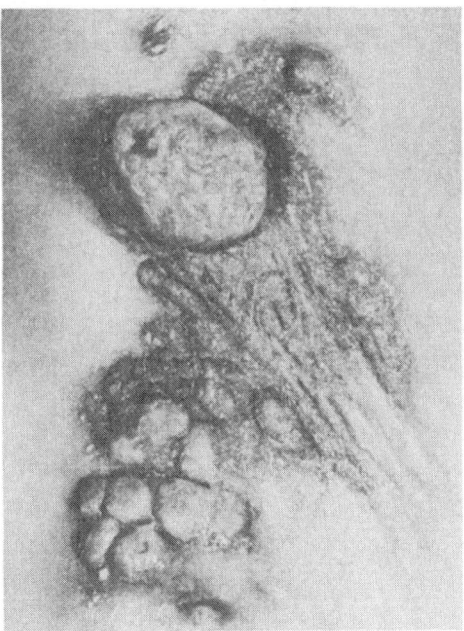

Fig. 58.  Giant condyloma acuminatum of Buschke and Loewenstein in
the axillary region of same patient as in Fig. 57.

axillae were found to contain epidermal staphylococci
sensitive to various antibiotics.

Histologic examination of a biopsy specimen from the
tumor in the left eye region (Figure 59) revealed a hyperplastic spinous layer showing irregularly shaped acanthotic
strands projecting into the dermis. In places, collections
of epidermal cells that had separated from the mass of the
proliferating epidermis were seen. There was moderate
hyperkeratosis of a parakeratotic structure. Horny cysts
were present in some areas. No cellular polymorphism was
noted. Thus, the biopsy specimen presented an appearance
of pseudocarcinomatous hyperplasia compatible with the
diagnosis of giant condyloma acuminatum. A similar histologic picture was seen in the biopsy specimen taken from an
axillary lesion.

In the Department of Ophthalmology, the left upper
eyelid was removed and a plastic operation was done to
repair the defect. The patient was then given intramuscular injections of cephaloridine in a total dose of
10 000 000 units and applications of 50% Prospidinum ointment to the axillary lesions.

The subsequent histologic studies of specimens from
various areas of the removed tumor were interpreted as
indicating "an epithelioma with local destructive growth",
but the clinical features (rapid evolution of the tumor,

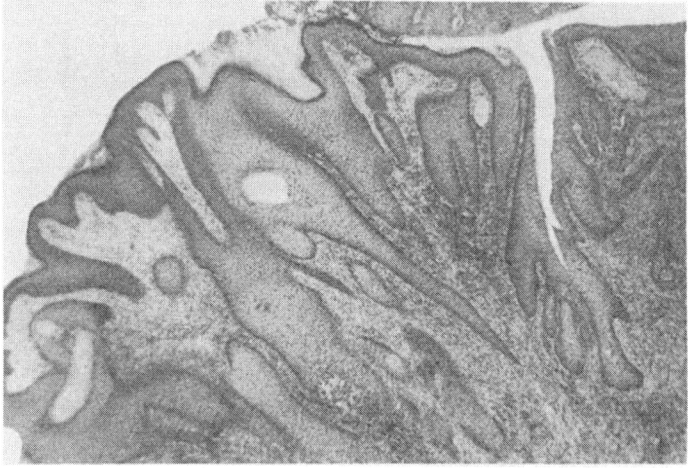

Fig. 59.   Giant condyloma acuminatum in the upper eyelid of same
           patient as in Figs. 57 and 58, showing striking acanthosis
           and pseudocarcinomatous epidermal hyperplasia. (50 X;
           hematoxylin and eosin.)

multiple condylomalike lesions, unaltered regional lymph
nodes) argued against this conclusion. The patient was
discharged in a good condition: the skin graft was successful and the lesions in the armpits had resolved. However,
1½ months thereafter, rapidly enlarging condylomata
acuminata reappeared around the postoperative scar on the
left upper eyelid to result, within a month, in the formation of a cauliflower lesion 2 x 3 cm in size. The lesion
was again excised and another plastic operation was performed.

Multiple biopsies from various areas of the excised
tumor showed papillomatosis accompanied by pseudocarcinomatous hyperplasia. Within the proliferations of acanthotic
epidermis, hyperchromic cells with signs of polymorphism
(incomplete individual cell keratinization) were noted in
places.

The histologic diagnosis was "papilloma undergoing
malignant degeneration". Again, it was decided to forgo
roentgen therapy. A course of nonspecific pyrogenic treatment with Prodigiosanum was carried out instead, as was a
repeat course of antibiotic therapy with cephaloridine for
a total dose of 12 000 000 units, which resulted in an
apparently complete cure. On two inspections 3 and 6
months after discharge, no recurrence of the disease was in
evidence.

This case of atypically localized giant condyloma acuminatum
with disseminated lesions suggests that serious problems may arise
with histologic differentiation of condyloma acuminatum and that its
clinically aggressive course is not necessarily attended by a histologic appearance which does not raise a suspicion of malignancy. The
histologic features of giant condyloma acuminatum, as well as its
nature, have been under discussion ever since the first description
of this condition.

Histologic appearance. It is held by most investigators that
the major points of similarity between the giant and ordinary kinds
of condyloma acuminatum include regularity of cellular structure,
striking acanthosis, and, in some cases, vacuolation of epidermal
cells (e.g. Machacek and Weakley, 1960; Montgomery, 1967; Nazzario
and Tosti, 1968; Anderson, 1971; Vulcan, 1972; Kovi et al., 1974;
Lever and Schaumburg-Lever, 1975; Marghescu et al., 1976), and that
the important differences between these two types are hyperkeratosis
and pronounced pseudocarcinomatous epidermal hyperplasia in the giant
type, with the epidermis showing a tendency to grow deeply and to
displace the underlying tissues, which closely mimics the invasion of
tissues seen in carcinomas of low grade malignancy (Machacek and
Weakly, 1960). Also, there may be a degree of cellular atypia and

enhanced mitotic activity in giant condyloma acuminatum (Marghescu et al., 1976).  The dermis usually shows a rather dense chronic inflammatory infiltrate and many dilated blood vessels and lymphatics (Lever and Schaumburg-Lever, 1975).

The histogenesis of giant condyloma acuminatum remains unclear. Buschke and Loewenstein (1925) and Loewenstein (1939) emphasized the benign nature of the condition, pointing out that although the neoplasm infiltrated and destroyed deep tissues, there were no accompanying histologic signs of malignancy and no metatases.  More recently, however, the view has often been expressed that giant condyloma acuminatum of Buschke and Loewenstein may represent the so-called verrucosus carcinoma described by Ackerman in 1948 which is frequently located on the glans penis (Kraus and Perez-Mesa, 1966; Willis, 1967; Lever and Schaumburg-Lever, 1975; South et al., 1977; Ruppe, 1981).  Bruns et al. (1975) have even gone as far as to state that virtually all of the reported cases of giant condyloma acuminatum fall into the verrucous carcinoma category.

Verrucous carcinoma is defined as a slowly growing fungating tumor causing ulceration and destruction of the adjacent tissues and presenting a histologic picture identical to that of giant condyloma acuminatum.  Thus, in verrucous carcinoma as well as in giant condyloma acuminatum, there is a discrepancy between the aggressive clinical course and the "benign" histologic appearance.  Bruns et al. (1975) consider this condyloma as an intermediate phase in viral carcinogenesis between an absolutely benign condyloma and an anaplastic epidermoid carcinoma.  A number of authors have reported cases both of giant condyloma acuminata and of ordinary condylomata acuminata, undergoing transformation into high-grade keratinizing squamous cell carcinoma, including its verrucous variety (Machacek and Weakley, 1960; Dawson et al., 1965; Rook, 1968; Kerl and Pickel, 1971; Helle, 1972; Vulcan, 1972; Kovi et al., 1974; Bruns et al., 1975; Netto et al., 1976; Mayenburg et al., 1977).  A giant condyloma acuminatum may, however, transform into a low-grade squamous cell carcinoma, as it did, for instance, in one of our five patients.

Patient K., a 41-year-old man, was admitted to our department complaining of an eruption on his penis of about 5 months' duration for which no treatment had been given. He had a history of tuberculosis in the past.

Physical examination showed a circumscribed raised cauliflowerlike warty lesion approximately 3.5 cm in diameter located on the prepuce and encroaching on the dorsal aspect of the lower third of the penis.  On the surface of the lesion, papillomatous growths covered with a sticky discharge were present, as were areas of hyperkeratosis. At the periphery of the lesion, small condylomatous elements were noted.  The inguinal and iliac lymph nodes were not enlarged. The clinical diagnosis was giant condyloma acuminatum of Buschke and Loewenstein.

Histologic examination of the skin biopsied from the margin of the lesional area revealed acanthosis, papillomatosis, and hyperkeratosis with a well-defined granular

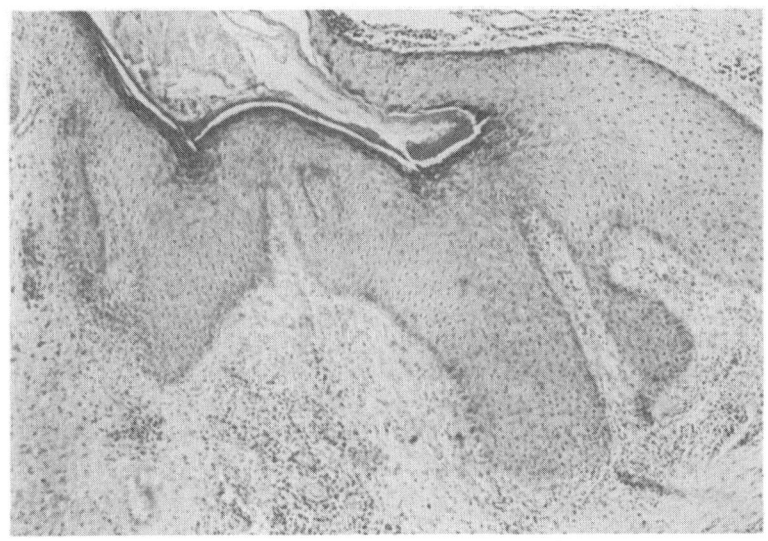

Fig. 60a. Giant condyloma acuminatum of the penis. Irregular epidermal proliferations (75 X; hematoxylin and eosin).

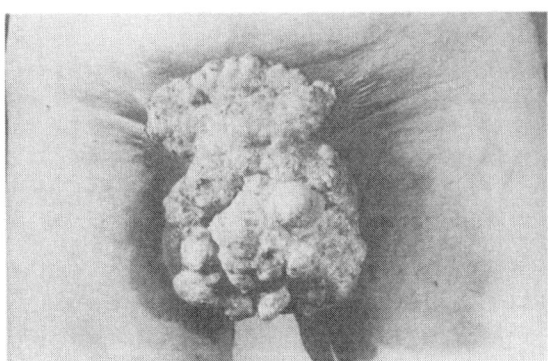

Fig. 60b. Giant condyloma acuminatum of the penis. Same patient after 5 years, diagnosed as having "squamous cell carcinoma of the penis of the fungating papillary type".

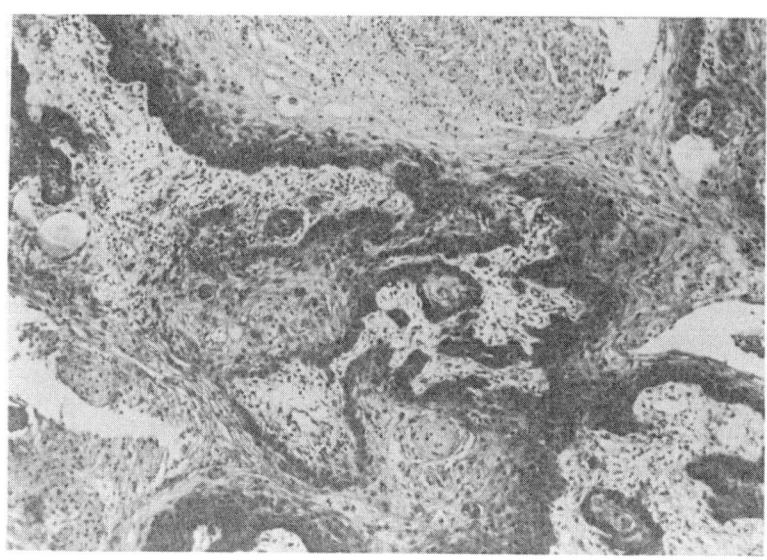

Fig. 60c.  Giant condyloma acuminatum of the penis.  Histologic
           specimen from same patient showing poorly differentiated
           squamous cell carcinoma (75X; hematoxylin and eosin.)


layer being present under the hyperkeratosis.  The
acanthotic epithelium showed an orderly arrangement of
spinous cells.  The basement membrane was intact.  The
dermis was slightly edematous, the lymphatics and blood
vessels were dilated, and a moderate infiltrate composed of
lymphocytes and histiocytes with some plasma cells was seen
(Figure 60a).  It was concluded that the histologic picture
was consistent with the clinical diagnosis.

     The patient was transferred to the Department of
Urology of our Institute where the lesion was excised.  He
had not sought medical advice after discharge, but a few
years later he was summoned for reexamination to the
Institute where it was found necessary to readmit him to
our department.  His general appearance was strikingly
cachectic.  The penis and scrotum were completely involved
by a huge tumorous conglomerate which showed, on its surface, multiple villous papillomatous growths with a foul
smelling discharge lying between them (Figure 60b).  The
base of the tumor was hard and its borders were accentuated
by pigmentation.  The penis was not apparent.  During
urination, which remained free, a small urethral orifice
was visible within the tumor mass.  On palpation, the
inguinal lymph nodes were firm and appeared fused with the
surrounding tissue.  The patient said that the tumor had

evolved during the previous year at the place of a wartlike
overgrowth that recurred as soon as 2 or 3 months after the
operation.

The histologic appearance was one of a slightly differentiated keratinizing squamous cell carcinoma. Sheets of
epithelial cells showing pronounced structural disarray and
nuclear polymorphism, had penetrated deep into the dermis
(Figure 60c) and were surrounded by a dense lymphohistiocytic infiltrate with an admixture of plasma cells. The
vessels around these epithelial proliferations were grossly
dilated. The PAS reaction revealed a greatly reduced
amount of glycogen in the proliferations. The PAS-positive
basement membrane appeared as a thin tortuous line only in
places and was absent elsewhere.

This case is an example of a squamous cell carcinoma developing
from a giant condyloma acuminatum which failed to show histologic
features that could alert to the possibility of malignant degeneration. Admittedly, the tumor was undergoing malignant transformation
from the beginning, but there was no way of establishing this clinically or histologically. The case just described is not unsimilar to
the one reported by Goldstein et al. (1977) where histologic studies
were undertaken on several occasions over a 5-year period in various
centers because of fungoid changes and tumor recurrences in the glans
penis, and each time giant condyloma acuminatum was diagnosed until a
low-grade invasive carcinoma was finally recognized.

Without attempting to offer any hypothesis regarding the true
nature of giant condyloma acuminatum, we disagree with those who feel
that it is in the patient's interests to apply the same therapeutic
approach to the giant type of condyloma as to a low-grade squamous
cell carcinoma.

Etiology and pathogenesis. Many investigators have suggested
that giant condyloma acuminatum has a viral genesis (e.g. Buschke and
Loewenstein, 1925; Loewenstein, 1939; Rook, 1968; Wilkinson, 1968;
Bruns et al., 1975; Vulcan and Pais, 1976). Vulcan and Pais (1976),
in an electron microscopic study of one case, identified spherical
intranuclear particles in the degenerate nuclei of surface epidermal
cells; in addition to these, allegedly "typical viral particles, "
they detected intranuclear particles of obscure origin in cells of
the basal layer. One factor predisposing to giant condyloma
acuminatum is considered to be phimosis (Netto et al., 1976), but a
causal association between the two is unlikely.

Differential diagnosis. Giant condyloma acuminatum of Buschke
and Loewenstein should be differentiated primarily from squamous cell
carcinoma and oral florid papillomatosis and then from ordinary
condylomata acuminata and from condylomata lata.

The greatest difficulties are encountered in distinguishing giant condyloma from squamous cell carcinoma of the penis. An indication of these difficulties is provided by Whitmore's (1970) report of 5 patients with tumors of the penis, in only one of whom the clinical diagnosis (squamous cell carcinoma) was fully consistent with histologic findings, whereas in three others the histologic diagnosis of what later found to be squamous cell carcinoma was benign giant condyloma acuminatum and in the fifth, who was diagnosed histologically as having recurring squamous carcinoma, a recurrence of giant condyloma acuminatum was recognized eventually.

As already pointed out, it is at times impossible to distinguish between a giant condyloma acuminatum and a low-grade keratinizing squamous cell carcinoma either clinically or histopathologically (e.g. Machacek and Weakley, 1960; Kraus and Perez-Mesa, 1966; Willis, 1967; Lever and Schaumburg-Lever, 1975; Ruppe, 1981). It may be no less difficult to differentiate a giant condyloma from a verrucous carcinoma of the penis.

According to Goldstein et al. (1977), a squamous cell carcinoma of the penis consists of an alternation of benign and malignant areas, so that the entire lesion needs to be excised with subsequent examination of several specimens from different areas of the tumor if the correct histologic diagnosis is to be arrived at. There are, however, clinical and histopathologic criteria that may help in the differential diagnosis. Thus, verrucous carcinoma of the penis differs from the giant type of condyloma by slow growth, ulceration of the warty surface, and the absence of condylomalike satellites at the periphery of the lesion. Histopathologically, an important differential feature of giant condyloma acuminatum is vacuolation of many cells of the spinous layer.

Giant condyloma acuminatum differs from keratinizing, but poorly differentiated squamous cell carcinomas by a much more rapid growth rate; by the absence of metatases to regional lymph nodes which often arise in carcinomas of the penis (Gottron and Nikolowski, 1960; Sanderson, 1968); and by the frequent presence of typically condylomatous elements at the tumor periphery. Histological similarities between these two conditions are evident only in the more superficial parts of the specimens, whereas the deeper portions of carcinoma specimens show cellular anaplasia and absence of cellular vacuolation. Diagnostic problems may occur with the giant or ordinary type of condyloma acuminatum undergoing malignant transformation. As pointed out by Kovi et al (1974), a distinguishing feature in such cases is the presence of areas in situ cancer showing typical cellular anaplasia that arises during carcinomatous transformation of Buschke-Loewenstein's tumor.

In rare instances, giant condyloma acuminatum has to be differentiated from the so-called oral florid papillomatosis. In recent years, evidence has been mounting to indicate that oral florid papillomatosis is identical to verrucous carcinoma (e.g. Bazex et al., 1972; Reiffers et al., 1976).  Reiffers et al. (1976) have stressed that giant condyloma acuminatum and oral florid papillomatosis both tend to show invasive growth coupled with a favorable histologic appearance that is not matched  by the aggressive clinical course. Bazex et al. (1972) described four types of florid papillomatosis affecting mucous membranes of the oral cavity, vagina, glans penis, and anus, with the type affecting the glans penis being virtually indistinguishable from giant condyloma acuminatum.

But, unlike the latter, oral florid papillomatosis is apt to undergo malignant change.  Accordingly, Kuffer and Fiore-Donno (1975) classify oral florid papillomatosis among premalignant ("nearly obligatory") dermatoses.

Giant condyloma acuminatum differs from ordinary condylomata acuminata by its much larger size, its capacity for invasive growth, and its unresponsiveness to topically applied cytostatics.

The same features distinguish giant condyloma acuminatum from pseudoepitheliomatous keratotic balanitis which is characterized by a slow, but relentless progression and tends to recur after excision (Read and Abell, 1981).

Lastly, the features which distinguish the condylomata lata of secondary syphilis from giant condyloma acuminatum include a much smaller lesional area, the absence of tendency to invasive growth, the presence of other manifestations of syphilis and of positive serologic tests for syphilis, and a characteristic histologic appearance marked by massive plasma cell infiltration of the dermis and by absence of vacuolated cells in the acanthotic epidermis.

# 9
# Skin Diseases with Facultative Development of Pseudocarcinomatous Hyperplasia

This chapter considers miscellaneous skin disorders which vary widely in etiology and pathogenesis, but which all tend to show atypical pseudocarcinomatous hyperplasia of the epidermis at some stage of their evolution.  Unlike the diseases discussed in the preceding chapter, the dermatoses to which pseudocarcinomatous epidermal hyperplasia is facultative, are many and varied.  They include granulomatous conditions of bacterial or mycotic origin, chronic ulcerative pyodermas, toxicodermas, and dermatoses of indeterminate etiology presenting ulcerative or ulcerative-vegetative, verrucous, and/or hyperkeratotic lesions.

Since the clinical manifestations and histologic appearances of these dermatoses are well known and described in detail in a number of fundamental works (e.g. Mashkilleison, 1960, 1965; Grzhebin and Tseraidis, 1960; Civatte, 1967; Montgomery, 1967; Lever and Shaumburg-Lever, 1975), the dermatoses of this category will be discussed here predominantly in relation to the pseudocarcinomatous epidermal hyperplasias to which they give rise.

## 9.1 TROPHIC ULCERS

Trophic ulcers occur most commonly on the lower extremities, mainly the shins.  The course of such an ulcer may extend over years or even decades (Sinyavskii, 1973).  Trophic ulcers have various causes, the most frequent causes being varicose veins (often in the presence of chronic thrombophlebitis) and traumas, resulting in circulatory disturbances and impaired nutrition of the affected part. According to Sinyavskii (1973), about two thirds of all trophic ulcers of the lower limbs arise in varicose veins in patients with the postphlebitic syndrome and a third are consequent upon damage to large vessels and nerves resulting from mechanical trauma, burn, or other insults to the skin.  Vascular factors also play an important part in causing trophic ulcers in certain syndromes such as Martorelle's (Potekaev and Konstantinov, 1966; Sinyavskii, 1973). Sinyavskii (1973), in reviewing his experience comprising some 1300 patients with trophic ulcers of the lower extremities, found that about 57% of the patients were women and that more than half of the women were beyond 60 years of age, whereas over 80% of the men were aged between 18 and 60.

Clinical manifestations.  Trophic ulcers are characterized by epidermal and dermal defects that vary in shape, size, and depth. More often than not, a round or oval ulcer discharging seropurulent material appears on a pigmented and hardened skin in relation to varicose veins.  Concurrently or after a short interval, several other ulcers may arise and coalesce to form a large lesion.

A trophic ulcer has irregular edges and is slightly raised above the level of the skin.  Depending on the reactivity of the tissue involved, the duration of the disease, the etiologic agents, and other factors, the granulations vary in appearance from bright red to grayish-pink and may be almost level with the surrounding skin (Grigoryan et al., 1972).  If the ulcer is very large, the healing process at its margin slows down with time, and the ulcer takes a chronic indolent course, comes to have elevated callous, hard edges and a pale floor devoid of granulation. The base of the ulcer becomes hardened as fibrosis develops.  Such ulcers show little tendency to heal and arouse suspicion of malignancy on clinical grounds, although they may remain benign for years or decades.  Trophic ulcers that have developed in scarred tissue and are accompanied by vegetations bear close resemblance to cutaneous squamous cell carcinoma.  Though benign in nature, these ulcers pose problems before clinicians, and the doubt is not always dispelled by histopathologic findings.  The case report which follows is an example of a pseudocancerous trophic ulcer.

Patient K., a man aged 43, presented with a long-lasting ulcer on the right shin with little tendency to heal. He considered himself to have been ill for some 20 years - ever since his left leg had to be amputated because of wounds caused by explosion of a grenade, and osteomyelitis developed in his right leg which had multiple fractures.  Somewhat later, trophic ulcers began to appear periodically on the right shin, the last ulcer having arisen about 3 years previously and having been increasing in size over the past 1½ years; hyperkeratosis had developed at the margin of the ulcer to spread later to the entire ulcerative surface.

His general condition was satisfactory. The cardiovascular system, respiratory organs, and gastrointestinal
tract were unremarkable; the liver and spleen were not
enlarged. The pulse was 78/min, rhythmic, and full. The
arterial blood pressure was 140/80 mm Hg. The blood and
urine tests showed no abnormalities.

An ulcer 11 x 7 cm in size with even edges that were
raised 0.7 to 1.5 cm above the plane of the skin was seen
on the scarred anterior surface of the middle third of the
deformed right lower leg (Figure 61). The central portion
of the ulcer was composed of vegetations covered by grayish
horny masses and purulent material. On palpation, the base
of the ulcer was firm while its edges felt doughy. The
horny masses could be easily lifted to reveal a surface
with seropurulent exudate. The skin around the ulcer was
pigmented, and a deep whitish scar was seen at its upper
pole. The inguinal and iliac lymph nodes were of kidney-
bean size, firm yet elastic in consistency, mobile, and
painless. The clinical appearance suggested malignant
degeneration of the ulcer because of its hyperkeratotic
elevated margin, the presence of hyperkeratosis on the
vegetations, the long duration of the ulcer and the fact
that it had arisen in scars. Before admission to our
clinic, the patient had been examined by an oncologist and
a traumatologist who did not rule out malignancy.

Histologic examination of a skin biopsy from the
margin of the ulcer revealed a picture of pseudocarcinomatous epidermal hyperplasia. There were considerable papillomatosis, acanthosis, and hyperkeratosis. The epidermal
ridges were bizarre in outline and penetrated deep into the
dermis. In places, aggregates of epithelial cells that had
separated from the acanthotic epidermis were seen, and some
of these cells showed incomplete keratinization. No
nuclear polymorphism or irregularly dividing cells were
noted, however. The dermis showed an inflammatory infiltrate.

Taking into consideration the histologic findings and
the patient's history (the ulcer had healed periodically),
it was decided to institute conservative therapy. After
removal of the hyperkeratotic structures, application of
lotions, lubrication of the vegetations with lunar caustic,
and combined treatment with antibiotics, group B vitamins,
aloe, and Complamin (xanthionol nicotinate), the ulcer
flattened and underwent epithelialization.

This case report suggests that diagnostic problems may occur if
a trophic ulcer shows a pseudocarcinomatous epidermal hyperplasia

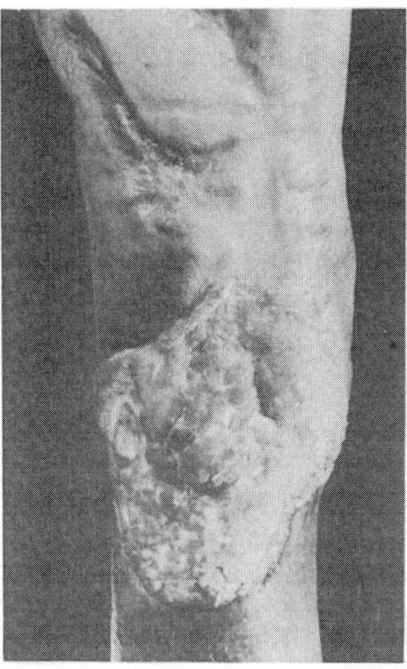

Fig. 61.  Trophic ulcer of the right shin mimicking squamous cell
          carcinoma.


histologically while presenting clinical features suggestive of
malignancy.

    Histologic appearance.  The histologic picture lacks strict speci-
ficity and may vary during the course of ulcer development.  If the
ulcerative process at the margin is of long standing, the acanthosis,
papillomatosis, and hyperkeratosis are usually pronounced and some
parakeratosis is present.  The dermis shows chronic inflammation and
a lymphohistiocytic infiltrate.  In some cases, the margins of
callous ulcers present an appearance of pseudocarcinomatous epidermal
hyperplasia.  Of 16 our patients with trophic (varicose or postthrom-
bophlebitic) ulcers, a pronounced pseudocarcinomatous hyperplasia was
noted in 9.  In most of these cases, however, a clinicopathologic
correlation left no doubt that the process was benign.  It is to be
noted, though, that malignant transformation of trophic ulcers
remains a real possibility.  There are many reports of squamous cell
carcinomas and even sarcomas supervening on long-standing trophic
ulcers of the lower extremities (e.g. Raichev and Andreev, 1965;
Shanin, 1969; Sinyavskii, 1973).

    Differential diagnosis.  In cases where the epidermal hyper-
plasia presented by a trophic ulcer mimics squamous cell carcinoma,

one should look for the following features which are usually shown by
ulcers undergoing malignant change: a flaccid floor of the ulcer
devoid of granulations and covered by hard grayish crusts; a callous,
cartilagelike edge of the ulcer fused with the subjacent tissue; a
protracted course of the ulcer without appreciable changes despite
vigorous local and systemic treatment; and, histologically, more
pronounced nuclear polymorphism and well-defined individual cell
keratinization.


9.2  CHRONIC PYODERMA ULCEROSUM VEGETANS

The term "chronic pyoderma ulcerosum vegetans" is used with
reference to a variety of clinical conditions, often not well delineated, which include, among others, chronic pyococcal ulcer,
pyodermia ulcerosa serpiginosa, papillomatous plaquelike pyoderma
with an epithelial reaction (inflammatory pseudoepithelioma of Azua),
and pyoderma gangrenosum.  Attempts to provide a consistent etiologic
classification of chronic pyodermas have failed, mainly because
identical microorganisms are often isolated in different clinical
forms of pyoderma (Trutnev, 1956; Mashkilleison, 1960; Rakhmanov,
1961; Chorążak et al., 1967).

The occurrence of particular clinical forms of chronic deep
pyoderma depends to a large extent on the general condition of the
body.  As pointed out by Mashkilleison (1960), some forms, primarily
the chronic ulcerative vegetating variety, arise in severely em-
aciated individuals, those with anemia, gastrointestinal disturbances, endocrine abnormalities, or so on.  In recent years great
importance has been attached to the state of the immune system which
shows reduced activity in most patients with chronic ulcerative
vegetating pyoderma (Haim and Friedman-Birnbaum, 1976; Delektorskii
et al., 1977; Brachtel and Lemmel, 1978).

Among the pustular disorders of the skin, which are many and
varied, chronic pyoderma ulcerosum vegetans is seen relatively seldom.  Most of the patients are men aged between 30 and 60 years, but
women are also affected occasionally, mainly in advanced and old age
(Mashkilleison, 1960).

Clinical manifestations.  These vary from one stage of the
disease to another.  Usually, a blue-red, tender infiltrate arises in
the presence of altered reactivity of the organism, in most instances
in relation to a preceeding trauma or at the site of a preexisting
pustular lesion (folliculitis, furuncle, ecthyma, etc.).  The infiltrate rapidly enlarges, and as a result of tissue breakdown, its
central portion develops an ulceration which is round or oval first
and irregularly shaped later because of nonuniform expansion of the
necrotic zone at or around the ulcer.  The floor of the ulcer is
uneven and covered with multiple granulations.  These soon assume the

character of vegetations with necrotic tissue fragments and purulent material on their surfaces. The edges of the ulcer are elevated and rather firm to palpation. Near the ulcer (within the infiltrate) and on its floor, there are many fistulous openings from which pus can be expressed. The most common sites of lesions are the lower extremities, but the process may involve virtually any area of the skin.

Apart from the clinical features just described, there may develop plaquelike soft lesions of cyanotic-red appearance with vegetations and areas of ulceration covered by seropurulent exudate that dires up to form loose crusts.

The process is long-lasting and may extend over years. The lesion heals leaving behind a scar of irregular outline. Frequently, the lesion scars in one area while slowly progressing in another. At the periphery of the lesional skin, pustular elements may be present.

Histologic appearance. The histologic appearance of chronic pyoderma ulcerosum vegetans has been studied in detail (Kozhevnikov, 1946, Trutnev, 1956; Mashkilleison, 1960; Il'ina and Vasil'eva, 1963; Chorażak et al., 1967; Montgomery, 1967; Bazyka and Lesnitskii, 1975; Lever and Schaumburg-Lever, 1975; Rutshtein et al., 1982) and is characterized by the presence in the dermis of an inflammatory infiltrate (often granulomatous) and of secondary proliferative epidermal changes which often produce the picture of pseudocarcinomatous hyperplasia. The histologic features depend to a great extent on the clinical ones and on the duration of the disease. Initially, changes are seen chiefly in the dermis and include dilation of vessels, edema, and a perivascular or diffuse inflammatory infiltrate; later on, the infiltrate, which is composed of lymphocytes, fibroblasts, histiocytes, and some plasma cells, involves the deeper layers of the dermis and hypodermis where overgrowth of granulation tissue occurs also (Mashkilleison, 1960). Epidermal hyperplasia is particularly marked at the edges of deep lesions. Bazyka and Lesnitskii (1975), in studying skin biopsies from 24 patients with chronic pyoderma ulcerosum vegetans, found in most a pseudocarcinomatous epidermal hyperplasia with extension of rete ridges deep into the dermis; areas of dyskeratosis; and regions with indistinct basement membrane.

Among our 35 patients with chronic pyoderma ulcerosum (20 men and 15 women aged 24 to 79), pronounced pseudocarcinomatous epidermal hyperplasia was observed in 26 cases.

As a typical example, here is one case report.

Patient I., a 46-year-old woman, was admitted to our department complaining of ulcerative lesions with purulent discharge. The lesions first appeared on the lower extremities and later on the arms and neck. She had not received any treatment.

On physical examination, erosive ulcerative infiltrated and crusted lesions of cyanotic appearance 2 to 6 x
9 cm in size were present on the left arm, neck, and left
shin.  On the lower third of the left shin, there was a
circumscribed lesion showing considerable infiltration and
long-standing hyperemia.  Almost the entire area of this
lesion was occupied by an irregularly shaped ulcer having a
knobby floor with papillary overgrowth and undermined edges
from which drops of pus could be expressed.  The clinical
diagnosis was chronic pyoderma ulcerosum vegetans (Figure
62).

Histologic examination of a specimen from the margin
of the ulcer revealed sheets of proliferating epidermis
deep in the dermis in the form of flask-shaped strands.
There were moderate hyperkeratosis and parakeratosis.  No
stratum granulosum was detectable beneath the areas of
parakeratosis.  In the center of the acanthotic epidermis
one could see concentrically arranged keratinous masses
containing nuclear remnants that resembled horn pearls.
The cytoplasm of spinous cells stained faintly.  There was
moderate exocytosis.  Islands of epidermal cells that had
separated from the epidermal overgrowths were observed.
Deep in the dermis, epidermal aggregates containing keratinizing cells in the center were present.  The stroma was
edematous and showed a diffuse lymphohistiocytic infiltrate
admixed with segmented and plasma cells (Figure 63).

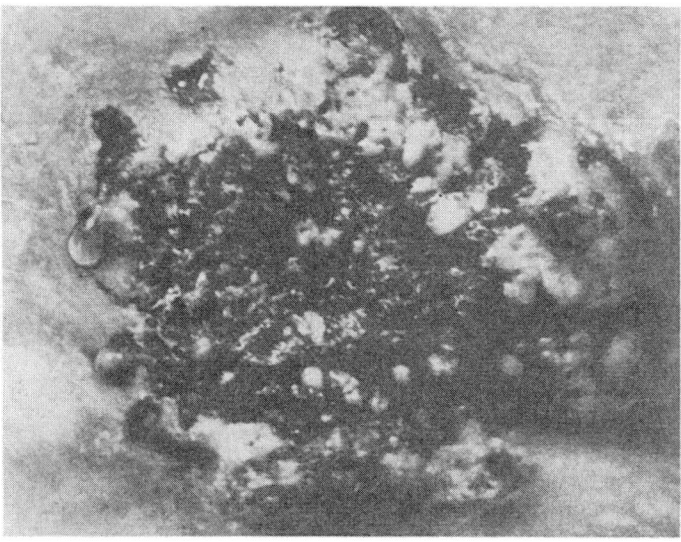

Fig. 62.  Chronic pyoderma ulcerosum vegetans.

Brachet's stain revealed more RNA in the cytoplasm of
proliferating basal cells than in that of the overlying
spinous cells.  In the basement membrane zone, the PAS-
positive, diastase-resistant material appeared as a thin
homogeneous band which was indetectable in places.  No
PAS-positive band was apparent around the epithelial cell
aggregates.  The bulk of Feulgen-positive substance
occurred in cells of the basal and suprabasal layers.  On
staining with toluidine blue, a slight degree of gamma-
metachromasia was noted in the basement membrane zone, in
vessel walls, and in the grains of mast cells.

It was concluded that the histologic appearance was
one of pseudocarcinomatous hyperplasia but that the
possibility of a differentiated squamous cell carcinoma in
its initial stage could not be ruled out.

Here, the histologic picture was so similar to that of highly
differentiated squamous cell carcinoma that the clinical evidence had

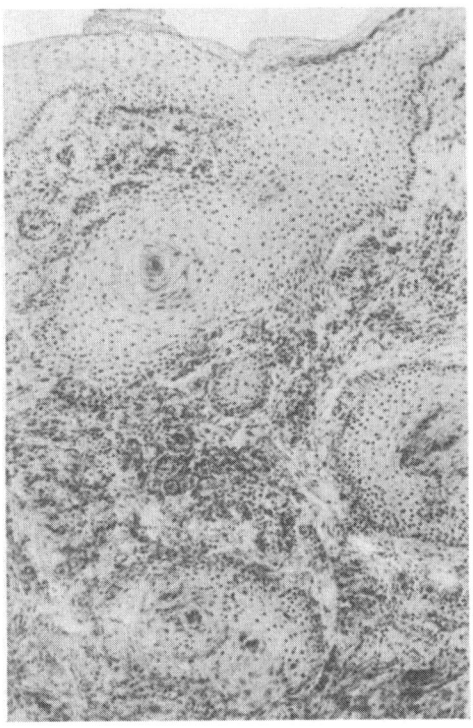

Fig. 63.  Chronic pyoderma ulcerosum vegetans of shin skin, showing
pronounced pseudocarcinomatous epidermal hyperplasia.
(75 X; hematoxylin and eosin.)

to be considered to exclude the latter.  The main criteria that led
to the diagnosis of chronic pyoderma ulcerosum vegetans in this
patient were the relatively short duration of the disease, presence
of multiple lesions with essentially similar clinical presentations,
profuse purulent discharge from the lesions, and pronounced inflammatory reactions in the lesional areas.  A combined treatment with
antibiotics, vitamins, autohemotransfusions, and with lotions and
other topical medicaments resulted in a striking improvement.  When
the patient was reexamined 3 years afterwards, atrophic scars were
seen at the sites of former lesions.

   Differential diagnosis.  Chronic pyoderma ulcerosum vegetans
must be differentiated from trophic ulcers, the deep mycoses, leishmaniasis, and scrofuloderma.  Trophic ulcers of the lower extremities
are difficult to distinguish from ulcerative vegetating pyoderma if
the latter does not develop pronounced vegetations and arises in
relation to varicose veins.  Usually, the lesions of deep pyoderma,
unlike trophic ulcers, arise in the absence of varicose veins, undergo rapid ulcerations, are cyanotic in appearance, are heavily infiltrated, and heal by forming a "creeping" scar.  Moreover, varicose
ulcers are seldom accompanied by vegetations and never show pustular
elements peripherally.

   In deep blastomycosis, in contrast to ulcerative vegetating
pyoderma, there is no tendency to self-healing of the lesions, and
the general condition of the patient is grave (the Busse-Buschke type
of blastomycosis).

   The lesions of cutaneous leishmaniasis differ from those of
pyoderma by showing inflamed lymph vessels arranged radially around
the ulcers, and the presence of Leishmania organisms in the discharge.  Moreover, an important consideration is the patient's history
of staying in an area endemic for leishmaniasis.

   In cases where chronic pyoderma is localized on the neck or
face, it can be distinguished from scrofuloderma by the characteristic features of the latter.  These include undermined soft edges of
the ulcers which arise in relation to lymph nodes and the development
of cordlike scars that bridge the ulcerative areas.

   In those less common cases where the lesions of chronic pyoderma
have greatly elevated borders and present a picture of pseudocarcinomatous epidermal hyperplasia, distinction from a well-differentiated squamous cell carcinoma may be difficult.  However, in pyoderma, in contradistinction to carcinoma, the lesions grow rapidly;
scar in some areas while continuing to expand in others; discharge
large amounts of purulent material; tend to have extensions in the
form of satellite pustular elements; and reveal the presence of
granulomatous infiltrate in the areas of invasive epidermal growth.

## 9.3  CUTANEOUS LEISHMANIASIS

Cutaneous leishmaniasis (synonyms: Borovsky's disease, Penjdeh ulcer, Turkestan ulcer, Oriental sore, and many more) is endemic in hot climates and is caused by two different Leishmania strains, each being responsible for a distinctive clinical form of cutaneous leishmaniasis.

Since the time when the nature of leishmaniasis was elucidated by the Russian investigator Borovskii (1898), a large body of information has been amassed covering in detail its clinical features, histopathology, epidemiology, and treatment (Martsinovskii, 1909; Gitel'zon, 1933; Mashkilleison, 1960; Kozhevnikov, 1961; Adler, 1965; Shuikina, 1969; Lever and Schaumburg-Lever 1975; Dobrzhanskaya, 1977; Rodyakin, 1982).

Clinical manifestations. Two distinct clinical forms are recognized: urban (late ulcerating) and rural (acute necrotizing) leishmaniasis. The principal vectors are mosquitos of the genus Phlebotomus.

With urban leishmaniasis, the incubation period is variable from 3 to 9 months or even longer. Thereafter a cyanotic tubercle 1 to 3 mm in diameter appears at the site of the infective mosquito bite. Very slowly (over a period of up to 6 months according to Koshevnikov (1961)), the papule transforms into an infiltrated plaque of livid pink color and variable size which becomes scaled and crusted. There may be one or more lesions depending on the number of infective bites. Approximately in 6 months (occasionally in 10-12 months) the lesion ulcerates. The margin of the ulcer is elevated above the level of normal-looking skin by a massive infiltrate and often overhangs the ulcer. The floor of the ulcer is granular and shows yellowish necrotic areas, hemorrhages, and serosanguinous exudate. Gradually, the necrotic mass detaches, the ulcer clears, and scarring begins. The duration of the disease from the appearance of the tubercle to the cicatrization of the ulcer is about a year.

Rural leishmaniasis has a much shorter incubation period lasting several days to between 1 and 2 months. At the site of the mosquito bite, a bright red tubercle appears, enlarges rapidly, and ulcerates in 2 to 3 weeks. The mature lesion is an irregularly shaped ulcer on an infiltrated base. The edges of the ulcer are sharply elevated and overhang it. The floor of the ulcer is usually covered with granulations and shows necrotic areas carrying serosanguinous material containing pus. Sometimes, its floor is covered by vegetations and its margin, by hard serosanguinous crusts. In some cases the center of the ulcer and its peripheral portions show fistula-like changes creating an appearance not unlike that seen in pyoderma ulcerosum vegetans. An important distinctive feature of leishmaniasis is the presence of nodular lymphangitis which usually spreads radially along

the periphery of the lesional area. The lesions of rural leishmaniasis persist for 3 to 4 months and heal with a scar.

Histologic appearance. The histologic picture depends on the
form and duration of leishmaniasis. The initial stage of late ulcerating (urban) leishmaniasis is characterized by a focal and then
diffuse infiltrate composed of histiocytes, fibroblasts, lymphocytes,
and macrophages. Kozhevnikov (1961) emphasizes that epithelioid and
giant cells are present in the infiltrate in small numbers only at
the height of the pathologic process, whereas later on macrophages
containing leishmania organisms are much more numerous and circumscribed foci of epithelioid cells appear in the infiltrate. The acute
necrotizing (rural) form is characterized by development of necrosis
inside the infiltrate which is similar in composition to that in the
late ulcerating form.

A feature of leishmaniasis noted by many investigators (e.g.
Gitel'zon, 1933; Mashkilleison, 1960; Montgomery, 1967) is deep
invasion of the infiltrate by proliferating epidermis. Foci of keratinization resembling horn pearls may be present within the acanthotic epidermal proliferations, and the dermoepidermal junction is
often completely obliterated by the infiltrate (Kozhevnikov, 1961).
Such a picture of pseudocarcinomatous hyperplasia was seen in two of
our patients with late ulcerating leishmaniasis. Here is one of these
cases.

Patient V., a man aged 26, was admitted to our department complaining of ulcerative lesions in the skin of about
5 months' duration that had appeared when he was staying in
Central Asia on an official assignment.

On physical examination, dark pink infiltrated lesions
with central ulceration and sharply defined borders were
seen on the dorsa of the right hand and arm, on the upper
third of the right shin, and in the region of the left
ankle joint; the lesional surfaces were covered by hard
grayish crusts and scales. At the base of the right thumb
there was a roundish ulcer 2 x 3 cm in size with an irregular border and a granular floor covered by a small amount
of sanguinopurulent exudate. A browinish-red infiltrate
was present at the ulcer base. The ulcer had elevated
rolled edges that were overhanging it (Figure 64).
Radially oriented inflamed lymphatic vessels were palpable
around the ulcer. The material discharged from the lesions
was found to contain Borovsky's bodies (leishmanias). The
clinical diagnosis was late ulcerating leishmaniasis.

Histologic examination of a biopsy specimen from the
margin of the ulcer showed considerable acanthosis with
proliferation of epidermal strands deep into the dermis.
The corneal layer was greatly thickened and showed foci of

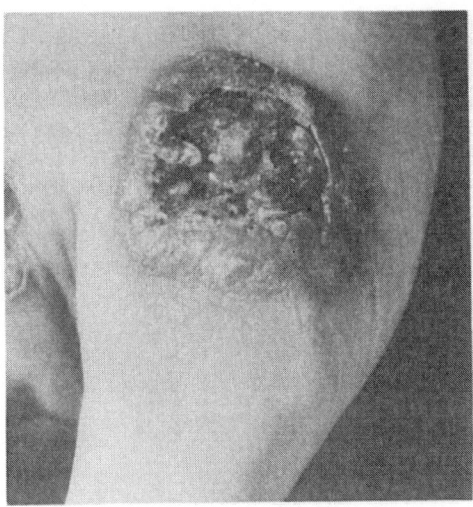

Fig. 64.   Cutaneous leishmaniasis of urban type.


a homogeneous substance in which destroyed cells with
pyknotic nuclei were seen.  Other areas showed moderate
hyperkeratosis with masses of horny material plugging the
dilated orifices of hair follicles which had produced
cystlike growths in places.  Under the corneal layer and in
regions of enhanced proliferation, cells undergoing vacuo-
lar degeneration were present.  The intercellular bridges
were widened.  The entire thickness of the dermis was
occupied by a diffuse infiltrate composed of lymphohistiocytic elements, plasma cells, some polymorphonuclear leukocytes, and occasional eosinophils.  In places, the proliferating epidermal strands were seen to have grown around
nuclear detritus to form cystlike cavities (Figure 65).  On
staining by Brachet's method, the cytoplasm of proliferating epidermal cells showed diminished pyroninophilia, thus
indicating a decreased level of cytoplasmic RNA.  Considerable amounts of PAS-positive, diastase-labile material were
found deposited within the acanthotic epidermis.  The
PAS-positive, diastase-resistant band was interrupted in
many places at the dermoepidermal junction, but was continuous in the blood vessel walls.

In the case just described, where cutaneous leishmaniosis presented a picture of pronounced pseudocarcinomatous epidermal hyper-
plaisia, neither the clinical features nor the histologic appearance
gave cause to doubt the benign nature of the condition.  In such
cases, the proliferating epidermal cells which grow around nuclear
detritus appear to perform an eliminative function by promoting the
separation and removal of foreign necrotic masses.

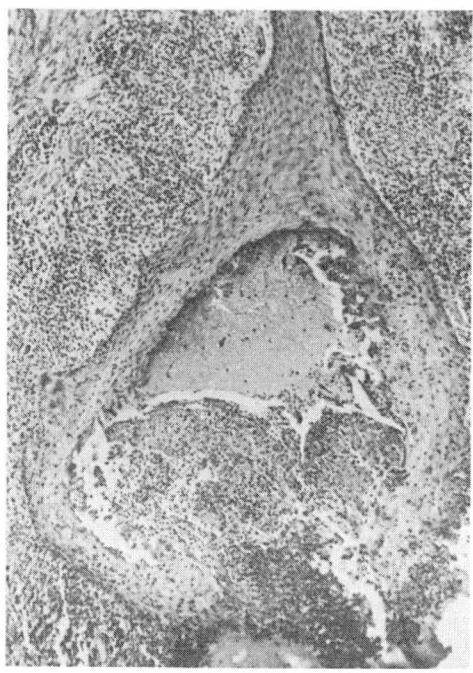

Fig. 65.  Cutaneous leishmaniasis.  Dorsum of the hand.  Prolifer-
          ating epithelial strands are seen to be growing over
          nuclear detritus thereby promoting its elimination.  (75 X;
          hematoxylin and eosin.)


        Differential diagnosis.  Diagnosis presents no problems in
typical cases.  The history (residence of the patient in an area
where leishmaniasis is endemic), the identification of leishmania
orgnaisms in discharges from the lesions, the clinical appearance of
these (a granular floor of the ulcer, lymphangitis at the periphery
of lesional skin), and its correlation with histologic findings will
make it possible to exclude chronic deep pyoderma ulcerosum vegetans,
tuberculosis, and the deep mycoses from all of which cutaneous leishmaniasis has to be differentiated.


9.4  CUTANEOUS TUBERCULOSIS

        The clinical features, histopathology, pathogenesis, and treat-
ment of tuberculosis luposa cutis (lupus vulgaris) have been described in great detail in numerous publications, and so will be
mentioned here only briefly, if at all.  Atypical epidermal proliferations that simulated squamous cell carcinoma were first observed in
tuberculosis luposa cutis by Unna (1894).  Pseudocarcinomatous epidermal hyperplasia is most commonly seen at the margins of ulcerative

areas, notably in the verrucous (hypertrophic) form of this condition (Shtein, 1938; Rossianskii and Smelov, 1947; Mashkilleison, 1960; Montgomery, 1967; Lever and Schaumburg-Lever, 1975; Wolff, 1979). Maskilleison (1960) has stated that the most common factor promoting the development of this clinical variant of lupus vulgaris is trauma and that the atypical epidermal growth is directly dependent on the arrangement and size of the infiltrate.

The verrucous form was present in four of our nine patients with lupus vulgaris (4 women and 5 men aged 21 to 56 years), and all four showed pronounced pseudocarcinomatous hyperplasia. Such hyperplasia was also noted in all of our nine patients with tuberculosis verrucosa cutis (2 women and 7 men aged 32 to 54 years).

Clinical manifestations. The verrucous form of lupus vulgaris is characterized by the presence of brownish plaques showing hyperkeratosis, warty growths on the surface, and individual lupomas at the periphery. Warty tuberculosis, which is known to be a much less common condition than lupus vulgaris, is characterized clinically by lesions appearing as dark red plaques in which three zones are distinguishable: (1) a central warty zone with a papillomatous surface covered by grayish scales; (2) a middle zone presenting a smooth bluish-red surface and encircling the warty center in a belt-like fashion; and (3) an outer inflammatory zone appearing as a halo at the periphery of the lesion. The lesions of tuberculosus verrucosa most often occur on the dorsa of the hands or on the extensor surfaces of the legs, run a protracted course (sometimes for decades), and heal with nonelevated, smooth scars.

Histologic appearance. Tuberculosis verrucosa cutis shows strongly marked epidermal changes, with the proliferating epidermis penetrating deep into the dermis to disturb the typical structure of the tuberculous inflammatory infiltrate (tubercle) which shows moderate caseation necrosis and is composed of polymorphonuclear leukocytes and of lymphocytes. Pseudocarcinomatous epidermal hyperplasia is a frequent finding. Here is one case report.

Patient K., a 42-year-old man, was admitted to our department with a diagnosis of tuberculosis verrucosa cutis. He considered himself ill for the past 15 years. He had been repeatedly and unsuccessfully treated with PAS, Phthivazidum (3-methoxy-4-hydroxyoxybenzylidenehydrazide of isonicotinic acid), and streptomycin; and topical applications of salicylic acid-containing ointments, pyrogallol ointment, etc. The eruptions had failed to resolve completely at any time during the 15-year period.

Physical examination showed a multitide (133) of round to oval, pink or dark bluish to purplish lesions from 1 to between 3 and 5 cm in size sharply delimited from the

normal-appearing skin and firm to palpation. The lesions
were distributed over the upper and lower extremities and
trunk and their surfaces were represented by papillomatous
overgrowths covered with dense grayish horny masses (Figure
66). On the feet, the warty nodules had coalesced to form
large plaques with irregular outlines. At the periphery of
such a plaque there was an infiltrated zone of cyanotic
appearance. The diagnosis of tuberculosis verrucosa cutis
was confirmed.

Histologic examination of a lesion on the right arm
revealed pronounced acanthosis with massive downgrowth of
epidermal strands which extended deep into the dermis
(below the sweat gland level). The interweaving epidermal
downgrowths formed cystlike cavities filled with horny
material. The epidermal growth had occurred through proliferation of spinous cells whose cytoplasm stained faintly
in the lower dermis. The basal layer was well defined. As
they passed into deeper portions of the dermis, the power-
ful sheets of epidermis thinned out into long strands made
up of more lightly stained spinous cells. In places, these
were arranged concentrically to form aggregates which had
partly keratinized central areas and resembled horn pearls

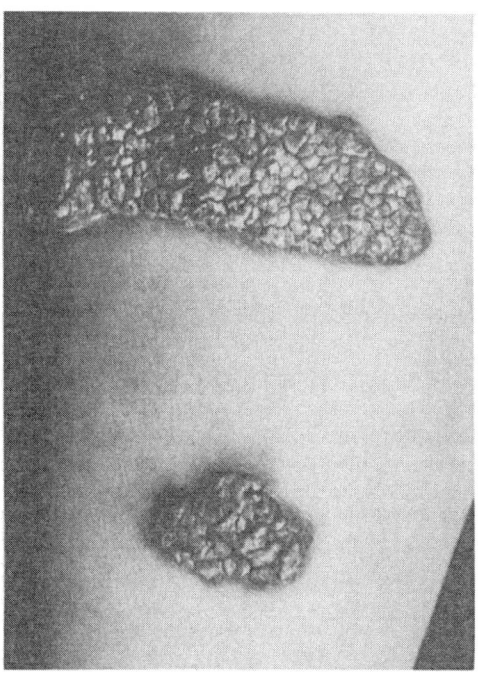

Fig. 66. Tuberculosis cutis verrucosa.

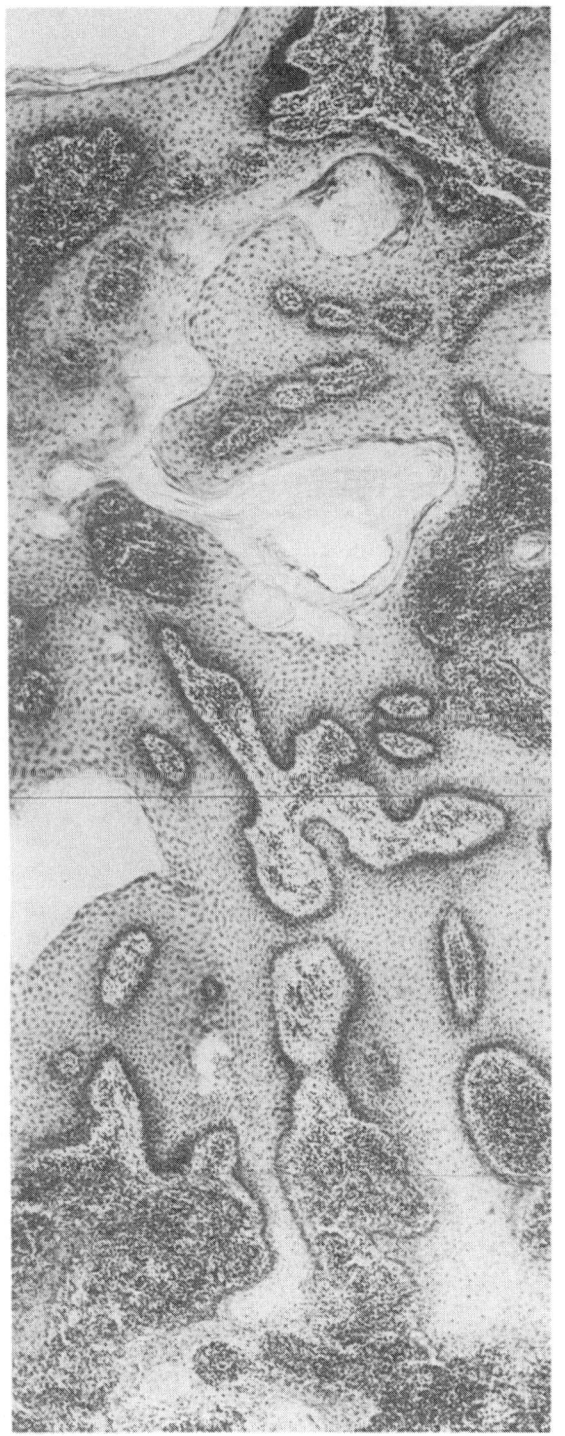

Fig. 67a.  Tuberculosis cutis verrucosa affecting the skin of an arm.  Pronounced pseudocarcinomatous epidermal hyperplasia (75 X; hematoxylin and eosin; montage.)

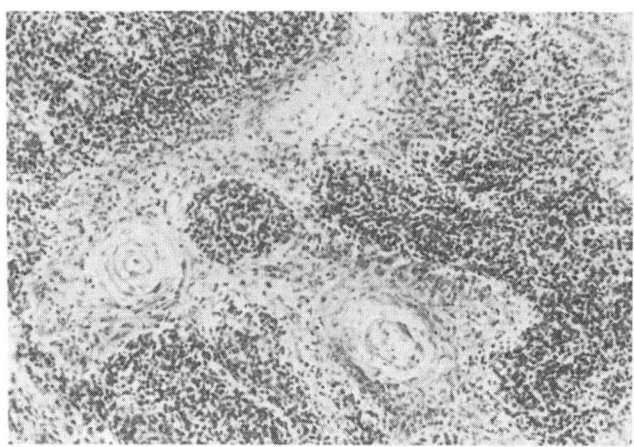

Fig. 67b.  Tuberculosis cutis verrucosa affecting the skin of an arm.
           Same biopsy specimen, showing epidermal proliferations
           that form horny pearls in the lower dermis.  (125 X;
           hematoxylin and eosin.)

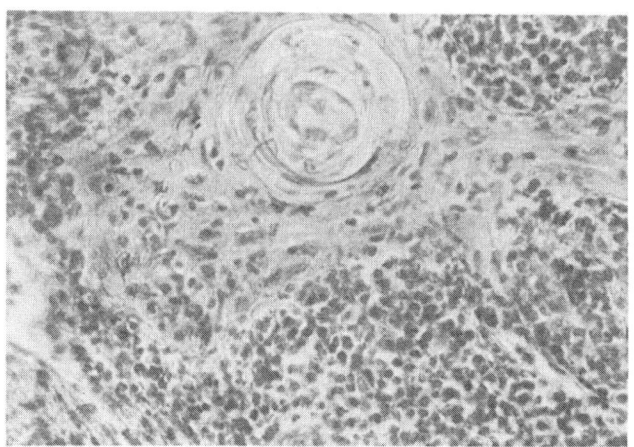

Fig. 67c.  Tuberculosis cutis verrucosa affecting the skin of an
           arm.  Same biopsy specimen, showing a horny pearl with
           partially keratinized center and concentrically arranged
           cells with nuclear remnants; the cells are in disarray and
           the basement membrane is indetectable; there is moderate
           exocytosis.  (250 X; hematoxylin and eosin.)


           (Figure 67a).  At higher magnifications (Figure 67b and c),
           one could clearly see the structure of such pearls with
           partly keratinized centers and concentrically arranged
           spinous cells which contained nuclei.  These epithelial

nests had processes with disorderly arranged spinous cells showing remnants of pyknotic nuclei, some edema, and moderate exocytosis. The basement membrane was indefinite. The dermis showed a dense diffuse infiltrate composed of lymphocytes, histiocytes, plasma cells, and some eosinophils. Staining by the Brachet method showed nonuniform distribution of cytoplasmic RNA in cells of the acanthotic epidermal strands, with the basal cells being more pyroninophilic and the overlying spinous cells staining more faintly. The more deeply Feulgen-stained nuclei were those of the basal layer and of the overlying two or three strata of the spinous cells; the overlying epidermal layers and the invasive epidermal proliferations showed poor staining. With the PAS reaction, glycogen occurred only in the cytoplasm of spinous cells of the upper epidermis; the invasive proliferations contained no glycogen. The PAS-positive basement membrane was rich in neutral mucopolysaccharides only in the upper portions of growing epidermal strands. Deep within the dermis, and especially around the sheets of spinous cells, the basement membrane was indetectable. On silver impregnation by the Foot method, the argyrophilic membranes were thinned out and were ruptured in places; they were absent around the epithelial nests. Staining with toluidine blue revealed gamma-metachromasia in the basement membrane zone. Mallory's stain showed no fibrin. Elastic fibers were absent in some areas and hypertrophic or fragmented in others.

In this case, warty tuberculosis was accompanied by considerable pseudocarcinomatous epidermal hyperplasia. The proliferating epidermal strands penetrated deep into the dermis, forming horn pearls. The epidthelial nests that resembled horn pearls were partly keratinized in the center; peripherally they were surrounded by concentrically arranged spinous cells containing nuclei. In such cases it is fairly difficult to distinguish pseudocarinomatous hyperplasia from a highly differentiated squamous cell carcinoma of the skin.

Differential diagnosis. Discrimination of the pseudocarcinomatous epidermal hyperplasias that develop in various clinical forms of cutaneous tuberculosis from squamous cell carcinomas of the skin is a matter of great practical importance. Indeed, true squamous cell carcinomas are known to arise in lesions of lupus vulgaris in some cases (e.g. Mashkilleison, 1960; Neradov, 1961; Kurlat, 1964; Raichev and Andreev, 1965:; Venkei and Sugar, 1965; Shanin, 1969), and at times it is impossible to distinguish lupus carcinoma from pseudocarcinomatous hyperplasia not only clinically but also histologically (Shanin, 1969). A number of authors (e.g. Kurlat, 1964; Shanin, 1969; Mashkilleison, 1970) believe that factors conducive to the development of squamous cell cancer in lupus vulgaris include inappropriate treatment and long duration of the pathologic process in

the skin.  It was considered by Bremener (1937) that the appearance
of a true carcinoma in lupus vulgaris is preceeded by a pseudocarcinomatous epidermal hyperplasia.  In our view, however, the pseudocarcinomatous hyperplasia arising in lesions of lupus vulgaris should
not be regarded as a precancerous condition.  Thus, although tuberculosis verrucosa cutis is likewise often accompanied by pronounced
psuedocarcinomatous epidermal hyperplasia, it is only in exceptional
cases that a cancer is seen to arise in this form of tuberculosis.
And the same is true of several other dermatoses (the deep mycoses,
pyoderma ulcerosum vegetans, vegetating toxicodermas, etc.).  We
agree with Golovin (1975) in that "an inflammatory-regenerative
hyperplasia is devoid of precancer significance and does not evolve
into a cancer.... Cancer begins with its own, specific precancerous
hyperplasis that has no adaptive importance."

The clinical picture of malignant transformed lupus vulgaris is
characterized by hardening of the normally soft margins of the ulcers
and by the appearance of vegetative growths both at the edges of the
ulcers and over the scars.  Such changes occur 30 to 40 years after
onset of the disease in elderly or old individuals with a history of
exposure to adverse factors (roentgen radiation, excessive insolation, etc).  Histologic criteria by which pseudocarcinomatous
epidermal hyperplasia can be distinguished from well-differentiated
squamous cell carcinoma of the skin include true dyskeratosis of
individual cells and, in advanced cases, invasion of the blood vessels by tumor cells.

Diagnostic differentiation of lupus vulgaris from other diseases
(syphilis, lupus erythematosus, etc.) does not usually present problems and rests on recognition of the typical and well-known characteristics of the lupus tubercle (the lupoma).

Tuberculosis verrucosa cutis can be separated from chromomycosis
and lichen ruber verrucosus on the basis of several signs peculiar to
each of these.  Thus, the lesions of chromomycosis are larger, have
no cyanotic halo around the warty centers, and contain the causative
organisms.  Lichen ruber verrucosus has as its distinctive signs the
presence of multiple lesions localized predominantly to the extremities; the absence of erythema at the periphery of the lesions;
itching; the presence elsewhere on the skin of elements typical for
lichen ruber planus; and, histologically, pronounced hypergranulosis.


9.5  THE DEEP MYCOSES

Of the various deep mycoses, pseudocarcinomatous hyperplasia
occurs more commonly in deep blastomycosis and in chromomycosis,
although it can also be encountered in sporotrichosis, coccidioido-
mycosis, and histoplasmosis (Montgomery, 1967).

### 9.5.1  Blastomycosis

Pseudocarcinomatous hyperplasia is seen predominantly in North American blastomycosis (Gilchrist's disease).

Clinical manifestations.  North American blastomycosis is characterized by the appearance, mainly on the extremities, of pleomorphic eruptions consisting of macules, nodules, and pustules which have a tendency to fuse, to ulcerate, and to develop vegetations. Shortly after onset of the disease, the individual lesions coalesce into extensive plaques that sometimes occupy the entire area of the extremity or buttock.  The plaques appear festooned in outline and have surfaces covered with soft vegetations, ulcerations, and crusts. Not infrequently, pustules with viscous sanguinopurulent contents can be found at the periphery of the lesions.  Later, such a lesion shows central scarring, while the infiltrate at the periphery of the lesion tends to spread further to produce elevated plaques.  The general condition of the patients remains satisfactory, even if the bones and internal organs are affected, as they are in some cases, although much less frequently than in European blastomycosis (Busse-Buschke's disease).

Histologic appearance.  This is not uncommonly marked by pronounced pseudocarcinomatous epidermal hyperplasia arising in the presence of an infiltrate which has a tuberculoid structure and contains many giant cells and a few fungal spores.  Characteristic features of the hyperplasia are multiple microabscesses and dyskeratotic cells arranged in groups that closely resemble horn pearls. However, because of the microabscesses and also because the number of mitoses is small, a squamous cell carcinoma is rarely suspected (Montgomery, 1967).

Differential diagnosis.  It is at times difficult to distinguish North American blastomycosis from warty tuberculosis.  However, the lesions of blastomycosis, unlike those of warty tuberculosis, lack distinct zones; have soft rather than hard warty vegetations; show miliary pustules at the periphery and, histologically, multiple microabscesses within the epidermis; and, finally, they contain the causative organism in the infiltrate.  These features are also helpful in discriminating between North American blastomycosis and chronic pyoderma ulcerosum vegetans.

### 9.5.2  Chromomycosis

Chromomycosis (chromoblastomycosis), like blastomycosis, is rather frequently accompanied by pseudocarcinomatous epidermal hyperplasia.  The disease usually results from contamination of wounds by the causative organisms (various species of fungi from Phialophora, Cladosporium, or Fonsecaea).

Clinical manifestations. Several days to months following trauma, wartlike nodules of dark pink color appear at the site of the trauma, slowly increase in size, and fuse to form tumorlike plaques of cyanotic appearance with warty vegetations on their surface that sometimes resemble a cauliflower (Mashkilleison, 1960). The lesions may ulcerate. Psoriasiform lesions consisting of flattened tumorlike plaques with massive strongly adherent serous scales and crusts may be present. When the papillomatous surfaces of the lesions ulcerate, laminated grayish-brown crusts are formed, from which pus can be expressed. Chromomycosis has been reported to occur more frequently in men aged between 30 and 50 years (Arievich, 1961). The sites of predilection are the lower extremities. The disease runs a protracted course (which extends for decades in some cases) and heals with scarring and fibrosis of the subcutaneous fat, which may sometimes cause lymphostasis (Minsker et al., 1975).

Histologic appearance. Chromomycosis is characterized by the presence in the dermis of a pronounced granulomatous infiltrate containing epithelioid cells and also lymphocytes, plasma cells, and eosinophils. Rather often, the epidermis displays pseudocarcinomatous hyperplasia and microabscesses, predominantly in the lower part of the spinous layer.

Differential diagnosis. Chromomycosis can be separated from other conditions by demonstration, in the exudate or histologic specimens from the lesional skin, of the causative organisms which appear as yellowish-brown spherical bodies with double septums. The presence of epidermal microabscesses and the tuberculoid structure of the infiltrate distinguish the pseudocarcinomatous hyperplasia arising in chromomycosis from a squamous cell carcinoma.

Clinically, chromomycosis bears similarities to warty tuberculosis (in both, the lesions have cyanotic appearance, tend to be localized to the extremities, and may have a cauliflower-like, firm, warty surface) and, in its ulcerative vegetating form, to chronic deep pyoderma ulcerosum vegetans. However, the correct diagnosis can always be established by demonstrating the causative agent of chromomycosis.

## 9.6   TOXICODERMAS

In toxicodermas, of which there exist many types, reactive pseudocarcinomatous epidermal hyperplasia is seen to arise mainly in cutaneous lesions showing vegetations and wartlike lesions, and these occur predominantly in bromoderma and iododerma.

### 9.6.1   Bromoderma

This results from prolonged ingestion of bromides and usually takes the form of bromide acne, papulomacular eruptions, or vegetat-

ing lesions.  It is in the latter type of lesion that pseudocarcinomatous epidermal hyperplasia is particularly apt to occur.

Clinical manifestations.  Vegetating bromoderma is characterized
by the appearance of wartlike papular eruptions of a vivid pink color
which fuse into lesions measuring 2-4 cm or more in diameter and
having surfaces covered with vegetations.  In some cases there appear
bullae with serous or serosanguinous contents; when the bullae rupture, they reveal vegetations which enlarge rapidly.  The favored
sites are the lower extremities.  Vegetating bromoderma is accompanied by a grave general condition of the patient and may be fatal.

Histologic appearance.  The dermis shows a massive granulomatous
infiltrate composed of lymphocytes, neutrophils, plasma cells, and
histiocytes.  There are many newly formed vessels, and areas of
hemorrhage are present.  Pseudocarcinomatous epidermal hyperplasia
is pronounced, with proliferating epidermal strands extending deep
into the dermis where islands of epidermal cells are often found.
Areas of incomplete individual cell keratinization resembling horn
pearls may be seen, and intraepithelial abscesses are frequently
present (Lever and Schaumburg-Lever, 1975).

Differential diagnosis.  Bromoderma should be differentiated
from iododerma, chronic pyoderma ulcerosum vegetans, pemphigus vegetans, and blastomycosis.  Of critical diagnostic importance may be the
history of long-term use of bromides.

Chronic pyoderma ulcerosum vegetans differs from bromoderma by
showing a profuse purulent discharge and the presence of isolated
pustules and inflamed follicles at the lesional periphery.

The lesions of pemphigus vegetans, unlike those seen in the
bullous form of vegetating bromoderma, are located in skin folds,
carry on their surfaces a thick serous material which is often malodorous, typically contain acantholytic cells, and show the presence
of Nikolsky's sign and a large proportion of eosinophils in the
granulamatous dermal infiltrate.

Blastomycosis can be separated from vegetating bromoderma by the
presence of giant cells and of the causative organisms in the infiltrate.

9.6.2  Iododerma

This may arise as a result of prolonged ingestion of iodides.

Clinical manifestations.  Iododerma is characterized clinically
by the appearance of vegetating papules which fuse to form rather

small, circumscribed lesions. These may occur in any area of the
skin, but are seen more commonly on the face, neck, and shoulders.
The surfaces of the vegetating plaques often ulcerate and become
covered with serosanguinous crusts. Along with ulcerative vegetating lesions, acneiform (iodide acne) or roseolous eruptions are
present in many cases.

Histologic appearance. This is frequently characterized by a
massive granulomatous infiltrate consisting predominantly of histiocytes. Often, the infiltrate destroys the acanthotic epidermis,
resulting in ulceration. At the margin of such an ulcer, intraepidermal abscesses and pseudocarcinomatous hyperplasia are frequently
seen (Lever and Schaumburg-Lever, 1975).

Differential diagnosis. Iododerma vegetans has to be differentiated from vegetating bromoderma, mycosis fungoides, and, rarely,
squamous cell carcinoma. In vegetating bromoderma, ulcerations
develop much less commonly than in the iododerma and the wartlike
plaques are much less prominent and occur·for the most part on the
lower extremities.

The tumor stage of mycosis fungoides may present a histologic
appearance similar to that seen in vegetating iododerma, but, unlike
the iododerma, it has a protracted course and is characterized by
multiple lesions with smooth or ulcerated surfaces that do not show
vegetations, so that the differentiation between the two can usually
be readily made on clinical grounds.

Occasionally, the lesions of vegetating iododerma resemble
cutaneous squamous cell carcinoma. For instance, Porters and
Zantkuyl (1975) described a 67-year-old woman who had been taking,
over a period of 2 years, a iodine-containing drug for stenosis
of the aorta and had developed ulcerated tumorlike lesions interpreted as cutaneous squamous cell carcinoma. However, the presence
of a nonspecific granulomatous infiltrate on histologic examination
coupled with the history of drug ingestion made it possible to
establish the correct diagnosis of iododerma.

The psuedocarcinomatous epidermal hyperplasia arising in vegetating iododerma, as well as that developing in vegetating bromoderma, differs from a squamous cell carcinoma by the presence of
multiple intraepidermal abscesses (Lever and Schaumburg-Lever, 1975).

## 9.7  Lichen Ruber Planus

Of the various clinical forms of lichen ruber planus (lichen
planus), epidermal hyperplasia is common only in lichen planus
verrucosus.

Clinical manifestations. The verrucous form of lichen planus (lichen planus hypertrophicus) is characterized by flat, wartlike papules that coalesce into irregularly shaped or ellipsoid plaques of dirty pink or, often, cyanotic appearance with well defined borders and covered by hard warty growths and small grayish scales. Along with the warty plaques, one often finds typical lichenoid papules of lichen planus. The sites of predilection are the anterior surfaces of the lower legs and, less often, the upper extremities. The disease occurs most commonly in individuals between the ages 30 and 60, more frequently in men (Mashkilleison, 1965).

Histologic appearance. The lesions of lichen planus verrucosus usually show hyperkeratosis, granulosis, and a striking acanthosis of a degree that often produces a picture of pseudocarcinomatous hyperplasia. The dermis displays a bandlike polymorphocellular infiltrate expressed to variable extent.

Among our 36 patients with this form of lichen planus, 23 were men and 13 women, ranging in age from 7 to 69 years, but most (26) were aged 30 to 60. In 22 of the patients, the lesions were confined to the anterior surfaces of the lower legs, in 10 they were located on the upper extremities, while in the remaining four patients the disease process was generalized, with involvement of the trunk as well as the limbs. The plaques on the trunk were small and flattened, whereas on the extremities they had a strikingly warty appearance. In a number of the cases, the warty elements had raised borders, thus giving grounds to suspect malignancy, and in some other cases the warty plaques on the lower extremities were accompanied by similar plaques on the vermilion border of the lip.

By way of example, one of these latter cases is described below.

Patient Kh., a man aged 50, presented with slightly itchy nodules on the shins. He said that he had been ill for about 10 years. Previous treatments with various agents (injections of groups B vitamins, corticosteroids, antibiotics, autohemotherapy, grenz-ray therapy, external applications of pure tar and salicylic acid-containing ointment, etc.) had resulted in only slight improvement of his condition. Later, further tumorlike formations covered with horny masses began to appear, with concurrent development of wartlike lesions on the lower lip.

Physical examination showed, on the anterior surfaces of both legs, faintly pink tumorlike structures 2 to 4 cm in diameter covered with horny matter. The margins of some of the tumorous formations were free from horny material and were elevated above the level of the skin. On palpation, the lesions were firm and fused with the subjecent tissue (Figure 68a). The glans penis showed a few glisten-

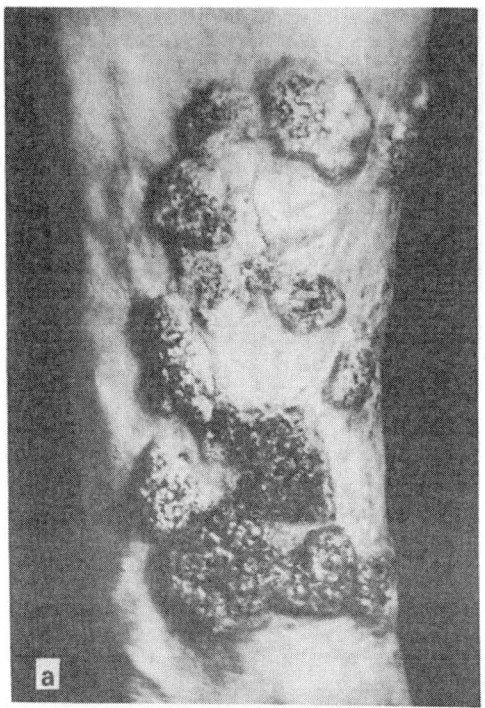

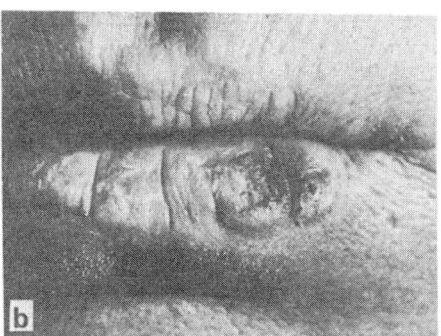

Fig. 68.  Lichen ruber verrucosus.  (a) On shin skin; (b) on the
          lower lip in same patient.


ing lichenoid elements.  The lower lip had a sharply demarcated plaque on the left covered with grayish-brown scales
and firm to palpation.  A deep fissure was seen in the
center of the plaque.  The submandibular lymph nodes were
not palpable (Figure 68b).  To ascertain the diagnosis and
exclude malignancy, histologic examination of biopsy specimens from lesions on the right leg and lower lip was undertaken.

The biopsy specimen from the lesion on the anterior surface of the right leg showed striking acanthosis and also hyperkeratosis with areas of parakeratosis. Horny material occurred in scalloped depressions of the epidermis as horny plugs which in places were arranged concentrically and resembled cysts. There was focal hypergranulosis in some areas. The acanthotic epidermal strands of bizarre shapes had penetrated deep into the dermis, and in these areas the cytoplasm of spinous cells stained more faintly in comparison with the overlying layers. The cell boundaries were ill-defined. There was some cellular disarray (Figure 69a). The dermis showed a diffuse lymphohistiocytic infiltrate containing some plasma cells, with elements of the infiltrate penetrating the epidermis in places. The blood vessels and lymphatics were dilated. On staining by the Brachet method, the cytoplasms of epidermal cells showed nonuniform pyroninophilia, staining more faintly at the lower extensions of the proliferating epidermis. On Feulgen staining, the nuclei of basal cells and of cells of the infiltrate, particularly lymphocytes, stained more deeply than did the nuclei of cells in the lower portions of the acanthotic strands. PAS-positive, diastase-labile substances had accumulated in small amounts in the spinous cells of the epidermal extensions deep in the dermis. No glycogen was detectable in the basal cells. In these areas the PAS-positive basement membrane presented as a thin, delicate fibrous structure that disappeared in places. Considerable deposits of PAS-positive material occurred in blood vessel walls. On staining by the Foot method, the argyrophilic basement membrane appeared thinned out and discontinuous in many places. No fibrin was demonstrated by Mallory's phosphotungstic acid-hematoxylin stain. It was concluded that the histologic picture was compatible with the clinical diagnosis of lichen ruber verrucosus and was one of pronounced pseudocarcinomatous epidermal hyperplasia.

Histologic study of the tissue biopsied from the plaquelike lesion on the lip revealed pronounced acanthosis and also hyperkeratosis with areas of parakeratosis. Stratum granulosum was absent under the parakeratotic masses and consisted of one or two rows of cells elsewhere. The epidermis had proliferated irregularly deep into the underlying tissue. In places, sheets of epithelial cells had separated from the acanthotic epithelial strands to appear as islands surrounded by cells of a massive infiltrate. In some areas the spinous cells stained more faintly than in others, and the boundaries between them were indistinct. The basal cells of the overlying epithelial strands were prominent in certain areas and

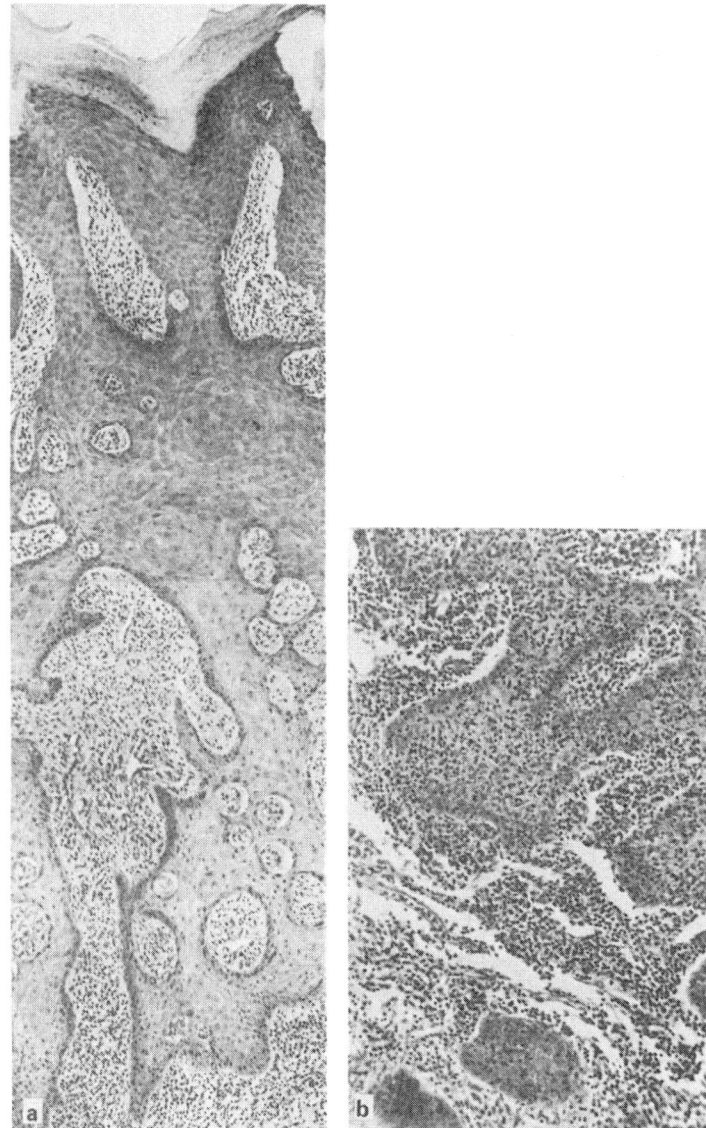

Fig. 69.  Lichen ruber verrucosus.  (a) Shin skin, showing moderate
          pseudocarcinomatous hyperplasia (montage); (b) lower lip,
          showing striking acanthosis with epithelial cells breaking
          away from the acanthotic epidermis to form aggregates which
          are surrounded by cells of a massive infiltrate.  (75 X;
          hematoxylin and eosin.)

indetectable elsewhere.   The epithelial islands were devoid
of basal layer.   There was pronounced exocytosis.   Cells of
the massive infiltrate, which was composed of lymphocytes,
histiocytes, and segmented cells, had invaded the epithelium everywhere.   There were marked cellular disorganization and polymorphism.   The lymphatics and blood vessels
were grossly dilated (Figure 69b).   The histologic diagnosis was lichen ruber verrucosus presenting a picture of
pseudocarcinomatous hyperplasia.

In the case just described, the clinical appearance of the
lesions on the lower extremities indicated lichen ruber verrucosus,
but the presence of elements which had markedly raised borders, were
fused with subjacent tissues, and were surrounded by atrophic scars,
aroused suspicion of malignant transformation.   The histologic examination of these lesions showed a pseudocarcinomatous hyperplasia
arising in lichen ruber verrucosus.   The cicrumscribed plaquelike
lesion on the vermilion border of the lower lip was interpreted
clinically as a manifestation of the underlying condition in view of
the presence of elements of the lichen on the buccal mucosa.   But
since the lesion was circumscribed, firm to palpaption, showed a deep
central fissure, and was of long duration (about 2 years), malignancy
had to be ruled out.   The histologic study revealed a picture of
pseudocarcinomatous hyperplasia, although it was not possible to
exclude completely an incipient squamous cell carcinoma of the lower
lip on the basis of the single biopsy.   The lesions improved considerably in response to a combined treatment (vitamins, sedatives,
and compresses containing salicylic acid ointment applied to the
lesions on the legs along with topical application of Flucinar [fluo-
cinolone acetonide] to the lips), with flattening of some of the
warty nodules on the legs and resolution of the lesion on the lip.
Followup of this patient confirmed the benignancy of the process.
When he was examined a year after discharge, no eruption was seen on
the vermilion border, but the warty nodules on the shins were still
persisting; however, after topical application of 30% Prospidinum
ointment, they became much flatter, and areas of erosion and ulceration covered with sanguinous crusts appeared at the sites of some of
them.

Differential diagnosis.   Diagnosis of lichen ruber verrucosus
poses no problems in typical cases and is based on recognition of its
distinctive features such as the presence, along with warty lesions,
of typical elements of the lichen (polygonal opalescent papules with
central umbilication, Wickham's striae) and, histologically, exaggerated granulation.   On occasion, however, the condition must be differentiated from squamous cell carcinoma which may arise in this
dermatosis (Mashkilleison, 1960; Shanin, 1969; Raichev and Andreev,
1965; Venkei and Sugar, 1965).

The surface of a malignant transformed warty plaque of lichen ruber planus is ulcerated. Such cases usually have a history of inappropriate treatment in the past (with x-rays, arsenic, tar, etc.). The pseudocarcinomatous epidermal hyperplasia that has developed in lichen ruber verrucosus, is almost indistinguishable from a well-differentiated squamous cell carcinoma histologically, and combined studies of the kind described in Chap. 4-6 above are then required.

Difficulties may arise at times in differentiating this form of lichen from tuberculosis verrucosa, verrucous neurodermatosis, prurigo nodularis and amyloidosis cutis.

Tuberculosis verrucosa cutis differs from lichen ruber verrucosus in that the lesions are usually solitary; have three zones; may show ulceration of the warty vegetations; tend to heal with non-elevated smooth scars; and, histologically, contain a tuberculoid infiltrate with moderate caseation necrosis from which <u>Mycobacterium tuberculosis</u> can be recovered.

Lichen ruber verrucosus differs from verrucous neurodermatosis by showing opalescent polygonal papules elsewhere on the skin and also on mucous membranes, by less pronounced itching, and by the lilac color of the lesions.

Prurigo nodularis of Hyde, unlike lichen ruber verrucosus, is accompanied by excruciating itching and shows multiple small round nodules covered with bloody crusts and, histologically, hyperplasia of neural elements and the absence of hypergranulosis in the acanthotic epidermis.

Lastly, cutaneous amyloidosis is characterized by hard hemispheric papules which frequently coalesce to form large plaques localized on the anterolateral aspect of the lower leg and accompanied by intense itching. In cases of doubt, staining for amyloid can help in establishing the correct histologic diagnosis.

## 9.8  Neurodermatoses and other Diseases

Among the various skin disorders included in the group of neurodermatoses (neurodermatitides), there are two conditions - giant lichenification of Brocq and Pautrier and prurigo nodularis of Hyde - in which pseudocarcinomatous epidermal hyperplasia is seen to arise much more commonly than in any other form this group (Zheltakov, 1964; Mashkilleison, 1965; Skripkin, 1967; Berenbein, 1971).

## 9.8.1  Giant Lichenification of Brocq and Pautrier

This is a variant of neurodermatitis circumscripta (giant hypertrophic neurodermatitis).

Clinical manifestations. Areas of lichenification occur pre-dominantly in the inguinal folds, in the perineal region, and on the inner surfaces of the thighs; are heavily infiltrated; often have nodular and wartlike elements on the surface; and are extremely itchy.

Another variety of neurodermatitis circumscripta is neuroderm-atitis verrucosa (Kreibic, 1915) in which the lesions are elevated, sharply delimited from the surrounding unaltered skin, and covered by closely packed wartlike structures all over their surface. They may occur in various areas of the skin, but are seen most commonly on the lower and upper extremities. They are solitary, as a rule.

These two forms of circumscribed neurodermatitis are rare, and most of the patients are men beyond the age 16-18 years.

Histologic appearance. The hypertrophic form of neurodermatitis circumscripta is characterized by a striking hyperkeratosis with formation of horny plugs in the orifices of hair follicles, and by acanthosis, often of a degree that produces a picture of pseudocarci-nomatous hyperplasia. In some cases, the acanthotic epidermis shows spongiosis. The dermis contains a diffuse infiltrate of lymphocytes, fibroblasts, and histiocytes, and shows some fibrosis. In most instances there are changes in nerve fibers, such as hyperplasia, irregular thickening, fragmentation, and degenerative changes (e.g. Zheltakov, 1964; Kaufman, 1968).

Differential diagnosis. Giant lichenification, and verrucous neurodermatitis in particular, should be differentiated from the verrucous form of lichen planus and secondarily lichenified eczema. Patients with such eczema, unlike those with giant lichenification, have a history of oozing or weeping lesions in certain stages of the disease.


9.8.2  Prurigo Nodularis of Hyde

This rare disorder is regarded by some as a variety of neuro-dermatitis circumscripta.

Clinical manifestations. There are firm, round, pink raised nodules 0.5 to 1.5 cm or, occasionally, 2 cm in size covered with sanguinous crusts. The favorite sites are the extensor surfaces of the arms and the anterior surfaces of the legs. The nodules do not coalesce and do not occur in groups. As a rule, the eruption is preceded by strong itching which becomes more intense after the lesions have appeared. This is a long disease, and the lesions seldom resolve spontaneously; if they do, they leave behind atrophic scars showing hyperpigmentation.

Both sexes may be affected, but there is a predilection for men
aged over 30 years.  There were 8 men and 4 women among our patients
with prurigo nodularis, ranging in age from 42 to 72 years.

Histologic appearance.  The histologic features of prurigo
nodularis have been studied by many authors (e.g. Pautrier, 1934;
Zheltakov, 1940; Thies, 1955; Mashkilleison, 1965; Kaufman, 1968;
Lever and Schaumburg-Lever, 1975) and include striking acanthosis,
often of a degree approaching pseudocarcinomatous hyperplasia; hyperkeratosis; and some parakeratosis.  The process of epidermal growth
involves hair follicles and the excretory ducts of sweat glands.
Acanthotic epidermal strands having bizarre outlines and showing
areas of mild spongiosis invade the dermis in the middle portion of
which there is a rather considerable infiltrate composed of lymphocytes and histiocytes with small numbers of plasma cells and eosinophils.  The older nodules display fibrosis.  Within the infiltrate,
the vessels are greatly dilated and have thickened and sclerotic
walls.

Many authors consider hyperplasia of neural elements as a diagnostic criterion for prurigo nodularis.  Pautrier (1934), for example, found large numbers of altered nerve fibers abutting the
epidermis within the lesions of prurigo nodularis.  Neurochisto-
logical studies carried out in our clinic have revealed, in all cases
of prurigo nodularis, various changes in neural elements such as
hyperplasia, thickening, and, often, degeneration of nerve fibers and
the presence of grains and of stellate inclusion bodies; many of the
neural elements were lying close to the acanthotic epidermis.

Differential diagnosis.  Prurigo nodularis of Hyde must be
separated from lichen ruber verrucosus, verrucous neurodermatitis,
and Kirle's disease.

The lesions of prurigo nodularis, in contrast to those of lichen
planus verrucosus, are more widespread, show sanguinous crusts, and
are not accompanied by typical polygonal papules or mucosal changes;
histologically, the distinctive signs of prurigo nodularis are the
absence of hypergranulosis or bandlike infiltrate and the presence of
hypertropic nerve fibers.

The hypertrophic form of neurodermatitis has as its distinctive
features lichenification and infiltration of the skin which produce a
continuous lesional area within which occasional nodules are present.

Prurigo nodularis differs from Kirle's disease (hyperkeratosis
follicularis et perfollicularis in cutem penetrans) by intense itching, by the type of morphologic elements of the eruption, and by
histopathologic features such as the absence of follicular hyperkeratosis extending into the dermis.

If a pronounced pseudocarcinomatous hyperplasia is present in prurigo nodularis, a well-differentiated cutaneous squamous cell carcinoma may be suspected histologically, but the suspicion can be readily dispelled clinically.

### 9.8.3  Miscellaneous Dermatoses

Occasionally, pseudocarcinomatous epidermal hyperplasia arises in secondarily lichenified eczema.  We have observed several such cases.  Here is one example.

Patient P., a 35-year-old man, was admitted to our department complaining of itchy eruptions on the face, trunk, and limbs that had appeared about 2 years before following exposure to sunlight.  He had been treated with desensitizing agents, vitamins, and antihistaminics, which resulted in only temporary improvement, with the disease recurring in springtime.

Physical examination showed the skin to be strongly hyperemic and edematous on the face, neck, and dorsa of the hands.  The surfaces of the lesions showed oozing vesicular elements that were coalescing into areas of erosion; serosanguinous crusts were seen in places.  The clinical diagnosis was "solar eczema."

The patient was administered a course of combined treatment (injections of vitamin $B_{12}$ and folic and nicotinic acids; dexamethasone, antihistaminic drugs, and steroid creams), which led to disappearance of the edema and oozing, but considerable lichenification appeared on the dorsa of the hands.  Topical application of naphthalene, hot baths, and compresses with steroid cream failed to eliminate or improve the lichenification; instead, circumscribed areas carrying wartlike elements appeared at the affected sites.  To ascertain the diagnosis, a biopsy specimen was taken from the dorsum of the right hand, and its histologic examination revealed irregular acanthosis and hyperkeratosis alternating with areas of parakeratosis. No stratum granulosum was in evidence in much of the specimen.  In certain regions, the epidermal ridges, some of which were thickened and some thinned, had penetrated the dermis (very deeply in places) in which cross-sectioned hypertrophic cystlike hair follicles with a well-defined granular layer surrounding the horny masses were seen.  In some areas, the lower dermis showed aggregates of epithelial cells which likewise were probably associated with the follicles.  Within these aggregates, the spinous cells were arranged regularly and were surrounded by rows of basal

cells that appeared blurred in places by the edema and
infiltrate.  The infiltrate was particularly pronounced
around the epithelial structures and consisted of lymphocytes, histiocytes, and some polymorphonuclear leukocytes.
Cells of the infiltrate had invaded the epithelial aggregates (Figure 70).  The lower dermis was somewhat sclerotic.
The collagen fibers were arranged in thick parallel bundles
and showed pronounced proliferation of fibroblasts.  The
lymphatics and blood vessels were dilated.  The blood
vessel walls were thickened and surrounded by perivascular
infiltrate.

In this case a lichenification secondary to chronic eczema was
attended by pseudocarcinomatous epidermal hyperplasia that was partially simulated by the cross-sectioned hypertrophic hair follicles.
That the disease process was benign was clear both histologically and
clinically.

Epidermal hyperplasia mimicking basal cell carcinomatous hyperplasia occurs rather frequently in the vegetating form of Darier's
disease.  Here is a case report to illustrate this.

Patient B., a 30-year-old woman, was admitted to our
department complaining of eruptions that had persisted
since the age 12 despite the administration of a variety of
treatments.  About 10 years prior to admission, areas of
erosion and ulceration covered with crusts and papillomatous growths began appearing on the lower extremities.

On physical examination, multiple papular growths
covered with horny crusts were seen on the upper and lower
extremities, neck, anterior chest, and interscapulum.  On
the lower extremities, notably the shins, many of these
growths had coalesced into diffuse lesions covered by
vegetations and seropurulent material that had dried up to
form firm crusts.  The clinical diagnosis was "Darier's
disease".

Histologic study of the skin biopsied from the right
shin showed acanthosis with hyperkeratosis and areas of
parakeratosis.  The granular layer was prominent.  The
proliferating epidermal strands thinned out downward and
produced, together with the cross-sectioned hair follicles,
an appearance of basal cell carcinoma.  The basal layer was
preserved throughout.  In many areas, clefts (lacunae) were
seen above the basal layer (Figure 71a).  Under high magnification, dyskeratotic cells appearing as round structures surrounded by a halo (corps ronds) could be clearly
seen, chiefly among cells of the granular layer.  In the
suprabasal lacunae, freely lying spinous cells undergoing

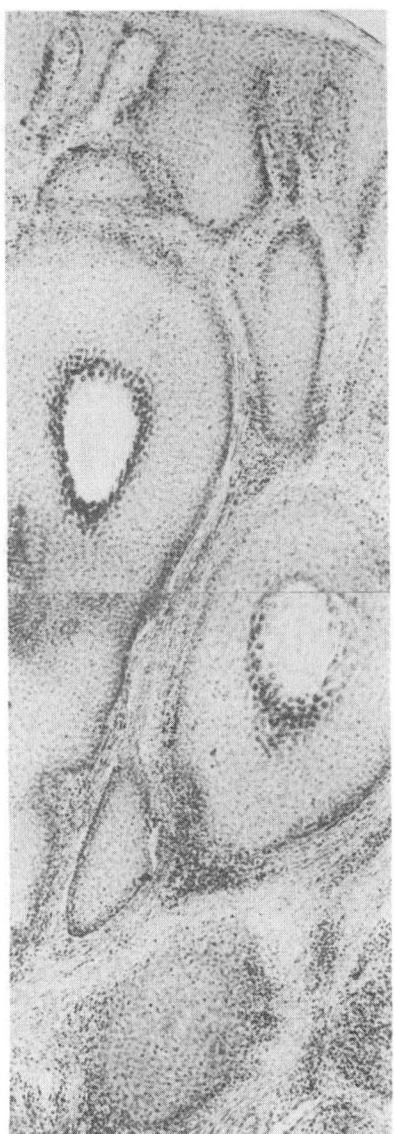

Fig. 70.  Eczema.  Dorsum of the hand.  There is pseudocarcinomatous
epidermal hyperplasia that has arisen in secondary
lichenification in a patient with chronic eczema.  (75 X;
hematoxylin and eosin.)


vacuolation and dystrophic changes were observed (Figure
71b).  The histologic picture was consistent with the
clinical diagnosis of Darier's disease.

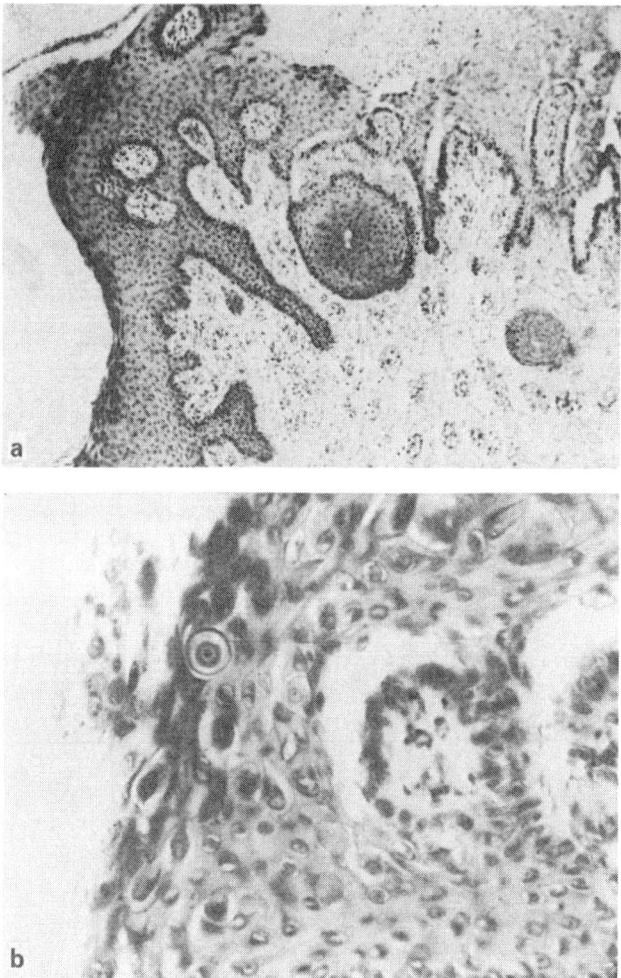

Fig. 71.  Darier's dyskeratosis (shin skin).  (a) Hyperkeratosis with
          areas of parakeratosis, showing proliferating epidermal
          strands that present an appearance of pseudobasaloid hyper-
          plasia; there are numerous lacunae (75 X); (b) same
          specimen:  the granular layer shows dyskeratotic cells
          surrounded by halo and containing homogeneous nuclei; in
          the suprabasal lacunae, freely lying spinous cells in a
          state of dystrophy are seen.  (250 X; hematoxylin and
          eosin.)


     In this patient, a prominent clinical feature of generalized
Darier's disease was the presence of vegetating lesions on the lower
extremitics, and these lesions were characterized histologically by a
moderate epidermal hyperplasia resembling basal-cell carcinomatous

growths. The major histopathologic signs of Darier's disease such as dyskeratotic cells (corps ronds) and suprabasal clefts, were well expressed. This case well exemplifies the difference in dyskeratotic cells between Darier's disease and keratinizing squamous cell carcinoma of the skin. Thus, in cancer the dyskeratotic cells, or cells with individual keratinization, appear as homogeneous formations present usually in the spinous layer of the acanthotic epidermis or within isolated spinous cell aggregates, whereas in Darier's disease such cells (the corps ronds) are most commonly found in the granular layer of the epidermis and are often surrounded by a halo.

## 9.9   SUMMARY

Although pseudocarcinomatous epidermal hyperplasias may arise in various dermatoses that differ in nature, these hyperplasias have much in common with each other and at the same time are closely associated with the clinicopathologic changes that occur in the particular dermatoses. Review of the literature and our personal observations indicate that the pseudocarcinomatous hyperplasia tends to occur most commonly in tumorlike and infiltrative ulcerative lesions showing pronounced vegetative growths. The decisive clues to the diagnostic differentiation between pronounced pseudocarcinomatous epidermal hyperplasia and keratinizing squamous cell carcinoma of the skin can often be provided by the clinical features of the dermatosis in question. In cases where clinical studies do not permit this differentiation, histologic examination or combined histologic, cytophysiologic, and cytogenetic investigations may be in order.

# 10
# Criteria for Diagnostic Differentiation Between Pseudocarcinomatous Epidermal Hyperplasia and Squamous Cell Carcinoma of the Skin

The availability of criteria for differentiating between pseudo-carcinomatous hyperplasia of the epidermis and squamous cell carcinoma of the skin which are known to present similar clinical and histologic appearances while being radically different in biologic nature, may be of great practical significance. It would be particularly important to be able to establish the nature of such a hyperplasia, that is, whether it will remain benign or is just a link in the complex chain of events leading up to malignant transformation of the epidermis.

Our followup studies (1 to 12 years in duration) of 103 patients with various dermatoses displaying pronounced pseudocarcinomatous hyperplasia, showed that a complete cure had occurred in 46 of them, but that in 54 other patients the process had been running an indolent course, with lesions failing to resolve completely in 45 of these cases. Transformation of the dermatitis into a keratinizing squamous cell carcinoma occurred in three of the patients (2.8%) — one with psoriasis, another with Buschke-Loewenstein's giant condyloma acuminatum, and one with trophic ulcer of the lower leg.

Thus, the dermatoses which we tentatively classify as pseudo-carcinoses, have in some cases proved to be premalignant conditions that progressed to malignancy. It can be inferred from this that a hyperplasia presenting as pseudocarcinomatous can be regarded as benign only at the time of examination of the patient. We therefore consider it too categorical a statement that a pseudocarcinomatous hyperplasia, even if it persists over a long time, will always remain such, that is benign. It seems that given certain circumstances (traumas, inappropriate treatment,, etc.), squamous cell carcinoma may supersede a hyperplasia originally considered pseudo-carcinomatous.

206

Table 14. Differences and Similarities Between Pseudocarcinomatous Epidermal Hyperplasia and Keratinizing Squamous Cell Carcinoma as Indicated by Clinical, Histopathologic, Cytogenetic, and Cytophysiologic Studies[1].

| Characteristics | Pseudocarcinomatous hyperplasia | Squamous cell carcinoma |
|---|---|---|
| **CLINICAL** | | |
| Tumorlike lesions | As a rule | Frequent |
| Infiltrative and ulcerative lesions | Rarely seen, mainly in chronic pyoderma ulcerosum vegetans, trophic ulcers of the lower leg, cutaneous leishmaniasis, and some deep mycoses | Frequent |
| Number of lesions | Often multiple | Solitary as a rule |
| Fusion of lesions with underlying tissue | Rare, but may occur in lesions of ulcerative-infiltrative type | Frequent |
| Firmness of lesions | Depends on underlying dermatosis, but firm lesions are rare | Usually firm |
| Surface of lesions: | | |
|   smooth | Very rare | Frequent |
|   warty | Frequent | Frequent |
| Growth rate of lesions: | | |
|   rapid | Frequent | In exceptional cases |
|   slow | Rare | As a rule |
| Enlarged and hardened regional lymph nodes | Only in cases of acute inflammation or infection of lesions | Usual in late phases of tumor evolution |
| Fused and immobile regional lymph nodes | Absent | Present in far advanced cases |

Table 14. (Continued)

| Characteristics | Pseudocarcinomatous hyperplasia | Squamous cell carcinoma |
|---|---|---|
| Clinicopathologic features of the dermatosis on which hyperplasia or carcinoma has supervened | Are retained | Are grossly distorted or nonexistent |
| Response to symptomatic therapy | Marked in most instances | None |
| **HISTOPATHOLOGIC** | | |
| Downward extension of epithelial strands to sweat gland level | Frequently seen | Usual in invasive growths |
| Horn pearl formation | Frequently seen, with incomplete cell keratinization | Usual |
| Individual cell keratinization | Rare | Present as a rule |
| Cellular disarray | Frequently seen | Usually seen |
| Nuclear polymorphism | Moderate | Usually pronounced in invasive carcinomas |
| Integrity of basement membrane | Often disrupted in areas of invasive epithelial cell proliferations | Usually disrupted in areas of invasive tumor cell proliferations |
| Invasion of epidermis by cells of the infiltrate | Seen as a rule | Very uncommon |

| | | |
|---|---|---|
| Presence of granulomatous infiltrate in dermis | Frequent | Exceptionally rare (only in cases of malignant transformation of pre-existing dermatosis) |
| Disintegration of infiltrate | Rare | Usual |
| Glycogen | Much in upper epidermis and little or none in invasive proliferations | Present in epidermis in well-differentiated carcinomas and absent in poorly differentiated ones |
| Neutral mucopolysaccharides | Unevenly distributed in the basement membrane zone | Unevenly distributed in the basement membrane zone |
| RNA | Occurs mostly in lower portions of spinous layer; little found in upper epidermis | Occurs mostly in lower portions of spinous layer; little found in upper epidermis |
| Nuclear area | Greater than in normal epidermis or in sites of ordinary acanthosis | Greater than in pseudo-carcinomatous hyperplasia |
| CYTOGENETIC | | |
| DNA content of epidermal cell nuclei as measured by micro-cytospectrophotometry | Cells with paradiploid DNA values account for more than half of all cells (59.7±2.9%) and constitute the modal class. Index of DNA accumulation = 2.5 | Percentage of cells with paradiploid DNA values is low (6.6±2%), while those of paraoctoploid and hyperoctoploid cells are high (57% on average). Index of DNA accumulation = 5.5 |

Mitotic regime

| | | |
|---|---|---|
| Mitotic activity (no. of mitoses per 1000 cells) | 12.4 ± 1.5 | 28.1 ± 4.2 |

Table 14. (Continued)

| Characteristics | Pseudocarcinomatous hyperplasia | Squamous cell carcinoma |
| --- | --- | --- |
| Percentage of cells in metaphase | Higher than in normal epidermis (52.4 ± 2.5%) | Higher than in pseudo-carcinomatous hyperplasia (70.5 ± 4%) |
| Percentage of cells showing mitotic abnormalities, including | Higher than in normal epidermis (19.5 ± 2.5%) | Much higher than in hyper-plasia (44.4 ± 2.4%) |
| C-mitoses | 10.5 | 15.0 |
| lagging of chromosomes in metaphase | 6.5 | 8.0 |
| lagging of chromosomes in ana- and telophase | 1.8 | 3.1 |
| chromosome scattering | 0.3 | 11.8 |
| monocentric mitoses | None | 1.4 |
| three-group metaphases | None | 0.6 |
| **Chromosomes** | | |
| Percentage of diploid metaphases | 50.5 (range: 40 to 70 or more) | 23.4 (range: 10 to 37) |
| Percentage of aneuploid metaphases including | 49.5 (range: 30 to 60) | 76.6 (range: 32.5 to 90) |
| hypoploids | 20.7 (range: 4.7 to 26.6) | 11.3 (range: 5 to 17) |
| hyperploids | 28.8 (range: 12.5 to 38.5) | 65.3 (range: 50 to 85) |
| Marker chromosomes | None | Present |

| | | |
|---|---|---|
| Structural analysis | Significantly increased chromosome number in group B | Significantly decreased chromosome numbers in groups A and B and significantly increased numbers in groups C and D |
| Percentage of sex chromatin-containing nuclei: | | |
| women | Insignificantly decreased in areas of moderate acanthosis and pseudo-carcinomatous hyperplasia (average value: 21.2%) | Significantly decreased in tumorous proliferations (average value: 10.7%) |
| men | Insignificantly increased but remains within normal limits of variation | Increased compared to pseudocarcinomatous hyperplasia but remains within normal limits of variation |
| CYTOPHYSIOLOGIC | | |
| Growth pattern of primary skin cultures | Growth begins at days 2-8 of incubation and is characterized by formation of cell islands and slow expansion of monolayer cell sheet (over 4-5 weeks) | Growth begins at 24-27 hr of incubation with the explant growing out a sheet of epitheloid cells which shows rapid expansion (over 2 weeks) |

[1]All figures appearing in this table are based on the studies described in Chap. 4-6.

It should be emphasized that a number of well-known clinical and histopathologic characteristics of malignant change - such as among others exophytic or endophytic growth of the lesion, extent of invasive epidermal proliferation (to the sweat gland level), cellular disarray, nuclear polymorphism, frequent mitoses and presence of abnormal mitoses, and destruction of the basement membrane - are at times seen also in pseudocarcinomatous epidermal hyperplasia and therefore cannot be relied upon unconditionally in differentiating between hyperplasia and squamous cell carcinoma. Hence the importance, both practical and theoretical, of studying the nature and direction of epidermal proliferation in pseudocarcinomatous hyperplasia.

A review of the literature and the results of our own correlative studies in patients and in rabbits - clinical, histopathologic, cytophysiologic, and cytogenetic (see Chap. 3-6) - have enabled us to identify an informative set of criteria of difference and similarity between pseudocarcinomatous hyperplasia and squamous cell carcinoma. These criteria may be recommended for clinical use both in diagnostic differentiation between these conditions and in elucidating the character of epidermal proliferation and predicting the direction which it will take. The more important criteria are listed in Table 14.

# 11
# Management and Prevention of Cutaneous Pseudocarcinoses

As shown in the preceding chapters, the dermatologic entities included under cutaneous pseudomalignancies cover a great diversity of conditions which belong to several classification groups but which do or may show considerable clinical and/or histologic similarities to squamous cell carcinoma at some stage of their evolution or in response to certain provoking agents, Therefore, the efficacy of therapy in each particular case will of course largely depend on the disease in which the pseudocarcinomatous epidermal hyperplasia has arisen and thus on the identification of the relevant etiologic factors and pathogenetic mechanisms.

With some dermatoses (pyodermas, cutaneous tuberculosis, the deep mycoses, vegetating toxicodermas), identification of the etiologic factors may allow an efficacious purposive treatment to be instituted, but in most dermatoses the etiologic agents, once they have evoked particular pathologic changes, are pushed into the background by pathogenetic factors which come to the fore to become the major determinants of the clinical and histologic features shown by the dermatosis. Hence the great importance of pathogenetic therapy directed at normalizing the nervous system function, circulation, and cell proliferation at the sites of lesion.

Of much value in the selection of therapeutic agents or modalities appropriate for the dermatoses involving excessive epidermal growth, is history taking. Here it is particularly important to elicit information regarding the factors that have been conducive to the disease (exposure to sunlight or chemical agents; trauma; concomitant disorders); the age of the lesions, their course, their response to the treatments given previously, and their seasonal behavior; the use of medications in the past, including potent agents

(arsenic, tar, etc.); and the hereditary factors, notably the genetic
predisposition to neoplastic disease.

In every case, the treatment must be strictly individualized and
also comprehensive. It should be administered with due regard to the
general condition of the patient, the presence of concomitant
diseases, and the clinicopathologic characteristics of the lesions.
There are two broad categories of treatment methods; systemic and
external (topical), and the relative importance of these varies from
one cutaneous disorder to another. In some disorders (e.g. cutaneous
tuberculosis, the deep mycoses, pyodermas), systemic therapy has
precedence over the external therapy which plays only an ancillary
role. In others (e.g. keratoacanthoma, giant condyloma acuminatum of
Buschke and Loewenstein, trophic ulcers of the lower extremities),
methods of external therapy are of decisive importance.

## 11.1 SYSTEMIC THERAPY

Methods of systemic therapy are applied for the most part in
disorders in which pseudocarcinomatous hyperplasia is reactive, being
of the secondary or facultative type. In these dermatoses, the
dermis usually shows a pronounced inflammatory infiltrate, often
granulomatous. In this group one can encounter processes that can be
described as granulomatous bacterial (tuberculosis, syphilis, leishmaniasis), granulomatous mycotic (blastomycosis, chromomycosis, and
other deep mycoses), and toxic allergy (vegetating toxicodermas).
Moreover, as shown above, atypical reactive epidermal hyperplasia is
frequently seen in chronic pyoderma ulcerosum vegetans, trophic
ulcers of the lower extremities, certain forms of neurodermatoses,
and some other cutaneous ailments.

Because the dermatologic entities classified under facultative
pseudocarcinoses are many and varied, the methods of systemic therapy
differ accordingly.

Sedatives. The rhizome and roots of the herb Valeriana
officinalis is administered as an infusion (6 to 10 g of the herb to
180-200 ml of water) in an amount of 1 or 2 tablespoons 3 or 4 times
daily or as a decoction (2 to 3 teaspoons of the minced herb are
poured over 200 ml of cold water, allowed to boil for 5 min, and
strained through gauze) in the same dosage. Where appropriate, a
more concentrated infusion or decoction may be used (20 g to 200 ml
of water) to enhance the sedative effect. The herb is also used as
a 20% tincture (prepared by maceration with 70° alcohol in 1:5 ratio)
in a dose of 20-30 drops 3 to 5 times daily, or else as an extract
in tablets containing 0.02 g of the extract each, with 1 or 2 tablets
being taken 2 or 3 times daily.

Herbs of the genus <u>Leonurus</u> are administered as an infusion
(15 g to 200 ml of water) 1 tablespoon 3 or 4 times daily or as a
tincture (prepared by maceration with 70° alcohol in 1:5 ratio) in
doses of 30-40 drops 3 times daily.

The preparations of <u>Valeriana</u> and <u>Leonurus</u> have similar actions
and are employed to alleviate nervous excitation, insomnia, and
neuroses due to intense itching in various skin disorders such as
giant lichenification, prurigo nodularis, and lichen ruber verrucosus.

<u>Tranquilizers</u>, (trimetozine, chlordiazepoxide, diazepam,
oxazepam, etc.) which have calming actions on the central nervous
system, are used in protracted dermatoses accompanied by particularly
intense itching and insomnia (prurigo nodularis, the giant form of
neurodermatitis) and in other severe skin disorders accompanied by
pseudocarcinomatous hyperplasia and derangement of the nervous system
function (trophic ulcers of the lower extremities, chronic deep
pyoderma ulcerosum vegetans, etc.).

<u>Vitamins</u>, chiefly of the B group ($B_1$, $B_6$, and $B_{12}$), have found
wide application in various cutaneous diseases, including dermatoses
attended by pseudocarcinomatous hyperplasia, such as lichen ruber
verrucosus, giant verrucosus neurodermatitis, prurigo nodularis,
chronic deep pyoderma ulcerosum vegetans, and vegetating toxicodermas
(bromoderma and iododerma). Multiple lesions of pyoderma ulcerosum
vegetans are sometimes associated with ulcerative colitis, dyspro-
teinemia, and some other diseases (Brachtel and Lemmel, 1978), and in
such cases the combined use of group B vitamins, ascorbic acid, and
other medicaments may provide an effective method of pathogenetic
therapy. Vitamin A is used in the combined treatment of lichen ruber
verrucosus and of Darier's disease. In the latter disease, it is
advisable to administer Aevitum (a combination of vitamins A and E)
in capsules or injections. It should be remembered that vitamin A
may have side-effects, particularly in children (liver enlargement,
joint pain, itching, etc.). Since nicotinic acid (Vitamin PP) plays
a large role in oxidative and reductive processes, enhances the
hematopoetic function of bone marrow, intensifies diuresis, and
improves liver function, it is desirable to use the acid in persistent infectious or toxic processes in which pseudocarcinomatous hyperplasia is often seen to arise (lupus vulgaris, tuberculosis cutis
verrucosa, the deep mycoses, chronic pyoderma ulcerosum vegetans,
vegetating toxicodermas etc.). Vitamin $D_2$ is effective in the treatment of lupus vulgaris and chromomycosis and is administered over a
period of 5 to 6 months, preferably in combination with Ftivazidum,
sodium para-aminosalicylate, or other tuberculostatics. In chromomycosis, large doses of vitamin $D_2$ in combination with potassium
iodine are beneficial.

Antibiotics are widely used in granulomatous bacterial (tuberculosis, syphilis, leishmaniasis) and granulomatous mycotic (blastomycosis, chromomycosis, and other deep mycoses) processes, and also in chronic deep pyoderma ulcerosum vegetans and other dermatoses accompanied by reactive pseudocarcinomatous epidermal hyperplasia and complicated by secondary infection. In dermato-venereologic practices, extensive use is made of penicillin and its semisynthetic forms (methylcillin, oxacillin, ambicillin, etc.), monomycin, tetracyclines (Oletetrinum, etc.), and antifungal antibiotics such as griseofulvin, nystatin, amphotericin B, etc.

In deep pyoderma ulcerosum vegetans, the choice of antibiotic is dictated by the antibiogram, and it goes without saying that antibiotics must be used in conjunction with other treatments (vitamins, iodine preparations, antistaphylococcal plasma, antistaphylococcal gamma-globulin).

Penicillin has proved effective in the combined treatment of certain deep mycoses (actinomycosis, chromomycosis).

Streptomycin is used in combination with other tuberculostatics in the management of cutaneous tuberculosis in its various forms. It is particularly effective in lupus tuberculosus and tuberculosis cutis verrucosa (Skripkin and Sharapova, 1972), that is, in diseases which, as indicated above, often display a very pronounced pseudocarcinomatous hyperplasia.

Monomycin is especially effective in leishmaniasis.

Amphotericin B is widely used in conjunction with iodides and vitamin $D_2$ in the treatment of blastomycosis and chromomycosis.

Nonspecific stimulating therapy is employed extensively in the combined treatment of deep pyoderma ulcerosum vegetans, leishmaniasis, and the deep mycoses, and it is also useful in the giant form of neurodermatitis, prurigo nodularis, and lichen ruber verrucosus. Stimulants are administered in cases showing an indolent course, and also to debilitated patients. The more commonly used drugs include gamma-globulin, Pyrogenalum, and Prodigiosanum. Studnitsyn et al. (1967) propose starting intramuscular injections of Pyrogenalum with a dose between 50 and 100 MPD (minimal pyrogenic doses) and then raising the dosage in increments of 50 MPD to an amount which depends on the systemic and temperature responses. Treatment with Prodigiosanum is started with a dose of 25 to 50 µg (15 to 25 µg in children), slightly raising each subsequent dose.

Corticosteroid therapy is now recognized as the most efficient and widespread means of treating allergic and toxic allergic processes. Low doses of corticosteroid hormones are known to have desensitizing and antiinflammatory actions, to reduce vascular permeability, and to improve metabolic processes (Mashkilleison, 1964; Rozentul, 1970; Mashkovskii, 1977).  The corticosteroids which are most widely used in dermatologic practice include, among others, hydrocortisone, prednisolone, dexamethasone, and triamcinolone.  To avoid complications, they should be combined with vitamins, anabolic hormones, potassium preparations, and appropriate diet.

Corticosteroid therapy is indicated in severe toxicodermas (vegetating bromoderma and iododerma).  In very grave cases, prednisolone is given in an amount of 60 to 90 mg as intravenous drip in conjunction with detoxifying agents such as, for example, Haemodesum,[1] Rheopolyglucinum,[2] or an isotonic solution of sodium chloride.

In persistent diseases accompanied by intense itching (the giant form of neurodermatitis, prurigo nodularis, and lichen ruber verrucosus) intralesional injections of corticosteroids are indicated. For this purpose, prednisolone and hydrocortisone are used most commonly.  The injections are made intradermally and subcutaneously into the margin of the lesion in a total dose of 1 ml (30 mg) of prednisolone per session (2-3 injections), the complete course comprising 8 to 10 sessions depending on the lesional area.

Cytostatics.  Attempts have been made to use cytostatics (methotrexate) and antitumor antibiotics (bleomycin) in the treatment of multiple keratoacanthomas and giant condyloma acuminatum of Buschke and Loewenstein (e.g. Vollum, 1976; South et al., 1977).  Methotrexate may have side-effects (stomatitis, gastritis, thrombocytopenia, etc.) and is contraindicated in pregnancy and diseases of the liver, kidneys, and bone marrow (Ashmarin et al., 1973; Mashkilleison et al., 1973).  Parenterally administered bleomycin accumulates predominantly in the skin and mucous membranes and is therefore effective in squamous cell carcinomas of penal skin, oral mucosas, and the like (Vermel', 1972).  It is injected intravenously or intramuscularly in a dose of 15 mg on alternate days for a total of about 300 mg per treatment course.  Bleomycin evokes a number of adverse reactions, such as fever, nausea, vomiting, stomatitis, conjunctivitis, alopecia, focal hyperkeratoses, hyperpigmentation, and pneumonia (e.g. Khlebnov, 1975).

We have employed with much benefit the Soviet-made cytostatic Prospidinum (which has alkylating properties) in the treatment of papillomatosis cutis carcinoides of Gottron, administering the drug parenterally in a dose of 100 mg once daily for a total dose of 2.5 g.

---

[1] A water-salt solution of 6% low-molecular mass polyvinylpyrrolidone.
[2] A 10% colloidal solution of partially hydrolyzed dextran.

## 11.2  EXTERNAL THERAPY

As already stated, methods of external (topical) therapy play
the leading role in the management of cutaneous disease to which
pseudocarcinomatous hyperplasia is obligatory (keratoacanthoma,
papillomatosis cutis carcinoides of Gottron, and giant condyloma
acuminatum of Buschke and Loewenstein), and are of ancillary
importance in most instances of dermatoses with facultative development of such hyperplasia.

In keratoacanthoma, the most effective method is excision.
Opinions  differ, however, as to what approach is best to the management of keratoacanthomas.  Thus, because of the tendency of keratoacanthomas to resolve spontaneously, some authors recommend adopting
a wait and see attitude so as not to start active treatment until
after the keratoacanthoma has been in existence for a long time (e.g.
Burge and Winkelmann, 1969), especially if the age of the lesion is
known and its course is followed by seeing the patient regularly.
Others believe that since keratoacanthomas may undergo malignant
transformation, it is best to remove them in good time and submit for
histologic study (Pinkus, 1967).  Del Rossi et al. (1977) advocate
excising giant keratoacanthoma with subsequent plastic repair of the
defect.  Scraping off the lesions is considered advisable in multiple
keratoacanthomas (Vollum, 1976).  Along with surgical removal, some
authors have treated keratoacanthomas with liquid nitrogen or $CO_2$
(cryotherapy), compresses with 15% salicylic acid ointment, 5-fluo-
rouracil ointment, and so on (e.g. Ebner and Miescher, 1975; Del
Rossi et al., 1977; Green et al., 1977).  We have used to advantage
applications of 50% Prospidinum ointment (Figure 72).  The use of
Prospidinum is particularly indicated if the keratoacanthoma occurs
in an area (e.g. the face or an eyelid) where surgical intervention
is objectionable for cosmetic reasons.  The use of roentgen therapy
is undesirable for the same reasons.

In papillomatosis cutis carcinoides of Gottron, surgical excision followed by plastic repair or roentgen therapy is considered
the method of choice by most authors in view of the exceptionally
indolent course of the process (Gottron and Nikolowski, 1960;
Schuppener and Steinke, 1960; Khristin et al., 1963; Riboldi and Del
Pozzo, 1976; and others).  We, however, have successfully treated a
patient with this condition by intralesional injections of prednisolone (a total of 15 sessions with 30 mg of the drug per session)
in combination with cryosurgery.

Giant condyloma acuminatum of Buschke and Loewenstein not infrequently presents formidable therapeutic problems.  As discussed in
Chap. 8, this disease shows a particularly aggressive epidermal
growth and is apt to recur even after careful excision of the lesion.
Many authors (e.g. Whitmore, 1970; Bruns et al., 1975; Netto et al.,
1976; South et al., 1977) consider topical application of cytostatics

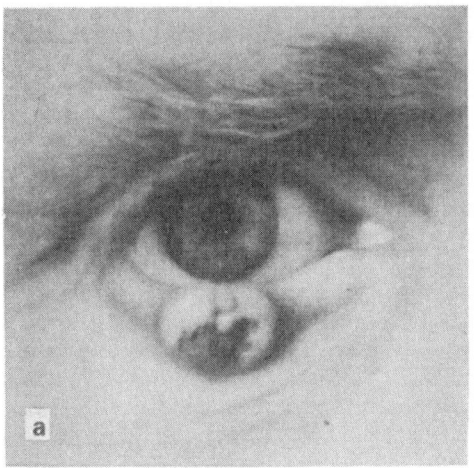

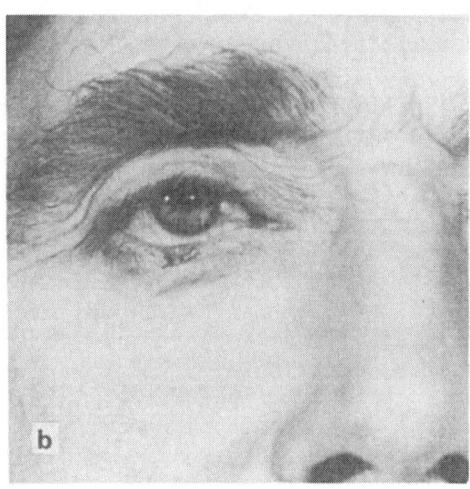

Fig. 72.  Keratoacanthoma.  (a) Before treatment;  (b) same patient
          3 weeks after applications of 50% Prospidinum ointment.


and roentgen irradiation ineffective.  Moreover, roentgen therapy may
be conducive to malignant transformation of the condyloma (Netto et
al., 1976).  In fact, the only method of treatment today remains
surgical excision, preferably with an electric knife.

     In lupus vulgaris, topical treatment is of auxiliary importance
and consists in destruction of the lupomas.  For this purpose, use is
made of electrocoagulation, applications of 30% resorcinol paste or
30% pyrogallol ointment, and cryocautery.  However, the method of
choice remains comprehensive systemic antituberculosis therapy.

In <u>verrucous tuberculosis</u>, topical therapy is more effective. It is advisable to remove individual small lesions by means of electrocoagulation and to deal with larger lesions by freezing them with carbon dioxide (Mashkilleison, 1964). In some cases, applications of an ointment containing 15% of salicylic or lactic acid in indicated.

In the <u>deep mycoses</u> (blastomycosis, chromomycosis), intralesional injections of amphotericin B (2-3 mg dissolved in 5 ml of a 20% procaine solution) done once a week (a total of 10 to 14 sessions) and applications of 5% amphotericin B ointment, 50% potassium iodide ointment, or aniline dyes are beneficial.

In <u>cutaneous leishmaniasis</u> (especially in its late ulcerating form), it is desirable to use, in conjunction with systemic therapy, diathermy to accelerate the healing of the ulcers and cryotherapy to destroy the nodules. For this purpose, plasters with a 10 to 20% pyrogallic acid are also used. We have successfully employed compresses with 30% Prospidinum or 5% methotrexate in an ointment base in the external treatment of leishmaniasis.

In <u>trophic ulcers</u>, proteolytic enzymes such as trypsin, chymotrypsin, and chymopsin (amorphous chymotrypsin) have been applied to advantage in a number of cases (Vilesov, 1967). Grigoryan et al. (1972), who used these proteolytic enzymes to treat 175 patients with trophic ulcers of the lower extremities, noted clearing of the ulcers and the appearance of granulations after 5 days of the treatment, on the average. Good results are obtainable with pressure or adhesive tape dressings. It is believed by many (e.g. Berkovskaya, 1958; Lapidus, 1959; Mashkilleison, 1964; Rozentul, 1970; Grigoryan et al., 1972) that an adhesive tape dressing creates physiologic conditions for tissue regeneration. Usually, the ulcer is first washed with hydrogen peroxide, and the adhesive tapes are placed like tiles all over the ulcer and are changed every 5 to 7 days. An important prerequisite for effective epithelialization of the ulcer is the satisfactory condition of its marginal zone. Trophic ulcers of the lower limbs tend to have callous, sharply elevated edges whose surface is covered by hard hyperkeratotic material, and it is such marginal zones of trophic ulcers which show pseudocarcinomatous epidermal hyperplasia. Therefore, in our view, the first stage of external therapy for trophic ulcers should consist in the use of a 10-15% salicylic acid or 10-15% resorcinol-containing ointment or paste applied in an occlusive dressing to the ulcer margin only. The healing of the ulcer margins proceeds at an accelerated pace after the horny material has detached. Cryotherapy has been reported effective in eliminating excessive epidermal growth at the margins of trophic ulcers (Apakidze, 1967).

In the giant form of circumscribed neurodermatosis, a pure tar applied for 20-30 min and followed by a hot compress or bath is beneficial. Skripkin (1967) has used, to considerable advantage,

intralesional injections of a 0.1 to 0.15% methylene blue solution in
1% or 2% Bencaine or procaine which prolong the itch-alleviating
action of the solution. Freezing the lesions with liquid
nitrogen has also been very effective in some cases. With this
method, a glass rod carrying a cotton pad soaked in liquid nitrogen
on its end is applied to the lesion for periods ranging from 10-15 s
to 1-2 min; this is followed by the appearance of a blister on the
lesional surface and by flattening of the warty growths and dimin-
ution of the infiltrate after the blister has resolved. Intralesional injections of prednisolone or hydrocortisone are also effective. In several cases, it is advisable to resort to grenz-ray
therapy.

Similar methods are used in prurigo nodularis of Hyde.
Mashkilleison (1965) has proposed destroying the nodules of this
dermatosis by means of diathermy or cryotherapy.


## 11.3  PREVENTIVE MEASURES

Prophylactic measures may be divided into two groups: those
directed at preventing diseases with obligatory or facultative
pseudocarcinomatous hyperplasia and those aimed to prevent precancerous changes in the lesions showing such hyperplasia.

As already indicated, the disorders classified tentatively under
cutaneous pseudocarcinoses vary widely in origin. In some of them
(keratoacanthoma, papillomatosis cutis carcinoides of Gottron,
chronic pyoderma ulcerosum vegetans, etc.), the major predisposing
factors include trauma, prolonged mechanical irritation, and
excessive exposure to sunlight, while in others (condylomata
acuminata including the giant type of Buschke and Loewenstein;
cutaneous tuberculosis; leishmaniasis; deep mycoses; etc.), important
etiologic considerations are viral, bacterial, and fungal infections.
Often, of critical importance in bringing about a particular disorder
is the state of the body as a whole, its immunologic reactivity,
metabolic status, and the condition of its vascular, neuroendocrine,
and other systems. Accordingly, the basic prophylactic interventions
should comprise a set of measures designed to improve the general
health, in particular through careful observance of personal hygiene
and diet; improvement of the working conditions and lifestyle; and,
if indicated, treatment in a sanatorium or health resort and placement of the patient under dispensary observation. Those measures may
take more specific forms depending on the dermatosis concerned. For
example, papillomatosis cutis carcinoides of Gottron arises most
often after a trauma or inadequate treatment of preexisting chronic
dermatosis localized on the skin of a lower limb, and therefore the
avoidance of trauma and the effective treatment of protracted,
chronic cutaneous diseases may be considered conducive to the prevention of this papillomatosis.

Local hygiene can possibly prevent the occurrence of giant condyloma acuminatum of Buschke and Loewenstein, since the untidy state of the genitals, for example accumulation of smegma on the inner surfaces of the prepuce, may predispose to this tumor.

Patients with varicose veins should avoid prolonged walking or standing, lifting weights, and incurring traumas, for any of these may precipitate the development of trophic ulcers on the lower limbs with the attendant pseudocarcinomatous epidermal hyperplasia.

Persons suffering from chronic ulcerative vegetating pyoderma should be examined by an internist to exclude gastrointestinal disease which may underlie the pyoderma.

In the USSR, much effort has been expended in the prevention of tuberculosis, and the extensive coverage of the population by preventive medical examinations; free medical care; dispensary services to patients; improved living standards; and establishment of an extensive network of sanatoria, spas, health resorts, prophylactoria, and other facilities have set the scene for the successful prevention of cutaneous tuberculosis or of its recurrence.

The prophylaxis of precancerous changes at the sites of pseudo-carcinomatous hyperplasia includes the following measures:  (1) dispensarization of all patients with long-lasting chronic granulomatous inflammatory lesions, benign epithelial tumors, and other skin disorders accompanied by atypical excessive epidermal growth; (2) early recognition of the clinical and histopathologic changes that are not typical for the dermatoses showing pseudocarcinomatous epidermal hyperplasia, for which purpose repeated histologic studies and, if need be, combined cytologic and cytogenetic analyses should be undertaken; (3) adequate treatment of the underlying disease and of precancerous changes at the earliest possible stage; (4) protection of the lesions showing pseudocarcinomatous epidermal hyperplasia, from repeated exposure to trauma, from excessive insolation, and from other adverse environmental factors; (5) appropriate job placement of the patients; and (6) genetic counseling.

It is particularly important to carry out the above measures in those skin diseases to which pseudocarcinomatous hyperplasia is obligate (i.e., keratoacanthoma, papillomatosis cutis carcinoides of Gottron, giant condyloma acuminatum of Buschke and Loewenstein).

In keratoacanthoma, even though the tumor tends to undergo spontaneous dissolution, early surgical treatment (excision, electro-desiccation, etc.) is indicated because otherwise undesirable disfiguring scars may result or malignancy may supervene (Burge and Winkelmann, 1969).  Also, patients with keratoacanthoma should undergo roentgen examination, since cases where this tumor was associated with primary multiple cancers of the stomach or large intestine have been reported (e.g. Bakker and Tjou, 1971; Poleksis, 1974).  In patients with multiple keratoacanthomas, the familial history must be taken.

Careful surgical treatment as early as possible in indicated in all cases of Buschke and Loewenstein's tumor - not only because the tumor may transform into a cancer, but also because it follows an exceptionally refractory and aggressive course, has a tendency to recur, and bears a close resemblance to verrucous carcinoma.  It must be borne in mind that roentgen therapy is not indicated in this condition.

In all disorders with facultative development of pseudocarcinomatous hyperplasia, adequate combined treatment of the underlying dermatosis is important if precancerous changes are to be avoided.

In recent years, the substance called "aromatic retinoid" has been suggested for use in the prevention of malignant transformation of the epidermis in a number of dermatoses accompanied by hyperplasia and excessive proliferation of the epidermis (Schnitzler et al., 1980).

Some of the dermatoses which we include in the group of disorders with facultative development of pseudocarcinomatous hyperplasia (verrucous tuberculosis, chronic pyoderma ulcerosum vegetans, deep mycoses, etc.), are regarded by certain authors as precancerous conditions (e.g. Raichev and Andreev, 1965; Venkei and Sugar, 1965; Shanin, 1969; Thambiah, 1969).  We, for our part, agree with Raben (1977) in that malignant transformation of these dermatoses is a very unlikely possibility.  It may be added that the improved cultural and living standards of the population, the large-scale health education activities in the field of cancer prevention, the extensive dispensary services available to the patients, and lastly, the expanding network of specialized medical facilities are all contributing to the successful prevention of precancerous conditions and to the reduced prevalence and incidence of malignant cutaneous neoplasms in our country.

# References

Abele, D. C., Dobson, R. L., and Graham, J. B., 1963, Heredity and psoriasis, Arch.Dermatol., 88:38–47.

Abell, C. W., and Monahan, T. M., 1973, The role of adenosine 3', 5'-cyclic monophosphate in the regulation of mammalian cell division, J.Cell Biol., 59:549.

Abercombie, M., and Ambrose, E. J., 1962, The surface properties of cancer cells, Cancer Res., 22:525–548.

Ackerman, L. V., 1948, Verrucous carcinoma of oral cavity, Surgery, 23:670–678.

Adachi, K., Yoshikawa, K., Halprin, K. M., and Levine, V., 1975, Prostaglandins and cyclic AMP in epidermis. Evidence for the independent action of prostaglandins and adrenaline on the adenyl cyclase system of pig and human epidermis, normal and psoriatic, Br.J.Dermatol., 92:381–388.

Adachi, K., Iizuka, H., and Halprin, K. M., 1977, Specific refractoriness of adenylate cyclase in skin to epinephrine, prostaglandin E, histamine and AMP, Biochim.Biophys.Acta., 497: 428–436.

Adam, W., Nikolowski, W., and Wiehe, R., 1956, Papillomatosis cutis carcinoides Gottron, Arch.Klin.Exp.Dermatol., 203:357–367.

Adler, 1965, Immunology of leishmaniasis, Isr.J.Med.Sci., 1:9–13.

Agroskin, L. S., 1962, On errors in cytophotometry, Tsitologiya, No. 5, 585–595. (In Russ.).

Agroskin, L. S., Brodskii, V. Ya., Gruzdev, A. D., and Korolev, N. V., 1960, Some aspects of quantitative spectrophotometric analysis of the cell, Tsitologiya, No. 3, 337–352. (In Russ.).

Alieva, I. G., 1967, Recurrence of skin cancer after radiation therapy at close range, Vest.Dermatol.Venerol., No. 6, 58–60. (In Russ.).

224

Allegra, F., and De Panfilis, G., 1974, An in vivo method of studying the kinetics of cell proliferation in normal human epidermis, Acta.Dermatol.Venereol.(Stockholm), 54:87-90.

Allen, A. C., 1954, "A Clinicopathologic Treatise," Mosby, St. Louis.

Alov, I. A., 1964, "Ocherki Fiziologii Mitoticheskogo Deleniya Kletki" [Essays on the Physiology of Cell Division by Mitosis], Meditsina, Moscow. (In Russ.).

Alov, I. A., 1965, Mitotic abnormalities, Vest.Akad.Med.Nauk SSSR, No. 11., 58-66. (In Russ.).

Alov, I. A., 1972, "Tsitologiya i Patologiya Mitoza" [Cytology and Pathology of Mitosis], Meditsina, Moscow. (In Russ.).

Alov, I. A., Braude, A. I., and Aspiz, M. E., 1966, "Oznovy Funktsional'noi Morfologii Kletki" [The Fundamentals of Functional Morphology of the Cell], Meditsina, Moscow. (In Russ.).

Anderson, N. P., 1957, Discussion, Arch.Dermatol., 75:219-223.

Anderson, W. A., 1971, Pathology, Mosby, St. Louis.

Andersson, G., and Kjellstrand, P. T., 1972, Influence of acid concentration and temperature on fixed chromatin during Feulgen hydrolysis, Histochémie, 30:108-114.

Andres, A. H., and Navaschin, M. S., 1936, Ein Beitrag zur morphologischen Analyse der Chromosomen des Menschen, Zellforsch-mikr.Anat., 24:552-558.

Apakidze, V. K., 1967, "Krioterapiya Troficheskikh Yazv Nizhnikh Konechnostei" [Cryotherapy for Trophic Ulcers of the Lower Limbs], Meditsina, Moscow. (In Russ.).

Apatenko, A. K., 1969, "Morphology, histogenesis, and classification of epithelial tumors of the skin", Doctoral dissertation. (In Russ.), Moscow.

Apatenko, A. K., 1973, "Epitelial'nye Opukholi i Poroki Razvitiya Kozhi" [Epithelial tumors and developmental anomalies of the skin], Meditsina, Moscow. (In Russ.).

Arievich, A. M., 1961, The deep mycoses, in: "Rukovodstvo po Dermatovenerologii" [A Handbook of Dermato-Venereology], Vol. 2, Leningrad, Medgiz. (In Russ.).

Arning, E., and Levandowsky, F., 1911, Noduli cutanei, eine bisher wenigbeobachtete Hautaffection, Arch.Dermatol.Syph., 10:3-14 (Berlin).

Arnold, J., 1879, Beobachtungen über Kerntheilungen in den Zellen der Geschwülste," Arch.Pathol.Anat., 78:279-301.

Arnold, H. L., and Tilden, J. L., 1943, Histiocytoma cutis, Arch. Dermatol.Syph., 47:498-516.

Arutyunov, V. Ya. and Golemba, P. I., 1959, A note on keratoacanthoma, Vopr.Onkol., No. 10, 480-483. (In Russ.).

Ashmarin, Yu. Ya., Kreinin, V. M., Alshtan, B. Ya., and Shatova, L. I., 1973, Treatment of psoriasis with antimetabolites: efficiency and complications, Vest.Dermatol.Venerol., No. 4., 14-20. (In Russ).

Aso, K., Orenberg, E. K., and Farber, E. M., 1975, Reduced epidermal cyclic AMP accumulation following prostaglandin stimulation:

its possible role in the pathophysiology of psoriasis, J. Invest.Dermatol., 65:375-378.

Aso, K., Rabinowitz, J., and Farber, E. M., 1976, The role of prost-aglandin E, cyclic AMP, and cyclic GMP in the proliferation of guinea pig ear skin stimulated by topical application of vitamin A acid, J. Invest.Dermatol., 67:231-234.

Atkin, N. B., 1962, The relationship between the deoxyribonucleic acid and ploidy of human tumors, Cytogenetics (Basel), 1:113-122.

Atkin, N. B., 1964, Die chromosomale Basis von Sexchromatinad-weichungen in menschilichen Tumoren, Wein.klin.Wochenschr., 76:859-862.

Atkin, N. B., Martinson, G., and Baker, M. C., 1966, A comparison of the DNA content and chromosome numbers of fifty human tumors, Br.J.Cancer, 20:87-101.

Atkin, N. B., and Baker, M. C., 1969, Possible difference between the karyotypes of preinvasive lesions and malignant tumors, Br.J.Cancer, 23:329-336.

Avrorov, P. P., and Timofeevskii, A. D., 1914, Experience with culti-vation of tissues outside the body, Imperatorskii Tomskii Universitet, Izvestiya. (Tomsk), 56:1-80, (In Russ.).

Avtandilov, G. G., 1970, Prospects for microspectrophotometric studies in pathology, Arkh.Patol., No. 9, 3-12. (In Russ.).

Avtandilov, G G., 1972, "Morfometriya v Patologii" [Morphometry in Pathology], Meditsina, Moscow. (In Russ.).

Avtandilov, G. G., and Chervonnaya, L. V., 1973, Comparative micro-spectrophotometric studies of DNA in cells from primary lesions of malignant melanoma and its metastases, Byull.Eksp.Biol.Med., No. 4, 77-79. (In Russ.).

Avtandilov, G. G., and Kazantseva, I. A., 1973, Microspectrophoto-metric studies of DNA content in the diagnosis of pretumorous lesions and of cancer, Arch.Patol., No. 1, 13-17. (In Russ.).

Avtandilov, G. G., Golbert, L. V., and Cervonnaja, L. V., 1972, Mikrospectrophotometrische Untersuchungen des DNA-Gehaltes in primären und metastatischen Melanomherden vor und nach Strahleneinwirkung, Radiol. Radiother., 13:675-679.

Avtsyn, A. P., and Shibaeva, S. M., 1960, Sex differences between nuclear structures in benign cutaneous tumors, Zh.Nevropatol.Psikh., No. 4, 426-433. (In Russ.).

Azua, J. and Suárez, J., 1894, Várices y neoplasias linfaricas der-micas, Rev.Med.Cirug.Pract. (Madrid), 34:372.

Babayants, R. S., Karpushkin, V. P., and Gribanov, Ya. G., 1973, On clinical features of skin cancer and comparative character-ization of various methods for its treatment, Vest.Dermatol. Venerol., No. 10, 3-9. (In Russ.).

Bakker, P. M., and Tjou, A. J., 1971, Multiple sebaceous gland tumors with multiple tumors of internal organs, Dermatologica (Basel), 142:50.

Barr, M. L., and Bertram, E. G., 1949, A morphologic distinction between neurones of the male and female, and the behavior of the nucleolar satellite during accelerated nucleoprotein synthesis, Nature, (London), 163:616-617.

Baruffi, I., Righetti, S., and Gondim, F., 1971, Topographical study of sex chromatin in breast cancer, Tumori, 57:1-4.

Baserga, R., 1965, The relationship of the cell cycle to tumor growth and control of cell division, Cancer Res., 25:581-595.

Baserga, R., 1971, "The Cell Cycle and Cancer," Marcel Dekker, New York.

Baserga, R., and Wiebel, F., 1969, The cell cycle of the mammalian cells," Int.Rev.Exp.Path., 7:1-30.

Bauer, R., 1977, Zyklische Nukleotide und Epidermisproliferation, Z.Hautkrankh, 52:81-85

Bazex, A., Deodati, E., Dupre, A., et al., 1972, Papillomatose conjonctivale profuse: rapports nosologiques avec la papillomatose orale profuse et avec le syndrome de Buschke-Löwenstein, Bull.Soc.franc.Derm.Syph., 79:180-183.

Bazyka, A. P., and Bashkirova, R. A., 1975, Focal epithelial hyperplasia, Vest.Dermatol.Venerol., No. 7, 55. (In Russ.).

Bazyka, A. P., and Lesnitskii, A. I., 1975, Histopathology of chronic deep pyoderma, Vest.Dermatol.Venerol., No. 10. 9-12.

Bedi, T. R., and Pandhi, R. K., 1977, Buschke-Loewenstein's tumor presenting with urinary fistula, Br.J.Vener.Dis., 53:200-202.

Bedner, B., and Stanova, M., 1976, Epithelial tumor-like changes in precancerous conditions and skin neoplasms, Cesk.Patrol., 12(2):104-112.

Belen'kii, G. B., 1963, Malignant tumors of the skin, in: "Posobie dlya Vrachei" [Physician's Manual], K. R. Astvatsaturov, ed., Medgiz, Moscow. (In Russ.).

Belen'kii, G. B., 1968, Parablastomatoses and pseudoblastomatoses in dermatology, in: "Sovremenniye Aspekty Klinicheskoi i Eksperimental'noi Dermato-Venerologii (Sbornik statei)" [Current Problems in Clinical and Experimental Dermato-Venereology (A collection of articles)], No. 5, pp.61-66, MONIKI, Moscow. (In Russ.).

Belen'kii, G. B., 1970, "Geneticheskiye Faktory v Dermatologii" [Genetic Factors in Dermatology], Moscow. (In Russ.).

Belen'kii, G. B., and Berenbein, B. A., 1967, Preliminary results of studies on pseudoepitheliomatous hyperplasia and skin cancer using cytogenetic methods, in: "Uspekhi Klinicheskoi i Eksperimental'noi Meditsiny" [Advances in Clinical and Experimental Medicine], pp. 341-342, Moscow. (In Russ.).

Belen'kii, G. B., Berenbein, B. A., Kryazheva, S. S., Kostrova, A. A., and Egorkina, D. A., 1968, Cytogenetic differential diagnosis of spinocellular cancer and chronic inflammatory processes of the skin, in "Sovremennyie Aspekty Klinicheskoi i Eksperimental'noi Dermato-Venerologii" [Current Problems in Clinical and Experimental Dermato-Venereology], No. 5, pp. 26-29, MONIKI, Moscow. (In Russ.).

Belisario, J. C., 1954, Discussion, Austral.J.Dermatol., 2:147.

Belisario, J., 1963, Precancerous changes in the skin (Russian translation), in: "Mezhdunarodnyi Protivorakovyi Kongress, 8-1"

[Eighth International Cancer Congress], pp.343-358, Moscow. (In Russ.).

Belisario, J., 1965, Keratoacanthoma and its incidence as affected by sunlight in the tropical and subtropical areas of Australia, Dermatol.Internat., 4:13.

Bellamy, E. D., Allen, J. H., and Hart, N. L., 1963, Keratoacanthoma of the bulbar conjunctiva, Arch.Opthalmol., 70:512-514.

Berenbein, B. A., 1971, "Zudyashchie Dermatozy (Neirodermatozy)" [Pruritic Dermatoses (Neurodermatoses)], Meditsina, Moscow. (In Russ.).

Berenbein, B. A., 1977, A comparative analysis of quantitative changes of chromosomes in karyotypic groups in reactive epidermal hyperplasia and in malignant epidermis, in: "Geneticheskiye Faktory v Dermatologii" [Genetic Factors in Dermatology], Vol. 15, pp. 14-17, MONIKI, Moscow.

Berenbein, B. A., and Egorkina, D. A., 1973, Alterations in the genetic apparatus of cells in atypical benign and cancerous proliferations of the epidermis, in: "VI Vsesoyuznyi S'ezd Dermato-venerologov" [Sixth All-Union Congress of Dermatologists and Venereologists], pp. 65-66. (In Russ.), Moscow.

Berenbein, B. A., and Egorkina, D. A., 1974, Epidermal tissue culture and cytogenetic features of epidermal cells in pseudoepitheliomatous hyperplasia, Vest.Dermatol.Venerol., No. 1., 37-41. (In Russ.).

Berenbein, B. A., and Kazantseva, I. A., 1973, Alterations in the mitotic pattern of epidermal cells in pseudoepitheliomatous hyperplasia and spinocellular skin cancer, Vest.Dermatol Venerol., No. 8, 25-27. (In Russ.).

Berkovskaya, L. M., 1958, Comprehensive treatment of slowly healing wounds and ulcers of the lower extremities, Vopr.Kurortol., No. 4, 358. (In Russ.).

Bertsch, S., Csontos, K., Schweizer, Y., and Marks, F., 1976, Effect of mechanical stimulation on cell proliferation in mouse epidermis and on growth regulation by endogenous factors (chalones), Cell Tissue Kinet., 9:445.

Beyreuther, K., 1960, Chromosomes in primary neoplastic growth, Nature (London), 186:6-9.

Biberstein, H., 1931, Fibrome mit atypischer Epithelwucherung, Arch. Dermatol.Syph. (Berlin), 164:69-81.

Birnbaum, J. E., Sapp, T. M., and Moore, J. B., 1976, Effects of reserpine, epidermal growth factor, and cyclic nucleotide on epidermal mitosis, J.Invest.Dermatol., 66:313-318.

Bissada, N. K., Cole, A. T., and Fried, F. A., 1974, Extensive condylomas acuminata of the entire male urethra and the bladder, J.Urol., 112:201.

Blinova, G. A., 1959, Keratoacanthoma, Vopr.Onkol., No. 8, 218-227. (In Russ.).

Blok, Yu. E., 1966, In vitro culture of adult human skin for purposes of cytogenetic studies, Byull.Eks. Biol.Med., No. 2, 117-120. (In Russ.).

Blokhin, N. N., 1976, Major lines of scientific research that should
    lead to success in cancer control, in: "38-ya Sessiya
    Obshchego Sobraniya AMN SSSR. Tezisy dokl." [38th General
    Meeting of the USSR Academy of Medical Sciences, Abstracts of
    papers]. (In Russ.), Moscow, pp. 25-29.
Blumenfeld, C. M., 1943, Studies of normal and abnormal mitotic
    activity, Arch.Pathol., 35:667-678.
Bochkov, N. P., and Nemtsova, L. S., 1962, In vitro incubation of
    tissues for studies on mammalian karyotypes, Tsitologiya, No
    3, 365-367. (In Russ.).
Bochkov, N. P., Kozlov, B. M., Saven'kaev, A. V., et. al., 1966,
    Analysis of aneuploidy in human embryonal fibroblast and
    leukocyte cultures, Genetika, No. 10, 120-124. (In Russ.).
Borovskii (Borovsky), P. F., 1898, On the Saratov Ulcer, Vienno-
    Meditsinskii Zhurnal, No. 11. (In Russ.).
Brachtel, R., and Lemmel, E. M., 1978, Chronisch vegetierende Pyo-
    dermie bei zellulärem Immundefect, Hautarzt, 27:488-491.
Braun-Falco O., 1960, in: "Dermatologie und Venerologie," Vol.2, Part
    2, H. A. Gottron and W. Schönfeld (eds.), Thieme, Stuttgart.
Bray, 1973, Leishmaniasis: epidemiology, Ethiop.Med.J., 11:197-198.
Bremener, M. M., 1937, "Tuberkulez Kozhi" [Cutaneous Tuberculosis],
    Moscow. (In Russ.).
Broders, A. C., and Dublin, W. B., 1939, Rhythmicity of mitosis in
    the epidermis of human beings, Proc. Staff Meet.Mayo Clinic
    14:423-435.
Brodskii, V. Ya., 1963, Polyploidy of somatic cells of animal
    tissues, in: "Vtoroe Soveshchanie po Poliploidii, 14-18 yan-
    varya 1963 g.," [Second Meeting on Polyploidy. January 14-18,
    1963]. (In Russ.). Leningrad, p.9.
Brodskii, V. Ya., 1966, "Trofika Kletki" [Nutrition of the Cell],
    Nauka, Moscow. (In Russ.).
Brodskii, V. Ya., Faktor, F. M., Milyutina, P. A., and Uryvaeva, I.
    V., 1969, Studies of DNA synthesis and of mitoses in re-
    generating mouse livers with the aim of identifying the $G_2$
    population of hepatocytes, Dokl.Akad.Nauk SSR, 189:639-642.
    (In Russ.).
Brodskii, V. Ya., Vasil'ev, Yu. M., Gel'fand, I. M., Gel'shtein, V.
    I., Domina, L. V., Kleminer, L. B., and Marshat, T. L., 1971,
    Proliferation kinetics of cultured mouse embryonal fibroblast-
    like cells, Tsitologiya, No. 11, 1369-1378. (In Russ.).
Bruns, T., Lauvetz, R., et al., 1975, Buschke-Loewenstein giant
    condylomas: pitfalls in management, Urology, 5:773-776.
Bullough, W. S., 1964, Mitotic activity in the adult female mouse
    (Mus musculus L.). A study of its relation to the oestrous
    cycle in normal and abnormal conditions, Philosoph.Trans.Roy
    Soc., 585:453-516, London.
Bullough, W. S., 1967, "The Evolution of Differentiation," Acad.
    Press, London and New York.

Bullough, W. S., and Laurence, E. B., 1960, The control of epidermal mitotic activity in mouse skin, dermis and hypodermis, Exp. Cell Res., 21:394-404.

Bullough, W. S., and Laurence, E. B., 1968, Epidermal chalone and mitotic control in the V x 2 epidermal tumor, Nature 220:134-135, London.

Burdette, W. J., 1962, "Methodology in Human Genetics", San Francisco.

Burge, K. M., and Winkelmann, R. K., 1969, Keratoacanthoma. Association with basal and squamous cell carcinoma, Arch.Dermatol., 100:306-311.

Buschke, A., 1896, Condylomata Acuminata, in: "Neisser's Stereoscopischer Atlas."

Buschke, A., and Loewenstein, L., 1925, Uber carcinomähnliche condylomata acuminata des penis, Klin.Wschr., 4:1726.

Butcher, R. W., Baird, Ch. C., and Sutherland, E. W., Effects of antilipolytic substances on adenosine 3',5'-monophosphate levels in isolated fat cells, J.Biol.Chem., 243:1705-1711.

Caro, M. R., 1959, Epidermal chalone associated with sclerosing hemangiomas, Arch.Dermatol., 80:793-799.

Caspersson, O., 1964, Quantitative cytochemical studies on normal, malignant, prelamignant and atypical cell populations from the human uterine cervix, Acta Cytol., 8:45-60.

Chambers, D. A., Martin, D. W., Jr., and Weinstein, G., 1974, The effect of cyclic nucleotides on purine biosynthesis and the induction of PRPP synthetase during lymphocyte activation, Cell, 3:375-380.

Chervonnaya, L. V., and Gladulova, Z. L., 1972, On the characterization of the ploidy of malignant melanomas and nevi, Vopr. Onkol., No. 1, 9-11, (In Russ.).

Cheung, W. J., 1972, Adenosine 3', 5'-monophosphate; on its mechanism of action, Perspect.Biol.Med., 15:221.

Chorazak, T., Rasiewicz, W., and Slopek, S, 1967, Ropne choróby skóry [Pustular Diseases], Pánstwow y Zakład Wydawnictw Lekarskich, Warsaw. (In Polish).

Civatte, J., 1967, Histopathologie Cutanée, Paris.

Civatte, J., Schnitzler, L., and Belaich, S., 1973, Hyperplasia pseudo-epithéliomateuse du dos des mains, Ann.Dermat.Syph., 100:29-48, Paris.

Cobl, J. P., Walker, D. G., and Wright, J. C., 1961, Comparative chemotherapy studies on primary, short-term cultures of human normal, benign, and malignant tumor tissues, Cancer Res., 21:583.

Cohen, S., 1972, Epidermal growth factor, J.Invest.Dermatol., 59:13-16.

Connors, R. C., and Ackerman, A. B., 1976, Histologic pseudomalignancies of the skin, Arch.Dermatol., 112:1767-1780.

Cowdry, E. V., 1958, "The Cancer Cells," [Russian translation from English], Inostrannaya Literatura, Moscow.

Cowdry, E. V., and Paletta, F. X., 1941, Changes in cellular, nuclear, and nucleolar sizes during methylcholanthrene epidermal carcinogenesis, J.Nat.Cancer Inst., 1:745-759.

Cramer, R., and Cramer, H., 1963, Uber die pseudobasaliomatose epi-
    thelhyperplasie der Haut, Arch.Klin.Exp.Dermatol.,
    216:231-245.
Curric, A. R., and Ferguson-Smith, J., 1952, Multiple primary spon-
    taneous healing squamous cell carcinomata of the skin, J.Path.
    Bact., 64:827-839.
Darshkevich, Yu, N., 1952, Inflammatory growth of hepatic epithelium,
    Dissertation, Leningrad. (In Russ.).
Davidson, J., 1969, "The Biochemistry of the Nucleic Acids," 6th ed.,
    Methuen, London.
Davydovskii, I. V., 1969, "Obshchaya Patologiya Cheloveka" [General
    Human Pathology], Meditsina, Moscow. (In Russ.).
Dawson, D. F., Duckworth, J. K., Bernhardt, H., and Young, J. M.,
    1965, Giant condyloma and verrucous carcinoma of the genital
    area, Arch.Pathol., 79:225.
De, P., 1963, Results of quantitative determination of nucleic acids
    and protein in normal and malignant stratified epithelia
    during their growth and differentiation (Russian translation),
    in: "8-i Mezdhunarodnyi Protivorakovyi Kongress" [Eighth
    International Cancer Congress], Vol. 2, pp. 29-62, Moscow.
    (In Russ.).
Degos, R., 1958, "Dermatologie", Paris.
Dehuhard, F., Brein, H., Schüsler, and Wehler, V., 1975,
    Cytogenetische Untersuchungen an Precancerosen im Carcinoma
    der Cervix uteri, Arch.Gynecol., 220:101-117.
Del Rossi, C., Peserico, A., and Simonetto, D., 1977, Keratoacanthoma
    centrifugum marginatum, Arch.Dermatol., 113:110.
Delektorskii, V. V., Fedorovskaya, R. F., Masyukova, S. A., and
    Zimine, L. P., 1977, Subcellular mechanisms of phagocytosis in
    chronic pyodermas, Vest.Dermatol. Venerol., No. 5, 7-11. (In
    Russ.).
Dobrynin, Ya. V., 1968, On the characterization of the various types
    of human epithelial tumor growth in multilayer cultures, in:
    "Kul'tura Tkanei v Onkologii" [Tissue Culture in Oncology],
    Meditsina, Moscow, pp. 33-44. (In Russ.).
Dobrzhanskaya, R. S., 1977, Factors promoting the production of
    humoral antibodies in patients with cutaneous leishmaniasis,
    Vest.Dermatol.Venerol., No. 10, 83-88. (In Russ.).
Döring, H., 1961, Papillomatosis cutis carcinoides Gottron und Lues
    III tuberoserpiginosa, Dermatol.Wschr., 1:135.
Doyle, J. L., and Manhold, J. H., Feulgen 1975, Microspectrophoto-
    metry of oral cancer and leukoplakia, J.Dent.Res.,
    54:1196-1199.
Drummond, G. J., and Duncan, L., 1970, Adenyl cyclase in cardiac
    tissue, J.Biol.Chem., 245:976-983.
Dubinin, N. P., 1961, "Problemy Radiatsionnoi Genetiki" [Problems in
    Radiation Genetics], Nauka, Moscow. (In Russ.).
Dubinin, N. P., and Gol'dman, I. L., 1965, Radiation aspects of
    genetic differentiation of cells and problems of malignant
    growth, Vest.Akad.Med.Nauk SSSR, No. 3, 53-67. (In Russ.)

Duell, E. A., Relson, W. H., and Voorhees, J., 1975, Epidermal
    chalone - past to present concept, J.Invest.Dermatol.,
    65:67-70.
Dupont, A., 1930, Kysté sébacé atypique, Bull.Soc.Belge Dermatol.,
    July, p. 177.
Dupont, A., 1952, Kystés sébacés végétants, keratoacanthomes,
    verrucomes, Bull.Soc.Franç.Dermatol.Syph., 50:340.
Ebner, H., and Miescher, G., 1975, Lokalbenhandlung bei
    Keratoacanthoms mit 5-Fluoruracil, Hautarzt, 26:585-588.
Egorkina, D. A., 1970, "Lupus erythematosus: cytologic and immunologic
    aspects", Dissertation, Moscow. (In Russ.).
Egorkina, D. A., Khmel'nitskii, G. A., Ignat'eva, E. N., Tikhomirova,
    L. K., and Yudin, Yu. G., 1972, Chromatin in neoplasms of
    various origins, in: "Aktual'nye Voprosy Klinicheskoi i
    Eksperimental'noi Meditsiny" [Current Problems in Clinical
    and Experimental Medicine], Moscow, pp. 159-161. (In Russ.).
Ehlers, G., 1968, Vergeichende cytophotometrische Untersuchungen an
    metatypischen Baselzellepitheliomen und Plattenepithelcarcino-
    men der Haut, in: "The Thirteenth International Dermatological
    Congress," Vol. 1., pp. 38-43, Springer, Berlin.
Ehlers, G., 1971, Gehalt von Haut-Präkanzerosen. Ein Beitrag zur
    Frage der nosologischen Sonderstellung kutaner Präkanzerosen,
    Fortschr.Med., 39:1043-1043.
Elgjo, K. E., 1975, Epidermal chalone and cyclic AMP, J.Invest,
    Dermatol., 64:14-18.
Elgjo, K., Laerum, O. D., and Edgehill, W., 1971, Growth regulation
    in mouse epidermis. I. $G_2$-inhibitor present in the basal cell
    layer, Virch.Arch.Zell.Pathol., 8:277-283.
Elgjo, K., Laerum, O. D., and Edgehill, W., 1972, Growth regulation
    in mouse epidermis. II. $G_1$-inhibitor present in the different-
    iating cell layer, Virch.Arch.Zell.Pathol., 10:229-236.
Epifanova, O. I., 1965, On mitotic cycle periods and stages of in-
    creased sensitivity to external factors, Tsitologiya, 9, No.
    9, 1033-1055. (In Russ.).
Ereaux, L. P., Schopflocher, P., and Fournier, C., 1955, Keratoacan-
    thomas, Arch.Dermatol., 71:73-83.
Eversen, A., and Iversen, O. H., Rate of cell proliferation in a
    mouse squamous cell carcinoma, Nature (London), 196:383-384.
Ferguson-Smith, M. A., Mallace, D. C., James, Z. H., and Renwick, J.
    H., 1971, Multiple self-healing squamous epithelioma, in: "The
    Third Conference on the Clinical Delineation of Birth
    Defects," D. Bersma (ed.), Part XII: Skin, Hair, and Nails,
    The National Foundation Edit., Baltimore.
Field, E. O., 1972, Chromosomal loss and cancer, Lancet, 2:86-87.
Finnerud, 1955 (cited in: N. A. Torsuev, 1959).
Fischer, H., 1963, Präkanzerosen und Pseudocanzerosen der Haut,
    Med.Klin., 27:1097-1101.
Fischer-Wasels, B., 1927, Allgemeine Geschoulstlekere, Hbl.norm.
    pathol.Physiol., 14/2, Berlin.
Fischer-Wasels, B., 1933, "Wege zur Verhütung der Krebskrankheit",
    Springer, Berlin.

Fomin, K. E., Nikolaeva, L. P., and Golysheva, L. V., 1971, Differential diagnosis of papillomatosis cutis carcinoides of Gottron, Vest.Dermatol.Venerol., No. 6, 67-71. (In Russ.).

Ford, C. E., and Hamerton, J. L., 1956, A colchicine, hypotonic citrate, squash sequence for mammalian chromosomes, Stain Technol., 31:247-251.

Foulds, L., 1969, Tumor Development, London.

Fouracres, F. A., and Whittick, J. W., 1953, The relationship of molluscum sebaceum (kerato-acanthoma) to spontaneously healing epithelioma of the skin, Br.J.Cancer, 7:58.

Frankfurt, O. S., 1970, Distribution of DNA-synthesizing cells in the hyperplastic epidermis and in cutaneous papillomatosis in mice, Tsitologiya, No. 2, 245-247. (In Russ.).

Frankfurt, O. S., 1975, "Kletochnyi Tsikl v Opukholyakh" [The Cell Cycle in Tumors], Meditsina, Moscow. (In Russ.).

Freeman, R. G., Cloud, T. M., and Knox, J. M., Keratoacanthoma of the conjuctiva, Arch.Ophthalmol., 65:817-819.

Freutz, G., Muller, U., and Christensen, H., 1980, DNA flow cytometry of human epidermis. I. Methodological studies on normal skin, J.Invest.Dermatol., 74:119-121.

Friedländer, Uber Epithelwucherung und Krebs, Strasburg, 1877.

Ganina, K. P., 1970, Functional importance of sex chromatin in hormone-dependent human tumors, in: "Metabolizm Kletochnogo Yadra i Yaderno-Plazmaticheskiye Otnosheniya" [Metabolism of the Cell Nucleus and Nuclear-Cytoplasmic Relationships], Kiev, pp. 119-121. (In Russ.).

Ganina, K. P., and Loboda, V. I., 1969, The sex chromatin and chromosome complement in pretumor and tumor lesions, Patol.Genet., No. 1, 46-53. (In Russ.).

Ganina, K. P., and L. V., Polishchuk, 1968, Diagnostic value of mitotic activity determination in pigmented neoplasms of human skin, in: "3-aya Belorusskaya Nauchnaya Konferentsiya Onkologov" [Third Byelorussian Conference of Oncologists], Minsk, pp. 115-118. (In Russ.).

Ganina, K. P., Gudim-Levkovich, I. A., Lysyuk, L. P., Naleskina, L. A., and Loboda, V. I., 1968, Spectrophotometric measurement of DNA in epithelial cells of the human mammary gland in pretumorous conditions and in cancer, Tsitologiya, No. 8, 981-987 (In Russ.).

Ganina, K. P., Knysh, I. T., Polishchuk, L. Z., et al., 1976, Sex chromatin in the buccal epithelium of patients with pigmented neoplasms, in: "Nasledstvennost' i Rak" [Heredity and Cancer], Moscow, pp. 28-35. (In Russ.).

Gardat and Baseux, 1955, A propos de kératoacanthome Bull.Soc. Franç.Dermatol.Syph., 62:246.

Garshin, V. G., 1927, Experimental studies of atypical epithelial growths in aseptic inflammation induced by infusorial earth, Arkh.Biol.Nauk., No. 3, 101-120. (In Russ.).

Garshin, V. G., 1939, "Vospalitel'nye Razrastaniya Epiteliya, Ikh Biologicheskoye Znachenie i Otnoshenie k Probleme Raka" [Inflammatory Epithelial Growths: Their Biologic Implications and Relation to Cancer], Medgiz, Moscow and Leningrad. (In Russ.).

Gautier, M., 1961, Study of chromatin corpuscles on fibroblasts cultivated in vitro, Bull.Soc.Med.Hôp.Paris, 77:344-353.

Gaylarde, P. M., and Sarkany, J., 1975, Cell Migration and DNA synthesis in organ culture of human skin, Br.J.Dermatol., 92:375-380.

Gay Prieto, J., 1977, Eye color in skin cancer, Internat.J.Dermatol., 16:406-407.

Gay Prieto, J., and Cascos, M. A., 1951, Uber die Pyodermitis chronics vegetans von Azua, Dermatologica, 103:135-144, Basel.

Gay Prieto, J., Perez, P., Hurertos, M. R., and Jaquet, G., 1964, On the virus etiology of keratoacanthoma, Acta. Dermato-Vener, 44:180.

Gelfant, S., 1977, A new concept of tissue and tumor proliferation, Cancer Res., 37:3845-3862.

Gelfant, S., and Gandelas, 1972, Regulation of epidermal mitosis, J.Invest.Dermatol., 59:7-12.

Genes, I. S., 1971, On the value of chromosomal analysis in the diagnosis of human malignant tumors, Vopr.Onkol., No. 10, 13-21. (In Russ.).

Gitel'zon, I. I., 1933, "Kozhnyi Leishmanioz" [Cutaneous Leishmaniasis], Ashkhabad. (In Russ.).

Ghadially, F. N., Barton, B. W., and Kerridge, D. F., 1963, The etiology of keratoacanthoma, Cancer, 16:603-611.

Glazunov, M. F., 1947, The classification and nomenclature of tumors and tumorlike lesions, in: "Zlokachestvennye Opukholi," [Malignant tumors], N. N. Petrov (ed.), Vol.1, pp. 148-181, Medgiz, Moscow. (In Russ.).

Glazunov, M. F., 1962, Molluscum contagiosum-like changes in the epidermis of horny molluscum (keratoacanthoma), and some papillary formations of the lower lip, Vopr.Onkol., No. 6., 48-55. (In Russ.).

Glazunov, M. F., 1971, "Izbrannye Trudy" [Selected Works], Meditsina, Leningrad. (In Russ.).

Glazunov, M. F., and Blinova, G. A., 1960, Horny molluscum (keratoacanthoma) of the lower lop. 1. Benign horny molluscum, Vopr.Onkol., No. 12, 8-29. (In Russ.).

Goette, D. K., and Helwig, E. B., 1975, Basal-cell carcinomas and basal cell carcinoma-like changes overlying dermatofibromas, Arch.Dermatol., 111:589-592.

Goldberg, N. D., Haddox, M. K., Duncan, E., Lopez, and Hadden, J. W., 1974, in: "Control and Proliferation of Animal Cells," B. Clarkson and B. Baserga (eds.), Cold Spring Harbor Laboratory, Cold Spring Harbor, New York, p. 609.

Goldstein, A. B., Reynolds, W. E., and Terry, R, 1977, Diagnostic problems of epithelial tumors of penis, Urology, 9 79-82.

Golemba, P. I., 1968, On pseudosarcomatosco of the skin, In: "Sovremennye Aspekty Klinicheskoi i Eksperimental'noi

Dermato-Venerology" [Current Problems in Clinical and Experimental Dermato-Venereology], No. 5, pp. 72-76, (In Russ.).

Golovin, D. I., 1952, Inflammatory growths of mammary gland epithelium, Arkh.Patol., No. 1., 59-65, (In Russ.).

Golovin, D. I., 1958, "Opukholi Kozhi" [Tumors of the Skin], Kishinev. (In Russ.).

Golovin, D. I., 1970, Early forms of cancer in the light of the tumor-field concept, in: "Respublikanskaya Konferentsiya Onkologov. 5-ya. Materialy" [Fifth Republican Conference of Oncologists. Proceedings], pp. 219-223, Kishinev. (In Russ.).

Golovin, D. I., 1975, "Atlas Opukholei Cheloveka" [An Atlas of Human Tumors], Meditsina, Leningrad. (In Russ.).

Golovin, D. I., and V. E. Pigarevskii, 1952, Inflammatory growths of gall bladder epithelium induced by tar, Byull.Eksp.Biol.Med., No. 6, 67-70. (In Russ.).

Golovin, D. I., and Zus', B. A., 1981, Sex chromatin in oncologic histology, Arkh.Patol., No. 12, 3-7. (In Russ.).

Golovin, D. I., 1982, "Oshibki, i Trudnosti Gistologicheskoi Diagnostiki Opukholei" [Pitfalls in the Histologic Diagnosis of Tumors], Meditsina, Leningrad. (In Russ.).

Golubchik, I. S., and Yakimenko, L. N., 1971, Tuberculin-induced alterations in the mitotic pattern of human amnionic cells in culture, in: "Materialy 6-oi Konferentsii po Itogam Sovremennykh Issledovanii po Izucheniyu Protsessov Regeneratsii Kletok" [Proceedings of the Sixth Conference on Results of Recent Research into Processes of Cellular Regeneration], pp. 36-37, Moscow. (In Russ.).

Gol'tsman, L. L., 1965, Abnormalities of cell mitosis on the surface of a foreign body in the abdominal cavity, Arkh.Patol., No. 8, 72-73. (In Russ.).

Gotlib-Stematsky, T., Vaniv, A., and Cezith, A., 1966, Spontaneous malignant transformation of hamster embryo cells in vitro, J.Nat.Cancer Inst., 36:477-482.

Gottron, H. A., 1932, Berliner Dermatologische Gesellschaft, Derm.Z., 63:409-410.

Gottron, H. A., 1954, Präkanzerosen und Pseudokanzerosen der Haut, Dtsch.med.Wschr., 79:1250-1254.

Gottron, H. A., and Nikolowski, W., 1960, Pseudokanzerose, in: "Dermatologie and Venerologie," Vol.4, pp. 312-328, H. A. Gottron and W. Schönfeld (eds.), Thieme, Stuttgart.

Gougerot, H., 1917, Verrucome squameuse et exulcérant de la face etc., Arch.Méd.Pharmac.Militaire, 744.

Gougerot, H., Blum, P., and Cousin, J, 1929, Un nuveau cas de verrucome avec adénite d'origine indéterminée à structure épitheliomatiforme, curable par le 914, Bull.Soc.franç. Dermatol.Syph., 36:356-357.

Graciansky, P., 1964, "La Dermatologie", Paris.

Grafova, G. Ya., 1965, Fluctuating ploidy of somatic cells, Trudy Voenno-Meditsinskoi Akademii im. S. M. Kirove [Transactions of the S. M. Kirov Academy of Military Medicine], 165:179-183. (In Russ.).

Graham, J. H., and Helwig, E. B., 1963, Cutaneous precancerous con-
    ditions in man, in: "The First International Conference on
    Biology of Cutaneous Cancer", U. S. National Cancer Institute
    Monograph No. 10, pp. 323–346.
Granberg, J., 1971, Chromosomes in preinvasive, microinvasive and
    invasive cervical carcinoma, Hereditas, 68:165–218.
Green, H., and Ghadially, F., 1951, Relation of shock, carbohydrate
    utilization, and cortisone to mitotic activity in epidermis of
    adult male mouse, Brit.Med.J., 1:496–498.
Green, W. S., Underwood, L. J., and Green, R., 1977, Multiple kerato-
    acanthoma on upper extremities, Arch.Dermatol, 113:512–513.
Greengard, P., Rudolph, S. A., and Sturtevant, J. M., 1969, Enthalpy
    of hydrolysis of the 3'-bond of adenosine 3',5'-monophosphate
    and guanosine 3',5'-monophosphate, J.Biol.Chem.,
    244:4798–4800.
Greiter, A., 1969, Die Geschwülste und Krebse der Haut. Ein
    Uberblick über die Dignität des Hauttumoren, Mitt.-Dienst
    Gesellsch. z. Bekämpfung der Krebskrankheit, 5:19.
Grigoryan, A. V., Gostishchev, V. K., and Tolstykh, P. I., 1972,
    Troficheskie Yazvy [Trophic Ulcers], Meditsina, Moscow. (In
    Russ.).
Grinberg, K. N., 1969, The sex chromatin, in: "Osnovy Tsitogenetiki
    Cheloveka" [The Fundamentals of Human Cytogenetics], pp.
    86–96, Meditsina, Moscow. (In Russ.).
Grinspan, D., and Abulafia, J., 1955, Idiopathic pseudoepithelioma-
    tous hyperplasia, Cancer, 8:1047.
Grixoni, G., 1955, Su di un caso di papillomatosis cutis carcinoides,
    Minerva Dermatol., 130:406–409.
Grove, G. L., Anderton, R. L., and Smith, J. G., 1976, Cytophoto-
    metric studies of epidermal proliferation in psoriatic and
    normal skin, J.Invest.Dermatol., 66:236–238.
Grzhebin, Z. N., and Tseraidis, G. S., 1960, "Osnovy Gistopathologii
    Kozhi" [The Fundamentals of Cutaneous Histopathology], Medgiz,
    Moscow. (In Russ.).
Grzybowski, M., 1950, A case of peculiar generalized epithelial
    tumors of the skin, Br.J.Dermatol., 62:310.
Hadden, J. W., Hadden, E. M., Hadden, M. K., and Goldberg, N. D.,
    1972, Guanosine 3',5'-cyclic monophosphate: a possible
    intracellular mediator of mitogenic influences in lymphocytes,
    Proc.Nat.Acad.Sci.USA, 69:3024–3027.
Haim, S. Friedman-Birnbaum, R., and Cohen, Y., 1976, Mycosis fung-
    oides and involvement of the lymph nodes, Harefuen,
    90:266–267.
Halprin, K. M., Adachi, K, Yoshikawa, K., Levine, V., Mui, M. M., and
    Hsia, S. L., 1975, Cyclic AMP and psoriasis, J.Invest.
    Dermatol., 65:170–178.
Hamperl, H., and Kalkoff, K., 1954, Zur Kenntnis des Molluscum pseudo-
    carcinomatosum, Der Hautarzt, 5:440.
Hansemann, D., 1893, Studien über Spezitität den Altruismus und die
    Anaplasie der Zellen, Hirschwald, Berlin.

Hardnen, D. G., 1960, A human skin culture technique used for cyto-
    logical examinations, Br.J.Exp.Pathol., 41:31–37.
Hauschka, T. C., 1953, Trans.N.Y. Acad.Sci., 16: Ser.2, 66–73.
Hauscha, T. C., 1961, The chromosomes in ontogeny and oncogeny,
    Cancer Res., 21:957–974.
Hauschka, T. C., 1963, Chromosome patterns in primary neoplasia,
    Exp.Cell Res., 9 (Suppl:Proceedings of the American Cancer
    Society on Nucleus of the Cancer Cell), 86–98.
Heenen, M., Achten, G., and Galauf, P., 1972, Phase S normale et
    pathologique de l'épiderme human. Étude par la méthode de
    double marquage, Bull.Soc.franç.Dermatol.Syph., 79:137–139.
Heenen, M., Lambert, J. C., and Achten, G., 1975, Kinetics of cell
    proliferation in benign and premalignant tumors of the human
    epidermis, J.Nat.Cancer Inst., 54:825–827.
Heite, H. J., and Rüssmann, R., 1960, On the difference in frequency
    of sex chromatin in keratoacanthoma and spinocellular carcin-
    oma, Dermatol.Wschr., 141:33–37.
Helle, S., 1972, Condylom Therapie, Arch.Dermatol.Forsch.,
    244:411–413.
Helshan, R. W., and Buchunan, G., 1960, Keratoacanthoma of the oral
    cavity, Oral Surg., 13:844–845.
Hentzer, B., and Kobayashi, T., 1975, Suction blister transplantation
    for leg ulcers, Acta Dermatol.Venereol. (Stockholm),
    55:207–209.
Holley, R. W., 1972, A unifying hypothesis concerning the nature of
    malignant growth, Proc.Nat.Acad.Sci.USA, 69:2840–2841.
Holzer, F., and Marberger, E., 1957, "Zur mikroskopischen Geschlechts-
    bestimung an Leichenteilen, Ges.Ccrichtl.Med., 46:242–249.
Howard, A., and Pelc, S. P., 1953, Synthesis of DNA in normal and
    irradiated cells and its relation to chromosome breakage,
    Heredity (London), 6 (Suppl.), 261–283.
Hsu, T. C., 1961, Chromosomal evolution in cell populations,
    Internat.Rev.Cytol., 12:69–162.
Hundeiker, M., 1975, Die Differential Diagnose des Keratoakanthoms,
    Akt.Dermatol., 1:3–8.
Hundeiker, M., 1978, Klinische Varianten der Keratoakanthome, Z.
    Hautkrh., 53:563–574.
Huriez, C., and Desmons, F., 1957, Les faux cancers. A propos de 42
    cas de kérato-acanthomes, La revue du praticien, 7:969.
Il'in, I. I., 1970, Clinical features and course of keratoacanthomas,
    Vest.Dermatol., No. 11, 24–29. (In Russ.).
Il'in, I. I., 1974, A solitary keratoacanthoma in an unusual site,
    Vest.Dermatol., No. 5, 68–70. (In Russ.).
Il'ina, A. V., and Vasil'eva, N. N., 1963, Pathologic anatomy of
    major cutaneous diseases, in: "Rukovodstvo po Patologicheskoi
    Anatomii" [Handbook of Pathologic Anatomy], Vol. 1, p. 330,
    Medgiz, Moscow. (In Russ.).
Isaeva, V. S., Kaltgrad, S. M., and Kaufman, I. A., 1966, Giant
    keratoacanthoma in a patient with eczema, in: "Problemy
    Klinicheskoi Dermatologii (Trudy Kliniki Kozhnykh Boleznei

MONIKI)" [Problems in Clinical Dermatology. Transactions of
the Clinic of Skin Diseases of the Moscow Institute for Clinical Research], No. 4, pp. 126-134. (In Russ.).

Ishikara, T., Eikuchi, Y., and Sandberg, A. A., 1963, Chromosomes of
twenty cancer effusions. Correlation of karyotypic, clinical
and pathologic aspects, J.Nat.Cancer Inst., 30:1303-1361.

Iskra, F. G., 1938, Inflammatory outgrowths of the salivary gland
epithelium, Arkhiv Biologicheskikh Nauk, No. 3, 94-104. (In
Russ.).

Issa, M., Atherton, G. W., and Blank, C. E., 1968, The chromosomes of
the domestic rabbit, Oryctolagus cuniculus, Cytogenetics,
7:361-375.

Iversen, O. H., 1969, Chalones of the skin, in: "Homeostatic Regulators," G. F. W. Wolstenholme and J. Knight (eds.), pp. 29-56,
Churchill, London.

Jablonska, S., and Langner, A., 1968, The mechanism of precancerous
and pseudocancerous conditions. A comparative study, in: "The
Thirteenth International Dermatological Congress," Vol. 1, pp.
17-19, Springer, Berlin.

Jablonska, S., Jakubowicz, K., Langner, A., Biczysko, W., and
Dabrowski, J., 1969, Badania nad isotota epidermodysplasia
verruciformis Lewandowsky-Lutz jako stanem przedrakowym,
Przeglad, Dermatologiczny, 56:715-719. (In Polish).

Jackson, I. F., 1967, Chromosome analysis of cells in effusions from
cancer patients, Cancer, 20:537-540.

Jacobs, P., Brown, W., and Doll, R., 1961, Distribution of human
chromosome counts in relation to age, Nature, 191:1178-1180,
London.

Jaffurs, W. J., Marlow, J. L., Turner, T. R., and Khanizadeh, A.,
1970, Chromosomal aberrations correlated with the cytologic
and histologic findings in carcinoma of the cervix uteri,
Cancer Cytol., 10:27-36.

James, J. G., 1962, Synthesis of deoxyribonucleic acid during interphase, Lancet, 1:744.

James, J., 1964, Observations on the so-called sex chromatin, Z.Zell.
Forsch., 64:178-188.

Janeja, M. G., and Stich, H. F., 1965, Chromosomes of tumor cells.
IV. Cell population changes in thymus, spleen, and bone marrow
during X-ray-induced leukemogenesis in C57BL/6j mice, J.Nat.
Cancer Inst., 35:421-431.

Ju, D. M. C., 1967, Pseudoepitheliomatous hyperplasia of the skin,
Dermatol.Internat., 6:82-92.

Judge, J. R., 1969, Giant condyloma acuminatum involving vulva and
rectum, Arch.Pathol., 88:46.

Kahn, G., Weinstein, G., and Frost, P., 1968, Kinetics of human
epidermal cell proliferation, J.Invest.Dermatol., 50:459-462.

Kaiser, R., and Schneider, E., 1968, Funktionszustäde und mitotische
Aktivität des Endometrium bei Endometrium Carcinoma,
Arch.Gynäk, 205:151-161.

Kalkoff, K. W., Berger, H., and Hundeiker, M., 1968, Zur Histogenese
    des Keratoakanthomas, in: "The Thirteenth International Derm-
    atological Congress," Vol. 1, pp. 53-54, Springer, Berlin.
Kallenberger, A., Hagmann, A., and Descoeudres, G., 1968, The inter-
    pretation of abnormal sex chromatin incidence in human breast
    tumors on the basis of DNA measurements, Eur.J.Cancer, 3:
    431-448.
Karasek, M. A., 1967, In vitro culture of human skin epithelial
    cells, J.Invest.Dermatol., 47:533-540.
Karasek, M. A., 1972, Dermal factors affecting epidermal cells in
    vitro, J.Invest.Dermatol., 59:99-101.
Katajama, K. P., and Jones, H. W., 1967, Chromosomes of atypical
    (adenomatous) hyperplasia and carcinoma of the endometrium,
    Am.J.Obstet.Gynec., 98:978-983.
Katajama, K. P., Woodruff, Y. O., Jones, H. W., and Preston, E.,
    1972, Chromosomes of condyloma acuminatum, Paget's disease, in
    situ carcinoma, and invasive squamous cell carcinoma of the
    human vulva, Obstet.Gynecol., 39:434-376.
Kaufman, I. A., 1968, On the lability of neural elements of the skin
    in some inflammatory dermatoses, in: "Sovremennye Aspekty
    Klinicheskoi i Eksperimental'noi Dermato-Venerologii"
    [Current Problems in Clinical and Experimental Dermato-
    Venereology], No. 5, pp. 105-110, Meditsina, Moscow. (In
    Russ.).
Kayumov, E. G., and Dmitrieva, E. N., 1973, Quantitative and quali-
    tative characteristics of sex chromatin in women in relation
    to age, Tsitologiya, No. 3, 344-346. (In Russ.).
Kazantseva, I. A., 1967, Changes in mitotic patterns of the laryngeal
    stratified squamous epithelium during hyperplastic processes
    in tumors, in: "Materialy Konferentsii po Patologii Kletki"
    [Proceedings of a Conference on Cellular Pathology], pp.
    75-78, Moscow. (In Russ.).
Kazantseva, I. A., 1973, DNA content of the gastric mucosal epi-
    thelium in chronic gastritis, polyposis, and cancer,
    Vopr.Onkol., No. 6, 51-54. (In Russ.).
Kazantseva, I. A., 1981, "Patologiya Mitoza v Opukholyakh Cheloveka"
    [Mitotic Abnormalities in Human Tumors], Nauka, Novosibirsk.
    (In Russ.).
Kazantseva, I. A., and Rogachikova, T. A., 1970, Mitotic patterns of
    tumor cells in various cancers differing in their clinical
    course, Vopr.Onkol., No. 10, 21-25. (In Russ.).
Kerl, H., and Pickel, H., 1971, Malegue Umwandlung von Condylomata
    acuminata der Vulva, Z. Haut Geschl.kr., 46:155-162.
Khesin, Ya. E., "Razmery Yader i Funktsional'noe Sostoyanie Kletki"
    [Nuclear Size and Functional State of the Cell], Meditsina,
    Moscow. (In Russ.).
Khlebnov, A. V., 1975, "Clinical studies of the antitumor antibiotic
    bleomycin", Dissertation, Moscow. (In Russ.).
Khlopin, N. G., 1940, "Kul'tura Tkanei" [The Tissue Culture], Medgiz,
    Leningrad. (In Russ.).

Khlopin, N. G., 1947, The growth and movement of tissue tumor elements outside the body, in: "Zlokachestbvennye Opukholi" [Malignant Tumors], Vol. 1, pp. 64-74, Medgiz, Moscow. (In Russ.).

Khlystova, Z. S., 1960, Cultivation of tissues in denervated areas of the body, Arkh.Patol., No. 3, 24-27. (In Russ.).

Khristin, L. I., Tomashevskii, D. I., and Tshetsetskaya, E. K., 1963, On papillomatosis cutis carcinoides of Gottron, Vest.Dermatol., No. 3, 20-23. (In Russ.).

Krushchev, G. K., Andres, A. G., and Il'ina-Kukueva, V. I., 1931, Cultures of blood leukocytes for the study of human karyotypes, Zh.Eksp.Biol., 7:455-460. (In Russ.).

Kirkland, J. A., 1966, Chromosomes in uterine cancer, Lancet, 1:152.

Kirkland, J. A., Stenley, M. A., and Collier, K. M., 1967, Comparative study of histologic and chromosomal abnormalities in cervical neoplasia, Cancer, 20:1934-1952.

Knierer, W., 1947, Pseudorezidive nach Röntgenbestrahlung von Hautkarzinomen, Dermatol. Wschr., 119:272-274.

Knoblich, R., and Failing, J. F., 1967, Giant condyloma acuminatum (Buschke-Loewenstein tumor) of the rectum, Am.J.Clin.Pathol. 48:389.

Koller, P. C., 1947, Abnormal mitosis in tumors, Br.J.Cancer, 1:38-47.

Kopf, A. W., 1968, Unusual forms of keratoacanthoma, in: "The Thirteenth International Dermatological Congress," Vol. 1, pp. 54-57, Springer, Berlin.

Korelenshtein, R. Ya., 1970, Clinical manifestations and differential diagnosis of keratoacanthoma of the vermilion border of the lip, in: "Respublikanskaya Konferentsiya Onkologov, 5-ya. Materialy," [Proceedings of the Fifth Republican Conference of Oncologists], pp. 170-172, Kishinev. (In Russ.).

Korfsmeier, K. H., 1967, Interzellulare Verbindungen bein Plattenepithelcarzinom der menschlichen Haut in der Gewebekultur, Experientia, 23:946-948.

Korfsmeier, K. H., 1968, Epitheliale Hauttumoren und gesundes Hautepithelial in der Gewebekultur, Arch.Klin.Exp.Dermatol., 232:434-444.

Kovi, J., Tilman, R. L., and Lee, S. M., 1974, Malignant transformation of condyloma acuminatum, Am.J.Clin.Pathol., 61:702-710.

Kozhevnikov, P. V., 1946, "Atipicheskie Piodermii (paratravmaticheskie, khronicheskie, yazvennye i giperplasticheskie)" [Atypical pyodermas (traumatic, chronic, ulcerative, and hyperplastic)], Turkmengiz, Ashkhabad. (In Russ.).

Kozhevnikov, P. V., 1961, Borovsky's disease (cutaneous leishmaniasis), in: "Rukovodstvo po Dermato-Venerologii" [A Handbook of Dermato-Venereology], Vol. 1., pp. 410-425, Medgiz, Moscow. (In Russ.).

Kozlov, V. V., 1969, "Reactive changes in proliferative processes in health and disease", Doctoral dissertation, Leningrad. (In Russ.).

Kraevskii, N. A., and Smol'yanikov, A. V., 1971, in: "Rukovodstvo po
    Patologoanatomicheskoi Diagnostlike Opukholei Cheloveka [A
    Handbook of Pathologic Diagnosis of Human Tumors], pp. 3-11,
    Meditsina, Moscow. (In Russ.).
Kraus, F. T., and Perez-Mesa, C., 1966, Verrucous carcinoma, Cancer,
    19:26.
Kreibic, C., 1915, Neurodermatitis verrucosa, Arch.Dermatol.Syph.,
    121:307-312.
Kryazheva, S. S., 1971, "Opredelenie Urovnya Polovogo Khromatina v
    Protsesse Kortikosteroidnoi Terapii Nekotorykh Dermatozov
    (Metodicheskoe Pis'mo)" [Determination of Sex Chromatin Fre-
    quency during Corticosteroid Treatment of Dermatoses (A
    Methodologic Guide)], Moscow. (In Russ.).
Kuffer, R., and Fiore-Donno, G., 1975, Affections preepitheliom-
    ateuses de la muqueuse buccale. Essai de classification,
    Acta Stomatol.Belg. 72:385-391.
Kurilo, L. F., 1970, "Three-group metaphases: morphology and mode of
    origin", Dissertation, Moscow. (In Russ.).
Kurilo, L. F., 1973, Colchicine mitosis and its reversibility, Byull.
    Eksp.Biol.Med., No. 3 97-101. (In Russ.).
Kurlat, M. M., 1964, Malignant transformation of lupous lesions, in:
    "Voprosy Tuberkuleza Kozhi" [Some Aspects of Cutaneous Tuber-
    culosis], pp. 82-91, Kiev. (In Russ.).
Lalaeva, A. M., 1972, "Clinicopathologic characterization of cutaneous
    changes in chromosomal diseases", Dissertation, Moscow. (In
    Russ.).
Lamb, D., 1967, Correlation of chromosome counts with histological
    appearances and prognosis in transitional-cell carcinoma of
    bladder, Br.Med.J., 5535, 273-277.
Lane-Brown, M. M., and Melia, D. F., 1973, A genetic diathesis to
    skin cancer, J.Invest.Dermatol., 61:39-41.
Langan, T. A., 1968, Histone phosphorylation: stimulation by adeno-
    sine, 3',5'-monophosphate, Science, 162:579-580.
Lanné, T. K., 1969, Pseudoepitheliomatous hyperplasia and its re-
    lation to cancer, Trudy Leningradskogo Obshchestva Pato-
    logoanatomov, No. 10, 19-26, (In Russ.).
Lanné, T. K. "Pseudoepitheliomatous hyperplasia", Dissertation,
    Leningrad. (In Russ.).
Lapidus, R. I., 1959, On the treatment of varicose ulcers of the
    shin, Zdravookhranenie Belorussii, No. 8, 36. (In Russ.).
Lasser, O., 1893, Zur Therapie die Hautkrebs, Berlin Klin.Wschr.,
    30:537.
Lazarenko, F. M., 1934, Experience with a new method for experimental
    study of tissues (preliminary results), Arkh.Biol.Nauk, 34:
    707-720. (In Russ.).
Lazarenko, F. M. 1959, "Zakonomernosti Rosta i Prevrashcheniya
    Organov i Tkanei v Usloviyakh Kul'tivirovaniya Ikh v Organizme"
    [Patterns of Growth and Transformation of Organs and Tissues
    Cultivated inside the Body], Medgiz, Moscow. (In Russ.).
Lejkan, K., and Starzycki, L., 1977, Giant keratoacanthoma on the
    inner surface of the prepuce, Br.J.Vener.Dis., 53:65-67.

Lelikova, G. P., 1972, "Cytogenetic analysis of human testicular
    tumors", Dissertation, Moscow. (In Russ.).
Lenz, E., 1963, Zur Frage der differential-diagnostischen Verwert-
    barkeit des Geschlechtschromatins bei der histologischen
    Beurteilung einiger Hauttumoren (Spinoliem, Basaliem, Kerat-
    oakanthom, Akanthokerathom, Verruca senilis), Z. Haut.
    Geschl.Kr., 10:336-348.
Leuchtenberger, C., and Leuchtenberger, R., 1960, Quantitative cyto-
    chemical studies on the relation of deoxyribonucleic acid of
    cells to various pathological conditions, Biochem.Pharmacol.,
    4:128-163.
Leuchtenberger, C., Leuchtenberger, R., and Davis, A. M., 1954, A
    microspectrophotometric study of the desoxyribose nucleic acid
    (DNA) content in cells of normal and malignant human tissues,
    Am.J.Pathol., 30:65-85.
Levan, A., 1956, Chromosomes in cancer tissue, Ann.N.Y.Acad.Sci.,
    63:774-792.
Levan, A., 1967, Some current problems of cancer cytogenetics,
    Hereditas, 57:343.
Levan, A., and Biessele, J. J., 1958, Role of chromosomes in cancer-
    ogenesis as studied in serial tissue cultures of mammalian
    cells, Ann.N.Y.Acad.Sci., 71:1022-1053.
Lever, W. F., 1967, Histopathology of the skin, 4th ed., Lippincott,
    Philadelphia.
Lever, W. F., and Schaumburg-Lever, G., 1975, Histopathology of the
    Skin, 5th ed., Lippincott, Philadelphia.
Levi-Coblentz, G., 1937, Pseudoépithelioma traumatique, Bull Assoc.
    franç.Et.Cancer, 26:117-181.
Levine, M., 1972, The growth of adult human skin in vitro,
    Br.J.Dermatol., 86:481-490.
Liozner, L. D., 1966, "Kletochnoe Obnovlenie" [Cell Renewal],
    Meditsina, Leningrad. (In Russ.).
Loewenstein, L. W., 1939, Carcinoma-like condyloma acuminatum, Med.
    Clin.North Am., 23:799.
Logan, W. S., 1972, Vitamin A and keratinisation, Arch.Dermatol.,
    105:748-757.
Lovell, C. R., Harman, R. R., and Bradfeld, J. M., 1980, Cutaneous
    carcinoma arising in erosive pustular dermatosis of the
    scalp," Br.J.Dermatol., 103:325-328.
Lowry, W. S., Clark, D. A., and Hannemann, J. H., 1972, Skin cancer
    and immunosuppression, Lancet, 1:1290-1291.
Lund, H. Z., 1957, Tumors of the skin, Washington.
Lynch, H. T., 1969, Skin, heredity, and cancer, Cancer, 24:277-288.
Lyon, M. F., 1961, Gene action in the X-chromosome of the mouse,
    Nature (London), 190:372-373.
Machacek, G. F., and Weakley, D. R., 1960, Giant condyloma acuminatum
    of Buschke and Loewenstein, Arch.Dermatol., 82:41-47.
Macieira-Coelho, A., 1967, Relationship between DNA synthesis and
    cell density in normal and virus-transformed cells," Internat.
    J.Cancer, 2:297-303.

Maggiera, A., 1968, Beitrag zum keratoakanthomproblem, **Dermatologica**, (Basel), 137:263-270.

Makino, S., 1957, The chromosome cytology of the ascites tumors of rats with special reference to the concept of the stemline cell, **Intern.Rev.Cytol.**, 6:26-84.

Makino, S. T., 1959, Ishikara, and Tonomura, A., Cytological studies of tumors. XXVII. The chromosomes of thirty human tumors, **Z. Krebsforsch.**, 63:184-208.

Makino, S., Sasaki, M. C., and Tonomura, A., 1964, Cytological studies of tumors. XL. Chromosome studies in fifty-two human tumors, **J.Nat.Cancer Inst.**, 32:741-771.

Manocha, S. L., 1969, Microspectrophotometric studies of DNA in the epithelial tumors induced by 3-methyl-cholanthrene and croton oil treatment in mice," **Acta Histochem. (Jena)**, 34:201-211.

Mardakhiashvili, Sh. I., and Shats, V. Ya., 1969, "Problema Polovogo Khromatina v Onkologii" [The Provlem of Sex Chromatin in Oncology], Meditsina, Moscow, (In Russ.).

Marghescu, S., Braun-Falco, O., and Konz, B., 1976, Nature et traitement de la maladie de Buschke-Loewenstein, **Bull.Soc.franç. Dermatol.Syph.**, 83:293-294.

Mark, J., 1965, Chromosome analysis in Raus tumors in the rabbit, **Hereditas**, 53:165-170.

Marks, F., 1971, Direct evidence for two tissue-specific chalone-like factors regulating mitosis and DNA synthesis in mouse epidermis, **Hoppe-Seylers Z. physiol.Chem.**, 352:1273-1274.

Marks, F., 1973, A tissue-specific factor inhibiting DNA synthesis in mouse epidermis, **Nat.Cancer Inst.Monogr.**, 38:79-90.

Martsinovskii, B. I., 1909, "Etiology of the Oriental ulcer (bouton d'Orient) and brief review of this disease", Doctoral dissertation, Moscow. (In Russ.).

Martynova, R. P., 1945, Heredity in the etiology of cancer, **Byull. Eksp.Biol.Med.**, No. 3, 12-14. (In Russ.).

Mashkilleison, L. N., 1960, "Infektsionnye i Parazitarnye Bolezni Kozhi" [Infectious and Parasitic Diseases of the Skin], Medgiz, Moscow. (In Russ.).

Mashkilleison, L. N., 1964, "Lechenie i Profilaktika Kozhnykh Boleznei" [Treatment and Prevention of Skin Diseases], Meditsina, Moscow. (In Russ.).

Mashkilleison, L. N., 1965, "Chastnaya Dermatologiya" [Specific Dermatology], Meditsina, Moscow. (In Russ.).

Mashkilleison, A. L., 1965, "Predrak Krasnoi Kaimy Gub i Slizistoi Obolochki Rta" [Precancer of the Vermilion Border of the Lip and of the Oral Mucosa], Meditsina, Moscow. (In Russ.).

Mashkilleison, A. L., Glebova, L. I., Kantsler, V. S., Kundel', L. M., and Klyavina, V. R., 1973, Treatment of dermatoses with Methotrexate: efficiency and adverse reactions, **Vest.Dermatol. Venerol.**, No. 10, 69-73. (In Russ.).

Mashkovskii, M. D., 1977, "Lekarstvennye Sredstva" [Pharmaceutical Preparations], Meditsina, Moscow. (In Russ.).

Masson, P., 1956, "Tumeurs Humanes. Histologie, Diagnostics et Techniques", 2nd ed., Maloine, Paris.

Mayall, B. H., and Mandelsohn, M. L., 1970, Deoxyribonucleic acid
     cytophotometry of stained human leukocytes, J.Histochem.Cyto-
     chem., 18:383-407.
Mayenburg, J., Ehlers, G., Mühlbaurer, W., and Stener, G., 1977,
     Condylomata acuminata gigantea (Buschke-Loewenstein-Tumoren)
     mit Vulva-Karzinom, Z.Hautkrh., 52:869-884.
Mazur, K. Ya., 1936, "Experience with the use of close-range roent-
     genography", Dissertation, Riga. (In Russ.).
McCarthy, W. C., 1936, Identification of the cancer cell, JAMA, 107:
     844-845.
McCormac, H., and Scarff, R. W., 1936, Molluscum sebaceum, Br.J.
     Dermatol.Syphil., 48:624-626.
McMichael, H., Wagner, J. E., Nowell, P. C., and Hungerford, D. A.,
     1963, Chromosome studies of virus-induced rabbit papillomas and
     derived primary carcinomas, J.Nat.Cancer Inst., 31:1197-1215.
Meier-Ruge, A., and Kallenberger, A., 1967, Das Mammacarcinom in
     seiner Relation zum pathologisch-anatomischen Bild und Sex-
     chromatingehalt, Med.Welt, 14:871-875.
Melczer, N., 1961, Präcancerosen und primäre Krebse der Haut,
     Akadémiai Kiadó, Budapest.
Mercer, E., 1962, The cancer cell, Br.Med.Bull., 18:187-192.
Miedzinski, F., Dratwinski, Z., Brozowski, J., and Sazankiewicz, B.,
     1973, Ein Beitrag zur nosologischen Stellun des Keratoakan-
     thoma centrifugum, Hautarzt, 24:120-123.
Miescher, G., 1950, Zur Frage der Papillomatosis cutis carcinoides,
     Dermatologica (Basel), 101:217-230.
Miles, C. P., 1967, Chromosome analysis of solid tumors. XI.XXVI.
     Epithelial tumors, Br.J.Cancer, 20:1274-1287.
Minsker, O. B., Agarunova, Yu. S., Malkina, A. Ya., Moskovskaya, M.
     A., and Panzur, G. S., 1975, Experience with the study of
     chromolysis, Vest.Dermatol.Venerol., No. 10, 40-45. (In
     Russ.).
Miyahara, M., 1913, Zur Frage der atypischen Epithelwunderung bei
     Lupus, Frankfurt Z. Pathol., 9:167-178.
Monacelli, M., 1967, Fibroepithelials Hauttumoren und Präkanzerosen,
     Med.Klin., 62:1154-1156.
Monastyrskaya, B. I., 1945, "Role of inflammation in the genesis of
     experimentally induced skin cancer", Dissertation, Leningrad.
     (In Russ.).
Montgomery, H., 1967, "Dermatopathology", Vol. 2, Harper and
     Row, New York.
Montgomery, H., and Holman, J. C., 1938, Pseudoepitheliomatous hyper-
     plasia in a case of sporotrichosis, Proc.Staff Meet.Mayo
     Clin., 13:465-469.
Moore, K. L., and Barr, M. L., 1954, Nuclear morphology according to
     sex in human tissues, Acta.Anat.(Basel), 21:197-208.
Moore, K. L., and Barr, M. L., 1957, The sex chromatin in human
     malignant tissues, Br.J.Cancer, 11:384-390.
Moore, K. L., Graham, M. A., and Barr, M. L., 1953, The detection of
     chromosomal sex in hermaphrodites from a skin biopsy, Surg.
     Gyn.Obstet., 96:641-648.

Moorhead, P. S., 1967, Comments on the human leukocyte culture, in:
    "Human Radiation Cytogenetics," J. H. Evans, W. M. Brown and
    A. S. McLeon (eds.), pp. 1-5, Elsevier, Amsterdam.
Morozov, Yu. E., Nikolaeva, N. V., and Pereverzov, B. D., 1971, The
    nucleic acids (quantitative analysis by the method of cyto-
    spectrophotometry), in: "Printsipy i Metody Gistotsitokhimi-
    cheskogo Analiza v Tsitologii" [Principles and Methods of
    Cytohistochemical Analysis in Cytology], A. I. Strukov and B.
    B. Fuks (eds.), pp. 336-360, Meditsina, Moscow. (In Russ.).
Muer, E. G., Yates-Bell, A. J., and Barlow, K. A., 1967, Multiple
    primary carcinomata of the colon, duodenum and larynx associ-
    ated with keratoacanthoma of the face, Br.J.Surg., 54:191.
Naleskina, L. A., 1971, DNA and sex chromatin in pigmented neoplasms
    of human skin, Vopr.Onkol., No. 4, 8-14. (In Russ.).
Nazzario, P., and Tosti, A., 1968, Le pseudo-cancerose cutané,
    Minerva Dermatol., 43:617-657.
Nebl, A. J., and Ghadially, F. N., 1966, Massive or giant keratoacan-
    thoma, J.Pathol.Bacertiol., 91:505-509.
Neradov, L. A., 1961, Tuberculosis of the skin, in: "Rukovodstvo po
    Dermato-Venerologii" [A Handbook of Dermato-Venereology], pp.
    332-408, Medgiz, Moscow. (In Russ.).
Netto, N. R., Chade, J., and Camaro, F. P., 1976, Giant condyloma or
    Buschke-Loewenstein tumor, Internat.Surg., 61:105-197.
Niemi, K. M., 1970, The benign fibrohistiocytic tumors of the skin,
    Acta Dermatol.Venereol.(Stockholm), 50 (Suppl.63): 1-66.
Nierman, H., 1964, Zwillingsdermatologie, Berlin.
Nikolowski, W., and Eisenlohr, E., 1950, Papillomatosis cutis car-
    cinoides, Dermatol.Wschr., 238:121.
Odinokova, V. A., Egorkina, D. A., and Berebein, B. A., 1973, Role of
    sex chromatin studies in the diagnosis of neoplasms in various
    sites, in: "S"ezd Onkologov RSFSR. 1-yi. Trudy" [First Con-
    gress of Oncologists of the RSFSR. Proceedings], pp.123-125,
    Ufa. (In Russ.).
Ohno, S., Kaplan, W. D., and Kinosita, R., 1959, Formation of sex
    chromatin by a single X-chromosome in liver cells of Rattus
    norvegicus, Exp.Cell Res., 18:415-418.
Olenov, Yu. M., 1967, "Kletochnaya Nasledstvennost', Differentsirovka
    Kletok i Kantserogenez kak Problema Evolyutsionnoi Genetiki"
    [Cellular Heredity, Cell Differentiation, and Carcinogenesis
    in Their Relation to Evolutionary Genetics], Nauka, Leningrad.
    (In Russ.).
Ou Bau-syan, 1961, Histochemical studies of epithelial and connective
    tissue changes during the development of inflammatory epi-
    thelial outgrowth, Byull.Eksp.Biol.Med., 52:101-114. (In
    Russ.).
Palmer, C. G., 1959, The cytology of rabbit pepillomas and derived
    carcinomas, J.Nat.Cancer Inst., 23:241-249.
Pastan, I., 1975, The role of cyclic AMP in malignant transformation,
    Am.J.Clin.Pathol., 63:669-670.
Pastan, I., and Johnson, G. S., 1974, Cyclic AMP and the transform-
    ation of fibroblasts, Adv.Cancer Res., 19:303-329.

Pastan, I. H., Johnson, G. S., and Anderson, W. B., 1975, in: "Annual
    Review of Biochemistry," E. E. Snell (ed.), Vol. 44, p. 401,
    Annual Rev Inc., Menlo Park, Calif.
Patau, K., 1960, The identification of individual chromosomes,
    especially in man, Am.J.Human Genet., 12:250-276.
Pautrier, L. M., 1934, Le névrome de al lichenification circumscrite
    nodulaire chronique (lichen ruber planus corné, prurigo nodul-
    aris), Ann. Dermatol.Syph., 5:897-919.
Perroud, H., and Delacretaz, 1977, Végétantes iodides, Ann.Dermatol.
    Venereol., 104:154-156.
Petrov, N. N., 1947, Introduction. Definition of the term "tumor",
    in: "Zlokachestvennye Opukholi" [Malignant Tumors], Vol. 1, pp.
    1-7, Medgiz, Moscow. (In Russ.).
Pinkus, H., 1966, The basement membrane in relation to carcinoma of
    the skin, Arch.Dermatol., 94:715.
Pinkus, H., 1967, Differenzierung bösartiger und relatif gutartiger
    Spinaliome und Melanome, Med.Klin., 62:1160-1162.
Pinkus, H., 1968, The role of the mesoderm in basaliomas, in: "The
    Thirteenth International Dermatological Congress," Vol. 1,
    pp. 8-10, Springer, Berlin.
Pinkus, H., and Mehregan, A. H., 1969, "A Guide to Dermatopathology",
    Appleton-Century-Crofts, New York.
Pinkus, H., and Mehregan, A. H., 1976, "A Guide to Dermatopathology",
    2nd ed., Appleton-Century-Crofts, New York.
Pinkus, H., and Mehregan, A. H., 1980, Pseudomalignant skin lesions,
    Clinics Plastic Surg., 289-300.
Pogosyants, E. E., 1969, Cytogenetics of tumors, in: "Osnovy
    Tsitogenetiki Cheloveka" [The Fundamentals of Human
    Cytogenetics], pp. 447-471, Meditsina, Moscow. (In Russ.).
Pogosyants, E. E., and A. F., Zakharov, 1965, Cytogenetic character-
    istics of tumor cells, in: "Biologiya Zlokachestvennogo
    Rosta" [The Biology of Malignant Growth], pp.152-179,
    Meditsina, Moscow, (In Russ.).
Pogosyants, E. E., Gudina, A. N., and Rodkina, R. A., 1972, Vari-
    ations in karyotype in malignant tumors of the human testicle,
    Vopr.Onkol., No. 6, 3-9. (In Russ.).
Poleksis, S., 1974, Keratoacanthoma and multiple carcinomas, Br.J.
    Dermatol., 91:461-464.
Policard, A., and Bassis, M., 1970, "Elementy Patologii Kletki"
    [Elements of Cellular Pathology] (Russian Translation), Mir,
    Moscow.
Porters, J. E., and Zantkuyl, C. F., 1975, Iododerma caused by amio-
    darone, Arch.Dermatol., 111:656.
Potekaev, N. S., and Kostantinov, A. V., 1966, Hypertonic ulcers of
    the shin (Martorelle's syndrome), Vest.Dermatol.Venerol.,
    No.3, 72-78. (In Russ.).
Poth, D. O., 1939, Tumorlike keratosis, Report of a case, Arch.
    Dermatol.Syphilol., 39:229.
Pott, P., 1963, Quoted in: M. Potter, Percivall Pott's contribution
    to cancer research, Nat.Cancer Inst.Monogr., 10:1-5.

Prasad, K. N., and Sheppard, J. R., 1972, Inhibitors of cyclic
    nucleotide phosphodiesterase induce morphological different-
    iation of mouse neuroblastoma cell culture, Exp.Cell Res.,
    73:436-440.
Prescott, D. M., 1961, The growth-duplication cycle of the cell,
    Internat.Rev.Cytol., 11:255.
Pricl, F. M., Camalier, R. F., Goutt, R., Taylor, U. G., Smith, G.
    H., and Sanford, K. K., 1980, A new culture medium for human
    skin epithelial cells, In vitro, 16:147-158.
Prokof'eva, O. G., 1952, Effect of carcinogenic substances on in-
    flammatory epithelial outgrowths, in: "Trudy AMN SSSR" [Trans-
    actions of the USSR Academy of Medical Sciences], A. I.
    Serebrov and L. M. Shabad (eds.), No. 5, pp. 170-178.  (In
    Russ.).
Prokof'eva-Bel'govskaya, A. A., 1961, Radiation damage to the chromo-
    somes of the salmon in early stages of its development,"
    Tsitologiya, No. 4, 437-445.  (In Russ.).
Prokof'eva-Bel'govskaya, A. A., and Gandelis, V. M., 1965, The ident-
    ification of human chromosomes, Izv.Akad.Nauk SSR, Ser.Biol.,
    No. 2, 188-200.  (In Russ.).
Pruniéras, M., 1975, Culture of the skin: how and why, Internat.J.
    Dermatol., 14:12-22.
Prutkin, L., 1968, An ultrastructural study of the keratoacanthoma
    experimentally produced, in: "The Thirteenth International
    Dermatological Congress, Vol. 1, pp. 57-58, Springer, Berlin.
Raben, A. C., 1977, On precancer of the skin and on its classi-
    fication, Klin.Med., No.7, 123-128.  (In Russ.).
Rahrbach, R., Lau, M., Thomas, C., and Sandritter, W., 1972, Cyto-
    photometric measurements of DNA and histone protein content in
    experimentally induced skin tumors of the rat and hairless
    mouse, Beitr.Pathol.Anat., 146:111-121.
Raichev, R., and Andreev, V., 1965, "Zlokachestvennye Opukholi Kozhi"
    [Malignant Cutaneous Tumors] (Russian translation from
    Bulgarian), Izd. Meditsina i Fizkul'tura, Sofia.
Raichev, R., Krystev, B., Andreev, V., et al., 1964, Oshibki
    Diagnostiki i Lechenie Zlokachestvennykh Opukholei [Malignant
    Tumors: Diagnostic Errors and Treatment] (Russian translation
    from Bulgarian), Meditsina i Fizkul'tura, Sofia.
Rakhmanov, V. A., 1961, Pyodermia, in: "Rukovodstvo po Dermato-
    Venerologii" [A Handbook of Dermato-Venereology], pp. 183-231,
    Medgiz, Leningrad.  (In Russ.).
Ramond, L., Burnier, U, and Eliaschef, O., 1931, Un nouveau cas de
    verrucome avec adénite et à structure épitheliomatiforme
    curable par le 914, Bull.Soc.franç.Dermatol.Syph., 38:612.
Randazzo, S. D., 1966, Cheratoacantoma insorto in sogetto con lupus
    volgare dopo trattamento con isoniazide, G. Ital.Dermatol.,
    107:1195-1210.
Randazzo, S. D., and Tichera, G., 1963, Su un caso de cheratoacantoma
    gigante a rapido accrescimento, Minerva Dermatol., 14:38.

Rao, C. J. S., Delmonte, M., and Nadler, H. L., 1971, Adenyl Cyclase
    activity in cultivated human skin fibroblasts, Nature (New
    Biology), 232:253.

Rathjens, B., 1953, Zur Kenntnis der Papillomatosis cutis carcinoides
    Gottron, Dermatol.Wschr., 127:313-317.

Read, S. I., and Abell, E., 1981, Pseudoepitheliomatous keratotic and
    micaceous balanitis, Arch.Dermatol., 117:436-437.

Reiffers, J., Laugier, P., and Olmos, L., 1976, Papillomatose orale
    floride et syndrome de Buschke-Loewenstein; étude comparative
    chez deux malades, Bull.Soc.franç. Dermatol.Syph., 83:294-296.

Riboldi, A., and Del Pozzo, V., 1976, Contributo clinico alla pap-
    illomatosis cutis carcinoides di Gottron, G.Ital.Dermatol.,
    111:144-147.

Richart, R. M., and Corfman, P. A., 1964, Chromosome number and
    morphology of a human preinvasive neoplasm, Science,
    144:65-67.

Robison, G. A., Butcher, R. W., and Sutherland, E. W., 1968, Cyclic
    AMP, Ann.Rev.Biochem., 37:143-174.

Rodermund, O. E., 1956, Uber des "Gesehlechtschromatin" in:
    "Geschwülsten," Z. Krebsforsch., 61:259-262.

Rodyakin, N. R., 1982, "Kozhnyi Leishmanioz (epidemiologiya, klinika,
    lechenie i profilaktika)" [Cutaneous Leishmaniasis (epidermio-
    logy, clinical features, treatment, and prevention)], Ilym,
    Ashkhabad. (In Russ.).

Rook, A., 1968, Condyloma acuminatae, in: "A. Rook, D. Wilkinson and
    F. Ebling, Textbook of Dermatology," Vol. 1., p. 759,
    Blackwell, Oxford.

Rook, A., and Gronin, 1962, cited in: "The Yearbook of Dermato-
    logy 1962-63," R. L. Baer and A. W. Kopf (eds.), Yearbook
    Publishers, Chicago.

Rook, A., and Moffatt, J. L., 1962, Multiple self-healing epithelioma
    of Ferguson-Smith type: report of a case of unilateral dist-
    ribution," Arch.Dermatol.Syphilol., 86:44-53.

Rook, A., and Whimster, I., 1950, Le kerato-acanthoma, Arch.Belg.
    Dermatol.Syph., 6:137-146.

Rook, A., Whimster, I., 1979, Keratoacanthoma - a thirty year retro-
    spect, Br.J.Dermatol., 100:41-47.

Rossianskii, N. L., and Smelov, N. S., 1947, "Tuberkulezniye
    Zabolevaniya Kozhi" [Tuberculous Diseases of the Skin], Moscow.
    (In Russ.).

Rothberg, S., Nancarrow, G. E., Meydreck, E. F., Ivanik, M. J.,
    Bertsch, S., Csontos, K., Schweizer, J., and Marks, F., 1976,
    Extracellular stimulation of epidermal DNA synthesis, Cell
    Tissue Kinet., 9:439-444.

Rowe, L., and Dixon, W. J., 1972, Clustering and control of mitotic
    activity in human epidermis, J.Invest.Dermatol., 58:16-23.

Rowe, L., and Dixon, W. J., 1975, Mitosis in human epidermis,
    Clustering, sister cells, and findings suggestive of a spread-
    ing mitotic otimulus, Oncology, 31:133-138.

Rozentul, M. A., 1970, "Obshchaya Terapiya Kozhnykh Boleznei" [General
    Therapy for Skin Diseases], Meditsina, Moscow. (In Russ.).

Rushinskii, B. P., 1910, On the etiology of experimentally induced
    outgrowths of epithelial tissues, Russkii Vrach, 9:2080-2083.
    (In Russ.).
Ruppe, J. P., 1981, Verrucous carcinoma, Arch.Dermatol., 117:184-185.
Rutshtein, L. T., Golousenko, I. Yu, and Myskin, V. S., 1982,
    A case of chronic ulcerative pyoderma, Vest.Dermatol.Venerol.,
    No. 7, 72-74.
Ryabinina, Z. A., and Benyush, V. A., 1973, "Poliploidiya i
    Gipertrofiya Kletok v Protsessakh Rosta i Vosstanovleniya"
    [Polyploidy and Hypertrophy of Cells During Growth and Re-
    generation], Meditsina, Moscow. (In Russ.).
Sandberg, A. A., 1966, The chromosomes and causation of human cancer
    and leukemia, Cancer Res., 26:2064-2081.
Sandberg, A. A., 1970, Chromosomal abnormalities in human neoplasia,
    Ann.Rev.Med., 21:379.
Sandberg, A. A., Ishibara, T., Moore, G. E., and Lickren, J. M.,
    1963, Unusually high polyploidy in a human cancer, Cancer,
    16:1246-1254.
Sandberg, A. A., Yamada, K., Kikuchi, Y., and Takagi, N., 1967,
    Chromosomes and causation of human cancer and leukemia. III.
    Karyotypes of cancerous effusions, Cancer, 20:1199-1216.
Sanderson, K. V., 1968, Tumors of the skin, in: "Textbook of Dermato-
    logy," A. Rook, D. S. Wilkinson and F. Ebling (eds.), pp.
    1658-1748, Blackwell, Oxford.
Sanderson, K. V., and Mackie, K. V., 1979, Tumors of the skin, in:
    "Textbook of Dermatology," A. Rook, D. S. Wilkinson and F.
    Ebling (eds.). 3rd ed., pp. 2119-2223, Blackwell, Oxford.
Sandritter, W., 1965, DNA content of tumors. Cytophotometric measure-
    ments, Eur.J.Cancer, 1:303-307.
Sandritter, W., and Fischer, R., 1964, The DNA content of normal
    stratified epithelium, carcinoma, in situ, and tumors,
    Z.Krebsforsch., 66:333-348.
Santha Cruz, L. J., and Clausen, K., 1977, Atypical hyperplasia
    accompanying keratoacanthoma, Dermatologica (Basel),
    154:156-160.
Scafield, H. H., Werning, J. T., and Shukes, 1974, Solitary intraoral
    keratoacanthoma, Oral Surg., 37:889-898.
Scarpa, C., 1971, Sull'evolutione spinaliomatose dei cheratoacantomi,
    G.Ital.Dermatol., 106: 365-368.
Scarpelli, D. G., and Van Haam, E., 1957, A study of mitosis in
    cervical epithelium during experimental inflammation and
    carcinogenesis, Cancer Res., 17:880-884.
Scassellati, S. G., and Mastrandria, V., 1963, Temperatura di com-
    bustione delle sigarette in diverse condizione, Boll.Soc.Ital.
    Biol.Sperim., 39:1007-1010.
Scheicher-Gottron, E., 1958, Papillomatosis mucosae carcinoides der
    Mundschleimhaut bei gleichzeitigem Vorhandensein eines Lichen
    ruber der Haut, Z. Haut Geschl.Kr. 24:99-101.

Scherman, F. G., Quasler, H., and Wimher, D., 1961, Cell population
    kinetics in the ear epidermis in mice, Exp.Cell Res., 25,
    998-1002.
Schimpf, A., and Seller, H., 1963, Zum Formenkreis der papillomatosis
    cutis carcinoides Gottron, Arch.Klin.Exp.Dermatol.,
    217:377-393.
Schindler, R., 1965, "Die Tierische Zelle in Zellkultur", Springer,
    Berlin.
Schnitzler, L., Schubert, B., Verret, J. L., Emerian, M., and Brunet,
    A., 1977, Epitheliomatose familiale de Ferguson-Smith (á
    propos de 2 cas familiaux), Ann.Dermatol.Vénéréol. (Paris),
    104:206-216.
Schnitzler, L., Schubert, B., and Verret, J. L., 1980, Essai de
    prévention des épitheliomas cutanés par le rétinoide aromati-
    que, Ann.Dermatol.Vénéréol., 107:657-663.
Schnuder, H., 1966, Genetik der Psoriasis, Arch.Klin.Exp.Dermatol.,
    227:143-150.
Schumann, J., Ehring, F., Göhde, W., and Dittrich, W., 1971,
    Impulscytophotometrie der DNS in Hauttumoren, Arch.Klin.Exp.
    Dermatol., 239:377-389.
Schuppiner, H. J., and Steinke, W., 1960, "Großoflächig-
    papillomatöses Reizakanthom mit maligner Entartung," Dermatol.
    Wschr., 142:907-911.
Sealy, R., Immerman, A., and Shepstone, B., 1972, Mitotic index in
    human squamous cell carcinoma, Acta Radiol. (Ther.)
    (Stockholm), 11:59-64.
Seidel, A., and Sandritter, W., 1963, Cytophotometrische Messungen
    des DNA-Gehaltes eines Lungenadenoms und eine malignan
    Lungenadenomtose, Z.Krebsforsch., 65:555-559.
Seigel, A., 1962, Malignant transformation of condyloma acuminatum,
    Am.J.Surg., 103:613-617.
Seldam, R. E., 1970, Pseudo-malignant cutaneous amoebiasis, Trop.
    Georg.Med., 22:142-148.
Serov, S. F., 1973, Ovarian precancerous conditions, in: "Voprosy
    Patologicheskoi Anatomii Opukholevykh Protsessov" [Pathologic
    Anatomy of Tumors], pp. 44-46, Krasnodar. (In Russ.).
Severin, S. E., 1975, "Sovremennye problemy fiziko-khimicheskoi bio-
    logii. Doklad na yubileinoi sessii Akademii Nauk SSR,
    posvyashchennoi 250-letiyu Akademii" [Current problems in
    physicochemical biology. Report presented to a Jubilee
    Session of the USSR Academy of Sciences devoted to the 250th
    Anniversary of the Academy], Moscow. (In Russ.).
Severin, S. E., 1981, The mechanism of action and the biologic role
    of the adenyl cyclase system, in: "Fundamental'nye Nauki -
    Meditsine. Sovmestnaya Sessiya Obshchego Sobraniya AN SSR i
    Obshchego Sobraniya AMN SSSR, 19-20 Noyabrya 1980 g." [The
    Contribution of Basic Sciences to Medical Practice. A Joint
    Meeting of Members and Corresponding Members of the USSR
    Academy of Sciences and of the USSR Academy of Medical
    Sciences, November 19-20, 1980], pp. 189-195, Nauka, Moscow.
    (In Russ.).

Shabad, L. M., 1962, Some experimental findings regarding the relationship between inflammation and cancer, Vopr.Onkol., No.
6, 74-80. (In Russ.).

Shabad, L. M., 1967, "Predrak v Eksperimental'no-Morfologicheskom
Aspekte" [Precancer: Experimental and Morphologic Aspects],
Meditsina, Moscow. (In Russ.).

Shabad, L. M., 1977, The evolution of concepts regarding chemical
carcinogenesis, in: "Tezisy Dokladov Vyezdnoi Nauchnoi Sessii
Otdeleniya po Probleme Biologicheskie Aspekty
Zlokachestvennogo Rosta," [Abstracts of Papers Presented at a
Traveling Seminar on Biologic Aspects of Malignant Growth],
Tallin. (In Russ.).

Shanin, A. P., 1969, "Opukholi Kozhi, Ikh Proiskhozhdenie, Klinika i
Lechenie" [Skin Tumors: Origin, Clinical Features, and Treat-
ment], Meditsina, Leningrad. (In Russ.).

Shanov, D. M., 1961, Characterization of the inflammatory phenomena
accompanying the development of cancer in various anatomic
sites, Izv.Akad.Nauk.Kazakh.SSR, Ser.Med.i Fiziol., No. 2,
86-95. (In Russ.).

Shapiro, L., and Baraf, C. S., 1970, Subungual epidermoid carcinoma
and keratoacanthoma, Cancer, 25:141-152.

Shapot, V. S., 1973, Biologic characteristics of tumor progression,
Vopr.Onkol., No. 4, 89-92. (In Russ.).

Shapot, V. S., 1975, "Biokhimicheskie Aspekty Opukholevogo Rosta" [The
Biochemical Aspects of Tumor Growth], Meditsina, Moscow. (In
Russ.).

Shchelkunov, S. I., 1971, "Tsitologicheskii i Gistologicheskii Analiz
Razvitiya Normal'nykh i Malignizirovannykh Struktur" [Cytologic
and Histologic Analyses of the Development of Normal and
Malignant Transformed Structures], Meditsina, Leningrad. (In
Russ.).

Shevchenko, I. T., 1976, Current problems in clinical oncogenetics,
in: "Nasledstvennost' i Rak" [Heredity and Cancer], pp. 5-10,
Meditsina, Moscow. (In Russ.).

Shmal'gauzen, I. I., 1946, "Factory Evolyutsii" [Factors of Evolution],
Moscow and Leningrad. (In Russ.).

Shtein, A. A., 1938, Inflammatory epithelial growths in some forms of
cutaneous tuberculosis, Arkh.Patol.Anat., No. 1. (In Russ.).

Shuikina, E. E., 1969, "Studies on the specific prophylaxis and
immunology of zoonotic cutaneous leishmaniasis", Dissertation,
Moscow. (In Russ.).

Silberberg, I. A., Kopf, A., and Baer, R. L., 1962, Recurrent
keratoacanthoma of the lip, Arch.Dermatol., 86:44-53.

Sinyavskii, M. M., 1973, "Troficheskie Yazvy Nizhnikh Konechnostei"
[Trophic Ulcers of the Lower Extremities], Izd. Belorus',
Minsk. (In Russ.).

Siracky, J., 1971, Nuclear size and sex-chromatin characteristics in
epidermoid cancer of the uterine cervix and endometrial
cancer, Neoplasma (Bratislava), 18:637-642.

Skripkin, Yu. K., 1967, "Neirodermit (voprosy étiologii, patogeneza i terapii" [Neurodermatitis (etiology, pathogenesis, and therapy)], Meditsina, Moscow, (In Russ.).

Skripkin, Yu. K., and Sharapova, G. Ya., 1972, "Kozhnye i Venericheskie Bolezni" [Skin and Venereal Diseases], Meditsina, Moscow. (In Russ.).

Skjaeggestad, O., 1964, Experimental epidermal hyperplasia in mice in relation to carcinogenesis, Acta Pathol.Microbiol.Scand. (Copenhagen), 169:125.

Sluzhinskaya, Z. A., Semkeev, I. I., and Yuzvenko, Yu. N., 1969, The content of sex chromatin in tumor cells, Vrach.Delo, No. 1., 59–61. (In Russ.).

Smelov, N. S., Mordovtsev, V. N., and Novikova, P. F., 1973, Role of genetic factors in psoriasis, in: "VI Vsesoyuznyi S"ezd Dermato-Venerologov" [The Sixth All-Union Conference of Dermatologists and Venereologists], A. A. Studnitsyn and N. M. Turanova (eds.), pp. 401–402, Kharkov. (In Russ.).

Socolov, E. L., Engel, E., Kantooth, L., and Stanbury, J. B., 1964, Chromosomes of human thyroid tumors, Cytogenetics, 3:394–413.

Söltz-Szöts, J., 1963, Soziales Verchalten von Zellen maligne entarteter Tumoren der menschen Haut in der Gewebekultur, Arch.Klin.Exp.Dermatol., 216:36–43.

Sommerville, J., 1953, Pseudoepitheliomatous hyperplasia, Acta Dermatol.Venereol., 33:236–261.

South, L. M., O'Sullivan, J. P., and Gazet, J.-C., 1977, Giant condylomata of Buschke and Loewenstein, Clin.Oncol., 3:107–115.

Sterlyuk, B. P., and Kaistrukova, D. S., 1973, Sex chromatin in cervical cancer cells, Vopr.Onkol., No. 7, 9–15. (In Russ.).

Stevanovič, D. V., 1968, Unusual in keratoacanthoma, in: "The Thirteenth International Dermatological Congress," Vol. 1, pp.51–52, Springer, Berlin.

Stich, H. F., Florian, S. F., and Emson, H. E., 1960, The DNA content of tumor cells. I. Polyps and adenocarcinomas of the large intestine of man, J.Nat.Cancer Inst., 24:471–482.

Stich, H. F., Van Hooster, G., and Trentin, J. J., 1964, Viruses and mammalian chromosomes. Chromosome aberrations by human adenovirus type V2," Exp.Cell Res., 34:400–421.

Studnitsyn, A. A., 1965, Cutaneous tumors, in: "Klinicheskaya Onkologiya Detskogo Vozrasta" [Pediatric Clinical Oncology], pp. 261–282, Meditsina, Moscow. (In Russ.).

Studnitsyn, A. A., Rozentul, M. A., Per, M. I., Ganyushina, E. Kh., Reznikova, L. S., Maslov, P. E., Ievleva, E. A., Alchyagyan, V. M., Dadiomova, V. G., Zheltakov, V. M., Kovalenko, G. P., Kundel', L. M., Semenova, N. I., Trofimova, E. M., and Kameneva, M. P., 1967, "Mechanism of action and therapeutic activity of pyrogenic drugs in the treatment of dermatoses, Vest.Dermatol.Venerol., No. 3, 8–13. (In Russ.).

Suss, R., Kinzel, V., and Seribuer, J. D., 1973, "Cancer Experiments and Concepts", Springer-Verlag, New York.

Sutherland, E. W., and Rall, T. W., 1957, The properties of an adenine ribonucleotide produced with cellular particles, ATP, Mg++, and epinephrine or glucagon, J.Am.Chem.Soc., 79:3608.

Sutherland, E. W., Rall, T. W., and Menon, T., 1962, Adenyl cyclase. 1. Distribution, preparation, and properties, J.Biol.Chem., 237:1220-1227.

Sutherland, E. W., Oye, I. J., and Butcher, R W., 1965, The action of epinephrine and the role of adenyl cyclase in hormone action, Recent Progr.Hormone Res., 21:623.

Suvorova, K. N., and Anton'ev, A. A., 1977, "Nasledstvennye Dermatozy" [Inherited Dermatoses], Meditsina, Moscow. (In Russ.).

Szodoray, L., and Vezekenyi, Cl., 1968, Histochemical and histo-enzymological studies in the precancerous conditions of the skin, in: "The Thirteenth International Dermatological Congress," Vol. 1, pp. 16-17, Springer, Berlin.

Tavares, A. S., 1955, On the sex of cancer and kerathoma cells, Lancet, 1:1948-1949.

Tavares, A. S., 1957, Nuclear sex in undifferentiated cell carcinomata, J.Pathol.Bacteriol., 74:25-29.

Tavares, A. S., 1968, Ploidy and histological types of mammary carcinomas, Cancer, 3:449-455.

Thambiah, A. S., 1969, Aetiology, natural course, pitfalls in diagnosis and prevention of skin carcinoma, Indian J.Dermatol., 14:65-69.

Therkelssen, A., and Lamm, L., 1966, Difference in the frequency of sex chromatin-positive cells in the different intermitotic phases of human cells in tissue culture, Exp.Cell Res., 44:636-644.

Thies, W., 1955, Neurohistologische Studie zur Differentialdiagnose des Prurigo nodularis Hyde und anderer Formen umschriebener Lickenifikation, Arch.Klin.Exp.Dermatol., 201:539-555.

Thies, W., and Hennies, T., 1968, Über Assoziation eines Histiocytoms mit einem Basalioma, Hautarzt, 4:163-167.

Tilgen, W., 1976, Pseudocancerosen der Haut, Ther.Umsch., 33:556-562.

Timofeevskii, A. D., 1934, Recent advances in tissue cultures, in: "Tomskii Gosudarstvennyi Meditsinskii Institut, Trudy" [Tomsk Medical Institute. Transactions]'," pp. 1-24. (In Russ).

Timofeevskii, A. D., 1947, "Eksplantatsiya Opukholei Cheloveka" [Explantation of Human Tumors], Medgiz, Moscow. (In Russ.).

Timofeevskii, A. D., 1971, Tissue and cell cultures in biology and medicine, Tsitologiya, No. 12, 1435-1442. (In Russ.).

Timofeevskii, A. D., and Dobrynin, V., 1967, Tumor cells in tissue culture: carcinogenesis and biologic features (advances made over the years of Soviet power), Vopr.Onkol., No. 5, 3-14. (In Russ.).

Timonen, S., and Therman, E., 1950, The changes of the mitotic mechanism of human cancer cells, Cancer Res., 10:431-439.

Tinyakov, G. G., and Tinyakov, Yu. G., Mechanisms of cell reproduction, and carcinogenesis, Arkh.Patol., No. 3, 9-25. (In Russ).

Tjio, J. H., and Puck, T. T., 1958, Genetics of somatic mammalian cells. II. Chromosomal constitution of cells in tissue culture, J.Exp.Med., 108:259-268.

Toews, J., Katayama, K. P., and Masukawa, 1968, Chromosomes of benign and malignant lesions of the breast, Cancer, 22:6.

Torsuev, N. A., 1959, On keratoacanthoma, in: "Sbornik Nauchnykh Rabot po Leprologii i Dermatologii Rostovskogo Eksperimental 'noklinicheskogo Leprozoriya Minzdrava RSFSR i Kafedry Kozhnykh i Venericheskikh Boleznei Rostovskogo Meditsinskogo Instituta" [Collection of Papers on Leprology and Dermatology of the Rostov Experimental and Clinical Leprosary (under the Ministry of Health of the RSFSR) and of the Department of Skin and Venereal Diseases of the Rostov Medical Institute], No. 12, pp. 98-132, Rostov-on-Don. (In Russ.).

Trofimova, L. Ya., and Mordovtsev, V. N., 1975, On warty psoriasis, Vest.Dermatol.Venerol., No. 7, 51-54.

Trutia, E., 1971, Spectrophotometric analysis of nucleic acids and their derivatives, Stud.Cercet.Ultramicrobiol., 22:434-442.

Trutnev, D. A., 1956, "Materialy k Etiologii, Patogenezu i Lecheniyu Khronicheskoi Glubokoi Piodermii" [Etiology, Pathogenesis, and Treatment of Chronic Deep Pyoderma], Voronezh. (In Russ.).

Unna, P. G., 1894, "Die Histopathologie der Hautkrankheiten", Hirschwald, Berlin. (English translation by N. Walker: P. G. Unna, "The Histopathology of the Diseases of the Skin", MacMillan, New York, 1965.)

Urbach, F., 1969, Geographic pathology of skin cancer, in: "The Biologic Effects of Ultraviolet Radiation," F. Urbach (ed.), pp. 635-650, Pergamon, Oxford .

Urbach, F., O'Brien, S., and Judge, P., 1970, The influence of environment and genetic factors on cancer of the skin in man, in: "Abstracts, Tenth International Cancer Congress," No. 174, p. 109.

Utkin, A. I., 1953, The role of environment in the regulation of mitotic activity. Communication 2. Effect of sound stimuli on the mitotic activity of corneal epithelium, Byull.Eksp. Biol. Med., No. 5, 52-55. (In Russ.).

Vakhtin, Yu. B., 1973, Selection in tumor cell populations, Vopr.Onkol., No. 4, 93-94. (In Russ.).

Vamaguchi, T., 1974, Hirobe, T., Kinjo, K., and Manaka, K., The effect of chalone on the cell cycle in the epidermis during wound healing, Exp.Cell Res., 89:247-254.

Vasil'ev, Yu. M., "Soedinitel'naya Tkan' i Opukholevyi Rost v Eksperimente" [Connective Tissue and Tumor Growth in Experiment], Moscow. (In Russ.).

Vasil'ev, Yu. M., 1965, Relationships of tumor cells with one another and with normal cells, in: "Biologiya Zlokachestvennogo Rosta" [The Biology of Malignant Growth], pp. 200-219, Meditsina, Moscow. (In Russ.).

Vasil'ev, Yu. M., 1967, Some characteristics of proliferative processes in tumor tissues, Tsitologiya, No. 9, 1121-1128. (In Russ.).

Vasil'ev, Yu. M., 1973, Patterns and mechanisms of alterations in cells during tumor evolution, Arkh.Patol., No. 1, 3-13. (In Russ.).

Vasil'ev Yu. M., and Gel'fand, I. M., 1973, Disturbance of morphologic responses of cells during neoplastic transformation, Vest.Akad.Med., Nauk SSSR, No. 4, 61-69. (In Russ.).

Vasil'ev Yu. M., Gel'stein, V. I., 1962, The relationship between precancerous changes and reactive proliferation, Vest.Akad. Med.Nauk SSSR, No. 5, 7-16. (In Russ.).

Vasil'eva, A. P., 1966, Variations in mitotic activity and in the number of pathologic mitoses during early carcinogenesis, Byull.Eksp.Biol.Med., No. 10, 83-86. (In Russ.).

Venkei, T., and Sugar, J., 1965, "Early Diagnosis, Pathohistology, and Treatment of Malignant Tumors of the Skin" (English translation from Hungarian), Adadémiai Kiadó, Budapest.

Vermel', E. M., 1972, Bleomycin: a new antibiotic possessing antitumor activity, Vopr.Onkol., No. 9, 85-93. (In Russ.).

Vikhert, A. M., Galil-ogly, G. A., and Poroshin, K. K., 1973, "Atlas Diagnosticheskikh Biopsii Kozhi" [An Atlas of Diagnostic Skin Biopsies], Meditsina, Moscow. (In Russ.).

Vilesov, S. P., 1967, "Proteoliticheskie Fermenty Podzheludochnoi Zhelezy i Ikh Primenenie v Meditsine" [Proteolytic Pancreatic Enzymes and Their Medical Applications], Kiev. (In Russ.).

Vincent, P. C., Vandenberg, R. A., Neate, R., and Nickolls, A., 1964, Chromosome analysis in the diagnosis of malignant effusions: report of a case, Med.J.Austral., 51:153-157.

Voitenko, V. P., 1976, Sex chromatin in epithelial cells of the oral cavity in men with malignant neoplasms, in; "Nasledstvennost' i Rak" [Heredity and Cancer], pp. 35-38, Meditsina, Moscow. (In Russ.).

Vollum, D. J., 1976, Multiple keratoacanthomas, Br.J.Dermatol., 95:78-79.

Voorhees, J. J., Marcelo, C. L., and Duell, E. A., 1975, Cyclic AMP, cyclic GMP and glucocorticoids as potential metabolic regulators of epidermal proliferation and differentiation, J.Invest. Dermatol., 65:179-190.

Voorhees, J. J., Chambers, D. A., Duell, E., Marcelo, C. L., and Kureger, G., 1976, Molecular mechanisms in proliferative skin disease, J.Invest.Dermatol., 67:442-450.

Vulcan, P., 1972, Consideratti asupra condilomazei acuminate gigante Buschke Löwenstein, Dermato-Venerol. (Bucharest), 17:101-108.

Vulcan, P., and Pais, V., 1976, Aspecte ultrastructurale in condilomatosa giganta Buschke-Löwenstein, Dermato-Vener., (Bucharest), 21:1-10.

Walker, D. G., Goldstein, N., Kopf, A. W., and Wright, J. C., 1964, Epithelial outgrowths from tissue cultures of basal cell epitheliomas, J.Invest.Dermatol., 42:435-441.

Walton, G. M., and Gill, G. N., 1973, Adenosine 3',5'-monophosphate and protein kinase-dependent phosphorylation of ribosomal protein, Biochemistry, 12:2604-2611.

Wao, Y. T., and Manery, J. F., 1973, Cyclic AMP phosphodiesterase
    activity of the external surface of intact skeletal muscles
    and stimulation of the enzyme by insulin, Arch.Biochem.
    Biophys., 154:510-519.

Watson, W., Cann, H. M., Farber, E. M., and Nall, M. L., 1972, The
    genetics of psoriasis, Arch.Dermatol., 105:194-207.

Weidman, F. D., 1955 - Cited in N. A. Torsuev, 1959.

Weinstein, G. D., 1979, Epidermal cell kinetics, in: "Dermatology in
    General Medicine", Th. B. Fitzpatrick et al. (ed.), pp. 85-95,
    McGraw-Hill, New York.

Weinstein, G. D., and Frost, P., 1968, Abnormal cell proliferation in
    psoriasis, J.Invest.Dermatol., 50:254-259.

Weinstein, G. D., and Frost, P., 1970, Cell proliferation in human
    basal cell carcinoma, Cancer Res., 30:724-728.

Weiss, P., and Kavanau, J. L., 1957, A model of growth and growth
    control in mathematical terms, J.Gen.Physiol., 41:1-47.

White, C., and F. D., Weidman, 1927, Pseudoepitheliomatous hyper-
    plasia at the margins of cutaneous ulcers, JAMA, 88:1959-1963.

Whitefield, J. F., MacManus, J. P., Braceland, B. M., and Gillan, D.
    J., 1972, The influence of calcium on the cyclic AMP-mediated
    stimulation of DNA synthesis and cell proliferation by prosta-
    glandin E, J.Cell.Physiol., 79:353-362.

Whiteley, H. J., 1957, The effect of the hair growth cycle on experi-
    mental skin carcinogenesis in the rabbit, Br.J.Cancer,
    11:196-205.

Whitmore, W. F., 1970, Tumors of the penis, urethra, scrotum, and
    testis, in: "Urologia," M. F. Campbell and J. H. Harrison
    (eds.), Vol.2, p. 1190, Philadelphia.

Wilkinson, D. S., 1968, Giant condyloma of Buschke-Loewenstein, in:
    "Textbook of Dermatology," A. Rook, D. S. Wilkinson and F. J.
    Ebling, Vol.2, p.1528, Blackwell, Oxford.

Williams, J. P. G., 1972, Interrelation of epithelial glycogen, cell
    proliferation, and cellular migration with cyclic adenosine
    monophosphate in epithelial wound healing, Cell Different.,
    1:317-323.

Willis, P. A., 1967, Pathology of Tumors, 4th ed., Butterworths,
    London.

Winder, S., Storer, J., and Lulhbaugh, C., 1951, The use of X-ray and
    nitrogen mustard to determine the mitotic and intermitotic
    times in normal and malignant rat tissue, Cancer Res.,
    11:877-883.

Winer, L. H., 1940, Pseudoepitheliomatous hyperplasia, Arch.Dermatol.
    Syph., 42:856-867.

Winkelmann, R. K., and Brown, J., 1968, Generalized eruptive keratoa-
    canthoma, Arch.Dermatol., 97:615-623.

Wiskemann, A., 1955, Über Pseudoepitheliome der Haut, Dermatol.Wschr.
    131:296-301.

Wodniansky, P., 1960, Die pseudoepitheliomatösen Hyperplasien in
    klinischer und differentialdiagnostischer Sicht
    (Papillomatosis cutis carcinoides Gottron, Pyodermitis

chronica vegetans von Azua, psuedoepitheliomatösen Hyperplasien), Dermatologica (Basel) 120:1-24.
Wolff, K., 1979, Mycobaterial diseases: tuberculosis, in: "Dermatology in General Medicine," Th. B. Fitzpatrick, A. Z. Eisen, K.
Wolff, I. M. Freedberg, and K. F. Austen (eds.), pp.
1473-1492, McGraw-Hill, New York.
Yamada, K., Takagi, N., and Sandberg, A. A., 1966, Chromosomes and
causation of human cancer and leukemia. II. Karyotypes of
human solid tumors, Cancer, 19:1879-1890.
Yamagiwa, K., and Ichikawa, K., 1915, Experimentelle Studie über die
Pathogenese der Epithelialgeschwülste," Mitt.Med.Fak,
15:295-344.
Yoshikawa, K., Adachi, K., Halprin, K. M., and Levine, V., 1975,
Cyclic AMP in skin: effects of acute ischaemia,
Br.J.Dermatol., 92:249-262.
Zalkind, S. Ya., 1954, Mitotic patterns in health and disease,
Uspekhi Sovr.Biol., No. 1, 68-85. (In Russ.).
Zalkind, S. Ya., 1972, Nuclear abnormalities in monolayer cell cul-
tures, in: "Mekhanizmy Regulyatsii Funktsii Kletochnogo Yadra
(Materialy IV Vsesoyuznogo Simpoziuma po Strukture i Funktsii
Yadra)" [Mechanisms Regulating the Function of Cell Nuclei
(Proceedings of the Fourth All-Union Symposium on Nuclear
Structure and Function)], pp. 49-51, Tbilsis. (In Russ.).
Zakharov, A. F., 1970, "Chromosomal variability and cell selection in
populations of long-cultured cells", Doctoral dissertation,
Moscow. (In Russ.).
Zavarzin, A. A., 1947, "Ocherki Evolyutsionnoi Gistologii Krovi i
Soedinitel'noi Tkani" [Essays on Evolutionary Histology of the
Blood and Connective Tissue], Moscow. (In Russ.).
Zavarzin, A. A., 1967, "Sintez DNK i Kinetika Kletochnykh Populyatsii
v Ontogeneze Mlekopitayushchikh" [DNA Synthesis and Cell
Population Kinetics in Mammalian Ontogeny], Nauka, Leningrad.
(In Russ.).
Zegarelli, D. J., Solitary intraoral keratoacanthoma, Oral Surg.,
40:785-788.
Zheltakov, M. M., 1964, Neurodermatosis, in: "Rukovodstvo po
Dermato-Venerologii" [A Handbook of Dermato-Venereology], pp.
120-161, Meditsina, Moscow.

# Index